Health Care USA

Understanding Its Organization and Delivery

Sixth Edition

Harry A. Sultz, DDS, MPH
Professor Emeritus
Social and Preventive Medicine
School of Medicine and Biomedical Sciences

Dean Emeritus
School of Health Related Professions
State University of New York at Buffalo
Buffalo, New York

Kristina M. Young, MS
Instructor
School of Public Health and Health Professions
State University of New York at Buffalo
Buffalo, New York

Instructor
Canisius College
Buffalo, New York

President
Kristina M. Young & Associates, Inc.
Buffalo, New York

JONES AND BARTLETT PUBLISHERS
Sudbury, Massachusetts
BOSTON   TORONTO   LONDON   SINGAPORE

World Headquarters

Jones and Bartlett Publishers
40 Tall Pine Drive
Sudbury, MA 01776
978-443-5000
info@jbpub.com
www.jbpub.com

Jones and Bartlett Publishers
Canada
6339 Ormindale Way
Mississauga, Ontario L5V 1J2
Canada

Jones and Bartlett Publishers
International
Barb House, Barb Mews
London W6 7PA
United Kingdom

Jones and Bartlett's books and products are available through most bookstores and online booksellers. To contact Jones and Bartlett Publishers directly, call 800-832-0034, fax 978-443-8000, or visit our website www.jbpub.com.

Substantial discounts on bulk quantities of Jones and Bartlett's publications are available to corporations, professional associations, and other qualified organizations. For details and specific discount information, contact the special sales department at Jones and Bartlett via the above contact information or send an email to specialsales@jbpub.com.

This publication is designed to provide accurate and authoritative information in regard to the Subject Matter covered. It is sold with the understanding that the publisher is not engaged in rendering legal, accounting, or other professional service. If legal advice or other expert assistance is required, the service of a competent professional person should be sought.

Production Credits
Publisher: Michael Brown
Production Director: Amy Rose
Associate Editor: Katey Birtcher
Production Editor: Tracey Chapman
Marketing Manager: Sophie Fleck
Manufacturing and Inventory Control Supervisor: Amy Bacus
Composition: Auburn Associates, Inc.
Cover Design: Kate Ternullo
Cover Image: © Nancy Brammer/ShutterStock, Inc.; © Cliff Deputy/ShutterStock, Inc.
Printing and Binding: Malloy, Inc.
Cover Printing: Malloy, Inc.

Library of Congress Cataloging-in-Publication Data
Sultz, Harry A.
  Health care USA : understanding its organization and delivery / Harry A. Sultz, Kristina M. Young. — 6th ed.
     p. ; cm.
  Includes bibliographical references and index.
  ISBN-13: 978-0-7637-4974-3 (pbk.)
  ISBN-10: 0-7637-4974-5 (pbk.)
     1. Medical care—United States. 2. Medical policy—United States. I. Young, Kristina M. II. Title.
  [DNLM: 1. Delivery of Health Care—United States. 2. Health Policy—United States. W 84 AA1 S96h 2008]
  RA395.A3S897 2008
  362.10973—dc22

                                                                                    2007044092
6048
Printed in the United States of America
12 11 10 09 08   10 9 8 7 6 5 4 3 2 1

This book is dedicated to our parents, William and Marabelle Sultz and Jacob Jay and Marie Young. Guiding these warm, loving, and dignified people through the health care system during the last years of their lives taught us more about the feats, functions, and foibles of medical care than all the research conducted, literature read, and services administered.

Contents

Foreword

The last few years have brought tremendous upheaval in the formerly tradition-bound and physician-dominated health care system in the United States. The widespread penetration of managed care, with its service management and cost-control strategies, and the resulting open market competitions among health care providers, have changed the face of the health care industry. In addition, medicine's most recent technological and pharmaceutical advances have altered the manner in which many diseases are treated and clinical services are delivered.

This volume, *Health Care USA*, has added significance in this period of enormous upheaval and turmoil affecting the health care professions and institutions. It offers a clear overview of the health care industry and the issues that confront it. It describes the changing roles of the components of the system as well as the technical, economic, political, and social forces responsible for those changes. Students of health care and related professions as well as neophyte practitioners, need a broad understanding of the U.S.'s new health care system. Critical insights into diverse health care topics and issues are necessary to function effectively and relate intelligently to the various segments of the health care sector.

This, the sixth edition of *Health Care USA*, brings the reader up to date on the significant developments that have occurred in health care during the past few years. The Balanced Budget Act of 1997 and related legislation are creating major changes in Medicare and other government-sponsored programs. Those changes, and the recognized dominance of managed care, have required major adjustments by the health care industry. In this edition, as in previous ones, the authors have meticulously screened for vast amounts of new information and included the most appropriate for updating this work. This text continues to retain its balanced population perspective, which allows the reader to understand the forces that are driving these rapid changes in the organization and financing of health care as well as the changes themselves.

The breadth of this book is ambitious, as is necessary for any text in a course that attempts to analyze the complex structures, processes, and relationships of health care in the United States. The authors have crafted an exceptionally readable text by balancing and integrating the diverse subject matter and presenting it in appropriate depth for an introductory course on this topic. Because a "population" rather than an "individual" health care perspective is clearly the wave of the future, the authors' public health orientation makes this text particularly valuable. Their combined experience in the public health and medical care fields has allowed them to interpret health care developments with objectivity. It is an important feature in an introductory text that strives toward analysis, not advocacy, thereby allowing the formulation of one's own position.

Michel A. Ibrahim, MD, PhD
Professor of Epidemiology
Editor-in-Chief, "Epidemiological Reviews"
Johns Hopkins Bloomberg School of Public Health
and
Dean and Professor Emeritus
School of Public Health
University of North Carolina at Chapel Hill

Acknowledgments

Because one of us has an academic base as a professor of social and preventive medicine and a former academic dean, and the other has served in a variety of executive positions in voluntary agencies, hospitals, and a managed care organization, we bring different experiences to our interpretations of health care developments. When we taught together, as we often did, our students were at first amused and then intrigued by the differences between academic and applied perspectives. They learned, by our willingness to debate the merits of different interpretations of the same information, to appreciate that health care is fraught with variance in understandings, dissonance in values, and contradictions in underlying assumptions.

We are grateful therefore to the students in the Schools of Medicine, Public Health and Health Professions, Management, and Law, and the Millard Fillmore College of the University at Buffalo, and Canisius College who contributed to our knowledge and experience by presenting challenging viewpoints, engaging us in spirited discussions, and providing thoughtful course evaluations. Over the years, their enthusiasm for the subject stimulated us to enrich our coursework constantly in an effort to meet and exceed their expectations.

We acknowledge with our sincerest gratitude Susan V. McLeer, MD, MS, Professor and Chair of the Department of Psychiatry, Drexel University College of Medicine, Philadelphia, Pennsylvania, who contributed the chapter on mental health services. A consummate clinician and academician, Dr. McLeer provided an exceptionally clear and insightful overview of the complex issues and service responses that characterize the field of mental health.

We are grateful to Michel Ibrahim, MD, PhD, Professor, Johns Hopkins Bloomberg School of Public Health and Dean and Professor Emeritus of the School of Public Health at the University of North

Carolina at Chapel Hill who encouraged us to write this book and has contributed the "Foreword" to each edition.

We also appreciate those who helped turn teachers into authors by providing the necessary editing, literature searches, word processing, and other support services. The early editions of this book benefited from the library and information science expertise of Karen Buchinger, the literary competence and editing skill of Alice Stein, and Ebrahim Randeree's service as our literature reviewer.

All manuscripts of the six editions of this book were word processed for submission to our publisher by Sharon Palisano. Sharon produced each edition with unparalleled attention to every aspect of the publisher's requirements. We are extremely grateful for her meticulous attention to the details of these very large texts.

We also wish to recognize the important contributions of the publisher's staff who encourage our efforts, help shape the results, and motivate us to improve the book's utility to its users. To each of you we offer our profound thanks.

About the Authors

Harry A. Sultz, DDS, MPH is Professor Emeritus of Social and Preventive Medicine at the University at Buffalo School of Medicine and Biomedical Sciences and Dean Emeritus of its School of Health Related Professions. Currently, he is an Adjunct Professor at the School of Law. He has also served as Adjunct Professor, Health Systems Management, School of Management and Clinical Assistant Professor, Department of Family Medicine.

Dr. Sultz has written five previous books, contributed chapters to several other books for professional audiences and published numerous articles for medical and allied health journals. An epidemiologist, health care services planner, and researcher, he established and, for 26 years, directed the Health Services Research Program of Buffalo's School of Medicine. His extensive research experience serves as background for the various editions of this book and for the courses that he teaches about health care and health policy. He also has long service as an expert consultant to several governmental and voluntary agencies and institutions.

Kristina M. Young, MS is an instructor at the University at Buffalo, School of Public Health and Health Professions, State University of New York, where she teaches graduate courses in health care organization and health policy for students in the fields of public health, law, and management. Ms. Young also is an instructor at Canisius College of Buffalo where she teaches graduate students in the Department of Health and Human Performance.

Ms. Young is the executive director of the Western New York Public Health Alliance, Inc., an organization that promotes public health activities in the western New York region. She also is president and owner of Kristina M. Young and Associates, Inc., a management consulting and training firm specializing in health and human services organizations. Previously, she served as president of a corporate training and development organization; as executive vice president of a not-for-profit organization dedicated to advancing the joint interests of a major teaching hospital and a health maintenance organization; and as the vice president for research and development for a teaching hospital system and executive director of its health, education, and research foundation.

Contributing Author

Susan V. McLeer, MD, MS
Professor and Chair
Department of Psychiatry
Drexel University College of Medicine

Introduction

In spite of its long history and common use, the evolving health care system has been a growing puzzle to many Americans. The prevention, diagnosis, and treatment of disease and injury, and the rehabilitation and maintenance of individuals challenged by the residual effects of those conditions have generated an enormously complex $2-trillion industry. It includes thousands of independent medical practices and partnerships; managed care and provider organizations; public and nonprofit institutions such as hospitals, nursing homes, and other specialized care facilities; and major private corporations. In dollar volume, the U.S. health care industry is second only to the manufacturing sector. For personal consumption, Americans spend more only on food and housing than they do on medical care. Furthermore, health care is by far the largest service industry in the country. In fact, the U.S. health care system is the world's eighth largest economy, second to that of France, and is larger than the total economy of Italy.[1]

More intimidating than its size, however, is its complexity. Not only is health care labor intensive at all levels, but also the types and functions of its numerous personnel change periodically to adjust to new technology, knowledge, and ways of delivering health care services.

As is frequently associated with progress, medical advances often create new problems while solving old ones. The explosion of medical knowledge that produced narrowly defined medical specialties has compounded a long-standing shortcoming of American medical care. The impressive capability to deliver sophisticated high-tech health care requires the support of an incredibly complex infrastructure that allows too many opportunities for patients to fall through the cracks between its finely tuned and narrowly defined services and specialists. In addition, our system has proven to be inept in securing even a modicum of universal coverage. Currently, over 47 million Americans are uninsured.

The increasing size, complexity, and technologic sophistication of health care in the United States have further complicated its long-standing problems of limited consumer access, inconsistent quality of services, and uncontrolled costs. In addition, the development of the health care system has done little to address the unnecessary and wasteful duplication of certain services in some areas, and the absence of essential services in others.

These problems have worried this country's political and medical leaders for decades and have motivated legislative proposals that are aimed at reform by seven successive U.S. presidents. One of the most highly publicized was the National Health Security Act of 1993, developed by President Clinton.

In 1994, the American public witnessed an unusually candid and sometimes acrimonious congressional debate over President Clinton's proposal to alter significantly how health care would be financed and delivered. Vested interests advocating change and those defending the status quo both lobbied extensively to influence public and political opinion. In the end, the stakeholders in the traditional system convinced a public—apprehensive about more governmental control over personal health services—that the Clinton plan was too much, too liberal, and too costly, and it was therefore defeated. More recently, the Balanced Budget Act of 1997 contained the most sweeping Medicare reforms to date, as well as other reforms affecting many other health care industry sectors. In a "universal coverage" initiative, it included funding for a program to provide health insurance for the nation's 11 million uninsured children. Besieged by health care industry opposition to Medicare reimbursement reductions and new regulations, the act was materially amended by the Balanced Budget Refinement Act of 1999, and other amendments.

Nevertheless, health care is undergoing a revolution. As evidenced by the failure of the National Health Security Act and the ongoing responses to the Balanced Budget Act of 1997, Congress is failing to enact health care reform legislation that is equal in strength to the market forces already altering the health care environment. Health care reform is occurring as a market-driven, not a policy-driven, phenomenon.

In a world of accelerating consolidation to achieve ever higher standards of effectiveness, the medical care system is a promising candidate for change. The result of this new environment has been a surge of health care facility and service mergers and acquisitions, new programs, new names, and new roles that signal the onset of fundamental changes throughout the system. Hospitals are competing for patients. Clinics have sprung up in shopping plazas, drug and department stores. Doctors have joined networks, and the public has been inundated with a confusing "alphabet soup" of PPOs, HMOs, and DRGs (Preferred Provider Organizations, Health Maintenance Organizations, and Diagnostically Related Groups).

The practice of medicine, long a cottage industry that valued individual entrepreneurship and physician control, has undergone dramatic change. Physicians have been most affected by recent health care system changes. Those who cherished the individual autonomy and privileged position afforded health care professionals now face the vexing oversight of case and utilization management, practice guidelines, disease management protocols, and clinical report cards. Unfortunately, the loss of professional control has also been accompanied by the loss of control over the allocation of health care dollars. The result has been a substantial decrease in annual physician incomes. Managed care organizations have controlled health costs by arbitrarily refusing reimbursement for certain medical procedures, reducing payments for others, and withholding a percentage of earned payments to physicians pending annual reviews of their practice performance.

Those physicians, hospitals, and other providers who resist the dramatic system alterations taking place are likely to be victims of their own unwillingness to adjust to the new reality. It is likely, therefore, that if legislated health care policy reform ever takes place, it will have little effect on the trends already in progress. Whatever the public and many health care professionals thought they knew about health care and its delivery system is no longer true. Much has already changed, and more changes are on the way.

That is why this book has been written. It is intended to serve as a text for introductory courses on the organization of health care for students in schools of public health, medicine, nursing, dentistry, and pharmacy, and in schools and colleges that prepare physical therapists, occupational therapists, respiratory therapists, medical technologists, health administrators, and a host of other allied health professionals. It provides an introduction to the U.S. health care system and an overview of the professional, political, social, and economic forces that have shaped it and will continue to do so.

To facilitate its use as a teaching text, this book has been organized into a succession of chapters that both stand alone as balanced discussions of discrete subjects, and when read in sequence, provide incremental additions of information to complete the reader's understanding of the entire health care system. Although decisions about what subjects and material were essential to the book's content were relatively easy, decisions about the topics and content to be left out were very difficult. The encyclopedic nature of the subject and the finite length of the final manuscript were in constant conflict.

Thus, the authors acknowledge in advance that nurses, dentists, pharmacists, physical and occupational therapists, and others may be disappointed that the text contains so little of the history and the political and professional struggles that characterize the evolution of their important professions. Given the centrality of those historical developments in students' educational preparation, it was assumed that appropriate attention to those subjects, using books written specifically for that purpose, would be included in courses in those professional curricula. To be consistent with that assumption, the authors tried to include only those elements in the history of public health, medicine, and hospitals that had a significant impact on how health care was delivered.

The authors had to make a similar set of difficult decisions regarding the depth of information to include about specific subjects in the text. Topics such as epidemiology, history of medicine, program planning and evaluation, quality of care, and the like, each have their own libraries of in-depth texts and, in many schools, dedicated courses. Thus, it seemed appropriate in a text for an introductory course to provide only enough descriptive and interpretive detail about each topic to put it in the context of the overall subject of the book.

This book has been written from a public health or population perspective and reflects the viewpoint of its authors. Both authors have public health and preventive medicine backgrounds, and long histories of research into various aspects of the health care system, have planned and evaluated innovative projects for improving the quality and accessibility of care in both the public and voluntary sectors, and have served in key executive positions in the health field.

The authors have used much of the material contained in *Health Care USA: Understanding Its Organization and Delivery* to provide students, consumers, and neophyte professionals with an understanding of the unique interplay of the technology, work force, research findings, financing, regulation, and personal and professional behaviors, values, and assumptions that determine what, how, why, where, and at what cost health care is delivered in the United States.

The first edition of this book was completed in 1996 and since then the magnitude of the changes taking place in health care, and the rapidity with which they have occurred, have been unprecedented. Although the forces reshaping the system are basically economic in nature, they impinge on every facet of health care from the education of the providers to the terminal care of the patients. Revered institutions, once thought immutable, have merged with others, completely altered their service missions, or just disappeared from the health care scene. Within incredibly brief periods of time, new organizations and corporations have become important influences in America's health care systems. Bending reluctantly to the cost-driven principles of expanding managed care, the practice of medicine has become significantly different from what it was only a few years ago. In this sixth edition, we have included important additions and updates to provide a current perspective on the health care industry's continuously evolving trends.

The authors hope that as this book's readers plan and expand their educational horizons and, later, their professional experiences, they will have the advantage of a comprehensive understanding of the complex system in which they practice.

Note

1. U.S. Bureau of the Census. *Statistical Abstract of the United States, 1995,* 115th ed. Washington, DC: United States Bureau of the Census, 1995.

CHAPTER 1

Overview of Health Care: A Population Perspective

This chapter provides a general overview of the U.S. health care industry, its policy makers, its values and priorities, and its various responses to health care diseases and problems. A template for understanding the natural histories of diseases and the levels of medical intervention is illustrated. Major influences in the continuing growth and change of the United State's health services system are briefly described in preparation for more extensive discussion in subsequent chapters. The conflicts of interest and ethical dilemmas resulting from medicine's technologic advances and the advent of managed care are also noted.

In recent years, health care, especially its medical or curative aspect, has captured as never before the interest of the public, political leaders, and an attentive media. News of medical miracles, breakthroughs, disasters, deficiencies, and rising costs attracts a consistently high readership. For many, the fortunes and foibles of health care take on deeply serious meanings. There is a widespread sense of urgency among employers, insurers, consumer groups, and other policy makers about the seemingly unresolvable need to correct problems of access and cost without compromising quality of care. The last decade's major economic and social changes in the United States have altered the way Americans think about the role health care plays in their lives and about the strengths and deficiencies of the complex labyrinth of health care providers, facilities, programs, and services.

There is growing concern that health care is a big, unmanageable business that consumes over 16% of the U.S. gross domestic product and exceeds $1.5 trillion in costs. The corporatization of the health care industry is creating major opportunities for megamergers and investors. Many health care providers and institutions have become commercial entrepreneurs beyond all expectations and to the concern of many. The commercialization of health care has created increasing conflicts between providers on one side and policy makers, managed care organizations (MCOs), and other third-party payers on the other.

Physicians are seeking public support for their concern that managed care may constrain expenditures without adequate regard for the quality of care. Policy makers and care managers assert that physicians expressing concerns over quality is a way to resist scrutiny and accountability without regard for economic efficiency. Against this contentious background, health care policy debates will likely continue to be unproductive. Recriminations from both sides block attempts at constructive dialogue.

Problems of Health Care

Although philosophical and political differences fuel the debates about health care policies and reforms, there is a general agreement that the health care system in the United States, as in most other countries, is fraught with problems and dilemmas. In spite of its impressive accomplishments, the U.S. health care system exhibits inexplicable contradictions in objectives; unwarranted variations in performance, effectiveness, and efficiency; and long-standing difficulties in its relationships with the public and governments.

The strategies for addressing the problems of cost, access, and quality over the last 30 years reflect the periodic changes in political philosophies. The government-sponsored programs of the 1960s were designed to improve access for older adults and low-income populations without regard for the inflationary effects on costs. These programs were followed by regulatory attempts to address first the availability and price of health services, then the organization and distribution of health care, and then its quality. In the 1990s, the ineffective patchwork of government-sponsored health system reforms was superseded by the emergence of market-oriented changes, competition, and privately organized MCOs.

The failure of government-initiated reforms created a vacuum that was filled quickly by the private sector. There is a difference, however, between recent governmental goals for health care reform and those of the market. Although the proposed government programs try to maintain some balance among costs, quality, and access, the primary goal of the market is to contain costs. As a result, there are serious concerns that market-driven reforms may not result in a health care system that equitably meets the needs of all Americans.

As Eli Ginzberg, writing in the *New England Journal of Medicine*, pointed out, as long as the dominant interest groups—government, employers, the public, and major provider groups—do not agree on how to change the system to accomplish widely desired reforms, the American people will continue temporizing. They are "unwilling to risk the strengths of our existing health care system in a radical effort to remedy admittedly serious deficiencies."[1]

Understanding Health Care

Health care policy usually reflects public opinion. Finding acceptable solutions to the perplexing problems of health care will depend on public understanding and acceptance of both the existing circumstances and the benefits and risks of proposed remedies. Many of the communication problems regarding health policy stem from the public's inadequate understanding of health care and its delivery system.

Early practitioners purposely fostered the mystique surrounding medical care as a means to set themselves apart from the patients they served. Endowing health care with a certain amount of mystery encouraged patients to maintain blind faith in the capability of their physicians, even when the state of the science did not justify it. When advances in the understanding of the causes, processes, and cures of specific diseases revealed that previous therapies and methods of patient management were based on erroneous premises, physicians were not held responsible. Although the world's most advanced and proficient health care system provides a great deal of excellent care, the lack of public knowledge has allowed much care to be delivered that was less than beneficial and some that was inherently dangerous.

Now, however, the romantic naiveté with which health care and its practitioners were viewed has eroded significantly. Since the revealing debates over President Clinton's health care reform proposal of 1993 and the public's increasing exposure to the concepts of managed care, attitudes toward health care and its practitioners have changed. Whether it was ever true, the long-held assumption by both health care providers and patients that their dictator–follower relationship was inviolate no longer exists.

Rather than a confidential contract between the provider and the consumer, the health care relationship now includes a voyeuristic collection of insurers, payers, managers, and quality assurers. Providers no longer have a monopoly on health care decisions and actions. Although the increasing scrutiny and accountability may be onerous and costly to physicians and other providers, it represents concerns of those paying for health care—governments, insurers, employers, and patients—about the value received for their expenditures. That these questions have been raised reflects the prevailing opinion that those who now chafe under the scrutiny are, at least indirectly, responsible for generating the excesses in the system while neglecting the problems of limited access to health care for many.

Cynicism about the health care system has grown as increasing information about the problems of costs, quality, and access has become public. People who viewed medical care as a necessity provided by physicians who adhere to scientific standards based on tested and proven therapies have been disillusioned to learn that major knowledge gaps contribute to highly variable use rates for therapeutic and diagnostic procedures that have produced no measurable differences in outcomes. Nevertheless, recent attempts at system-wide reforms have repeatedly demonstrated the enormously complex issues that underlie the health industry's problems and the ineptitude of the system's leadership in addressing them. Writing in a 2004 issue of *Health Affairs*, Nichols et al. described the situation as follows: "The quest for greater efficiency in the delivery of health care services is eternal in a country that spends far more on health care than any other, consistently has growth in spending that outstrips that of income, is unable to provide insurance coverage to at least 15% of its population, and ranks poorly among industrialized countries in system-wide measures such as life expectancy and infant mortality."[2]

Many health care system employees also have become discouraged. Institutional and agency administrators who say they care about patients but must reflect overriding budget considerations in every action confuse and demoralize health care workers. Most individuals in health care chose a health occupation not because of the income potential, but because they had a sense of caring and social justice. They made trade-offs and sacrifices for their values only to find that the reality is quite different. Nurses, the largest component of the health care workforce, are especially frustrated with their current role in hospitals. They feel overworked, unable to meet their own standards of quality care, and stressed to the point of leaving the profession. It is hoped that when the health care system again becomes stabilized in a more predictable economic environment those contradictory messages from higher administrative levels will cease.

Why Patients and Providers Behave the Way They Do

In Chapter 3, the evolution of the U.S. system of hospitals makes clear the long tradition of physicians and other health care providers behaving in an authoritarian manner toward patients. Hospitalized patients, removed from their usual places in society, were expected to be compliant and grateful to be in the hands of someone far more learned than themselves. The fact that submissive patient behavior has characterized even otherwise domineering individuals when they become ill has interested many researchers. Because the health beliefs and actions of patients have much to do with their timely and appropriate use of the health care system and their disposition and motivation to cooperate in their treatment, physicians, nurses, and social scientists have studied patient behavior for decades to try to understand the "sick role."

In 1951, Talcott Parson suggested that ill individuals in Western-developed nations demonstrate predictable behaviors, and his theories are still recognized as contributing to the understanding of illness behavior. Frederick Wolinsky stated that Parson's description of the sick role was "an integral part of the socio-cultural definition of health and illness."[3] Wolinsky reviewed the four major elements of Parson's assumptions. First, people who are ill believe that they are not solely responsible for their condition and that it is not within their power to get well. Second, by virtue of their diminished function, people who are ill are exempt from normal personal and social obligations in proportion to the severity of their illness. Third, because illness is undesirable, people who are sick are expected to take appropriate action and enlist the aid of others in getting well. Fourth, people who are sick are obliged to obtain competent assistance, usually from a physician, to aid recovery and to comply with the treatment and advice received.

Parson's description of the sick role explains why patients often abdicate personal responsibility for their condition and recovery to a health care system that is more than willing to accept the authority to decide what is best for them. More recently, however, recognizing the benefits of more proactive roles for patients and the improved outcomes that result, both health care providers and consumers are encouraging significant patient participation in every health care decision.

Indexes of Health and Disease

Although health care providers, researchers, analysts, and others in the health services industry have created a detailed and comprehensive taxonomy of diseases and disabilities, definitions of what constitutes "health" are frustratingly ambiguous. The 1958 World Health Organization definition—"a state of complete physical, mental and social well-being and not merely the absence of disease"—is hardly measurable and rarely achievable, certainly not for any extended length of time.[4] Thus, much of "health" is so subjective that for all practical purposes, it is determined clinically by the converse—whether individual physical, physiologic, and laboratory test values fall within or outside of "normal" parameters.

The body of statistical data about health and disease has grown enormously since the late 1960s, when the government began analyzing information obtained from Medicare and Medicaid claims and computerized hospital and insurance data allowed the retrieval and exploration of huge files of clinical information. In addition, there have been continuing improvements in the collection, analysis, and reporting of vital statistics and communicable and malignant diseases by state and federal governments.

Data collected over time and international comparisons reveal common trends among developed countries. Birth rates have fallen, and life expectancies have lengthened so that older people make up an increasing proportion of total populations. The percentage of individuals who are disabled or dependent has grown as the health care professions have improved their capacity to rescue moribund individuals.

Infant mortality and maternal mortality, the international indicators of social and health care improvement, have continued to decline in the United States but have not reached the more commendable levels of countries with more demographically homogeneous populations. In the United States, the differences in infant mortality rates between inner-city neighborhoods and suburban communities may be greater than those between developed and undeveloped countries. The continuing inability of the health care system to address those discrepancies effectively reflects the system's ambiguous priorities.

Natural Histories of Disease and the Levels of Prevention

For many years, epidemiologists and health services planners have used a matrix for placing everything known about a particular disease or condition in the sequence of its origin and progression when untreated; this schema is called the natural history of disease. Many diseases, especially chronic diseases that may last for decades, have an irregular evolution and extend through a sequence of stages. When the causes and stages of a particular disease or condition are defined in its natural history, they can be matched against the health care interventions intended to prevent the condition's occurrence or to arrest its progress after its onset. Because these health care interventions are designed to prevent the condition from advancing to the next and usually more serious level in its natural history, the interventions are classified as the "levels of prevention." Figures 1-1 through 1-3 illustrate the concept of the natural history of disease and levels of prevention.

The first level of prevention is the period during which the individual is at risk to the disease but is not yet affected. Called the "prepathogenesis period," it identifies those behavioral, genetic, environmental, and other factors that increase the individual's likelihood of contracting the condition. Some risk factors, such as smoking, may be altered, whereas others, such as genetic factors, may not.

When such risk factors combine to produce a disease, the disease usually is not manifest until certain pathologic changes occur. This stage is a period of clinically undetectable, presymptomatic disease. Medical science is working hard to improve its ability to diagnose disease earlier in

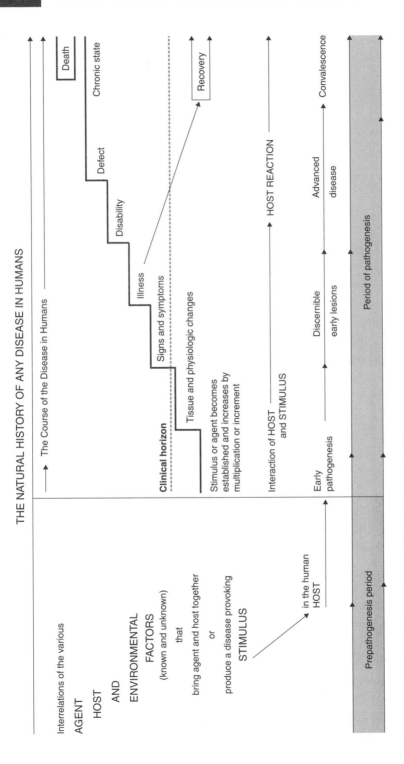

FIGURE 1-1 Natural History of Any Disease in Humans.

Source: Reprinted with permission from H. R. Leavell and E. G. Clark, *Preventative Medicine for the Doctor in His Community: An Epidemiologic Approach*, 3rd edition, p. 20, © 1965, The McGraw Hill Companies, Inc.

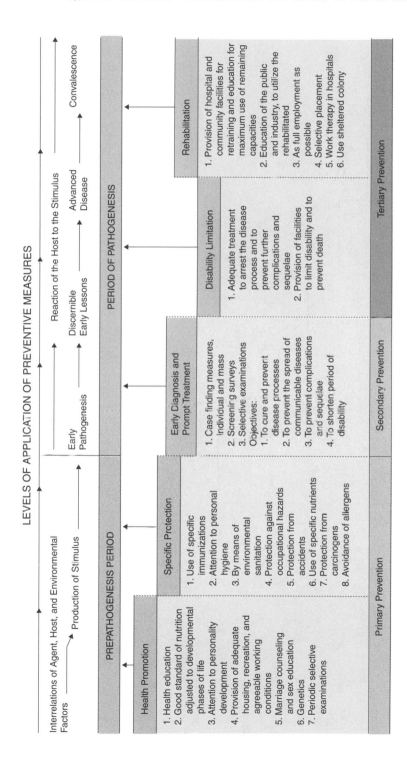

FIGURE 1-2 Levels of Application of Preventive Measures.
Source: Reprinted with permission from H. R. Leavell and E. G. Clark, *Preventative Medicine for the Doctor in His Community: An Epidemiologic Approach*, 3rd edition, p. 21, © 1965, The McGraw Hill Companies, Inc.

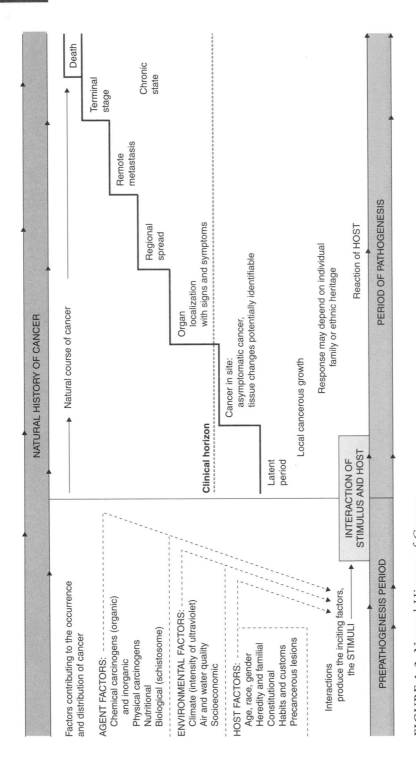

FIGURE 1-3 Natural History of Cancer.

Source: Reprinted with permission from H. R. Leavell and E. G. Clark, *Preventative Medicine for the Doctor in His Community: An Epidemiologic Approach*, 3rd edition, p. 272–273, © 1965, The McGraw Hill Companies, Inc.

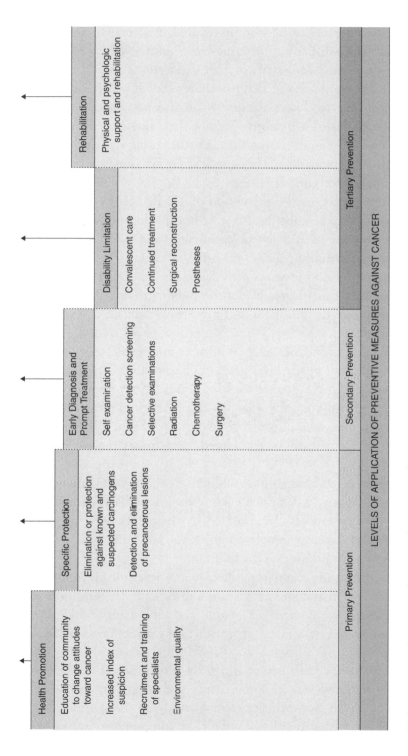

FIGURE 1-3 (continued) Natural History of Cancer.
Source: Reprinted with permission from H. R. Leavell and E. G. Clark, *Preventative Medicine for the Doctor in His Community: An Epidemiologic Approach,* 3rd edition, p. 272–273, © 1965, The McGraw Hill Companies, Inc.

this stage. Because many conditions evolve in irregular and subtle processes, it is often difficult to determine the point at which an individual may be designated "diseased" or "not diseased." Thus, each natural history has a "clinical horizon," defined as the point at which medical science becomes able to detect the presence of a particular condition. Because the pathologic changes may become fixed and irreversible at each step in the disease progress, preventing each succeeding step of the disease is therapeutically important. This concept emphasizes the preventive aspect of clinical interventions.

Primary prevention, or the prevention of disease occurrence, refers to measures designed to promote health (e.g., health education to encourage good nutrition, exercise, and genetic counseling) and specific protections (e.g., immunization and the use of seat belts).

Secondary prevention involves early detection and prompt treatment to achieve an early cure, if possible, or to slow progression, prevent complications, and limit disability. Most of preventive health care is currently focused on this area.

Sometimes the distinction between primary and secondary prevention is unclear. For instance, screening tests, such as colonoscopy and mammography are always considered secondary prevention procedures. But, they also may identify persons with precancerous conditions, which can be addressed to prevent the further development of cancers. Thus, such screening activities may also be considered "primary" as well as, "secondary" prevention.

Tertiary prevention consists of rehabilitation and maximizing remaining functional capacity when disease has occurred and left residual damage. This stage represents the most costly, labor-intensive aspect of medical care and depends heavily on effective teamwork by representatives of a number of health care disciplines.

Figure 1-4 illustrates the natural history and levels of prevention for the aging process. Although aging is not a disease, it is a condition that is often accompanied by medical, mental, and functional problems that should be addressed by a range of health care services at each level of prevention.

The natural history of diseases and the levels of prevention are presented to illustrate two very important aspects of the U.S. health care system. First, it quickly becomes apparent in studying the natural history and levels of prevention for almost any of the common causes of disease

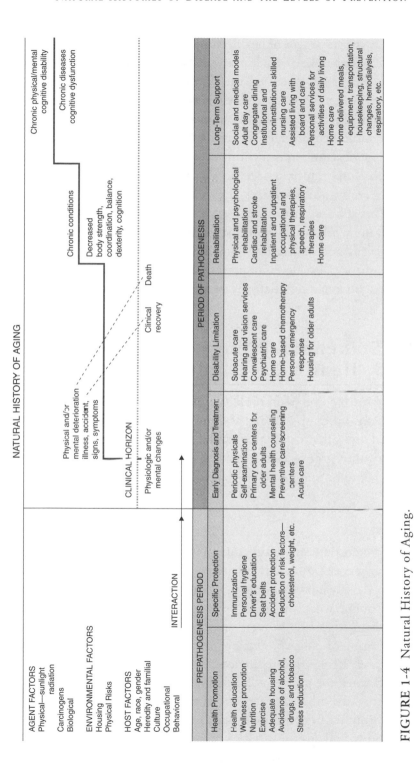

FIGURE 1-4 Natural History of Aging.

Source: Reprinted with permission from H. R. Leavell and E. G. Clark, *Preventative Medicine for the Doctor in His Community: An Epidemiologic Approach,* 3rd edition, p. 272–273, © 1965, The McGraw Hill Companies, Inc.

and disability that the focus of health care historically has been directed at the curative and rehabilitative side of the disease continuum. Serious attention has been paid to refocusing the system on the health promotion/ disease prevention side of those disease schemas only after the costs of diagnostic and remedial care became an unacceptable burden and the lack of adequate insurance coverage for over 40 million Americans became a public and political embarrassment.

The second important aspect of the natural history concept is its value in planning community services. The illustration on aging is a good example. That natural history and service levels blueprint provides the planning framework for a multidisciplinary health services planning group to identify and match the community's existing services with those proposed in the idealized levels of prevention. Within this framework, the group begins to plan and initiate the services necessary to fill the gaps.

Major Stakeholders in the U.S. Health Care Industry

It is important to come to an understanding of the health care industry and to recognize the number and variety of its stakeholders. The sometimes shared and often conflicting concerns, interests, and influences of these constituent groups cause them to shift alliances periodically to oppose or champion specific reform proposals.

The Public

First and foremost among health care stakeholders are the patients who consume the services. Although all are concerned with the issues of cost and quality, those who are uninsured or underinsured have an overriding uncertainty about access. It would be unrealistic to assume that the U.S. public will some day wish to treat health care like other inherent rights, such as education or police protection, but there is general agreement that some basic array of health care services should be available to all U.S. citizens. If and when the problem of universal access will be addressed politically in that or any other manner is open to conjecture. In the meantime, however, consumer organizations, such as the American Association of Retired Persons, and disease-specific groups, such as the American Cancer

Society, the American Heart Association, and labor organizations, are politically active on behalf of various consumer constituencies.

Employers

Employers constitute an increasingly influential group of stakeholders in health care because they not only are paying for a high proportion of the costs but are also taking more proactive roles in determining what those costs should be. Large private employers, coalitions of smaller private employers, and public employers now wield significant authority in managed care and other insurance plan negotiations. In addition, employer organizations representing small and large businesses wield considerable political power in the halls of Congress.

Providers

Health care professionals are the core of the industry and have the most to do with the actual process and outcomes of the service provided. Physicians, dentists, nurses, nurse practitioners, physician assistants, pharmacists, podiatrists, chiropractors, and a large array of allied health providers working as individuals or in group practices and staffing health care institutions are responsible for the quality and, to a large extent, cost of the health care system.

Hospitals and Other Health Care Facilities

Much of the provider activity, however, is shaped by the availability and nature of the health care institutions in which providers work. Hospitals of different types—general, specialty, teaching, rural, profit or not-for-profit, and independent or multifacility systems—are central to the existing health care system; however, they are becoming but one component of more complex, integrated delivery system networks that also include nursing homes and other levels of care, medical practices, and MCOs.

Governments

Since the advent of Medicare and Medicaid, federal and state governments, already major stakeholders in health care, have become the dominant authorities over the system. Governments serve not only as payers but also as regulators and providers through public hospitals, state and local health departments, Veterans Affairs medical centers, and other facilities. In addition, of course, governments are the taxing authorities that generate the funds to support the system.

Alternative Therapies

Unconventional health therapies—those not usually taught in established medical and other health professional schools—contribute significantly to the amount, frequency, and cost of health care. In spite of the scientific logic and documented effectiveness of traditional, academically based health care, it is estimated that one in three adults uses alternative forms of health interventions each year and that more office visits are made to alternative care providers than to primary care physicians.

It is estimated that over $10 billion per year is spent on such alternative forms of health care as rolfing, yoga, spiritual healing, relaxation techniques, herbal remedies, energy healing, megavitamin therapy, the commonly recognized chiropractic treatments, and a host of exotic mind–body healing techniques.[5]

The public's willingness to spend so much time and money on unconventional therapies suggests a substantial level of dissatisfaction with traditional scientific medicine. The popularity of alternative forms of therapy also indicates that its recipients confirm the effectiveness of the treatments by referring others to their practitioners. Whether or not these methods can be rationalized scientifically, if people feel better with their use and they do not deter individuals with treatable diseases from seeking conventional therapy, the methods serve a beneficial purpose. Insurance companies and MCOs are now considering alternative therapies as less expensive and probably equally effective options for keeping their beneficiaries feeling well.

In January 1995, the Wall Street Journal reported that several of the largest individual health insurance companies, including Mutual of Omaha and Prudential Insurance Company of America, began paying for selected unconventional therapies for heart disease and other chronic conditions.[6] In addition, the National Institutes of Health has established an Office of Alternative Medicine to fund studies of the efficacy of such therapies. Thus, as a somewhat paradoxical development, some of the most ancient concepts of alternative health care are gaining broader recognition and acceptance in an era of the most innovative and advanced high-technology medicine.

More for monetary than therapeutic reasons, a number of hospitals are now offering their patients some form of alternative medicine. According to an American Hospital Association survey, over 15% of U.S. hospitals had opened alternative or complimentary medicine centers by the year 2000. With a market estimated to be over $27 billion and patients willing to pay cash for alternative medicine treatments, hospitals are willing to rationalize the provision of several "unproven" services.[7]

Managed Care Organizations and Other Insurers

The insurance industry has long been a major stakeholder in the health care industry and probably has had more to do with defeating the Clinton health care reform plan than any other group. Although the traditional, indemnity-type plans such as Blue Cross and Blue Shield are being replaced rapidly by managed care plans, they still are very much in evidence. Managed care plans may be owned by insurance companies just as the indemnity plans are, or they may be owned by hospitals, physicians, or consumer cooperatives. MCOs and the economic pressures they can apply through the negotiation of capitated fees have produced much of the change that has occurred in the regional systems of health care during the last few years.

Long-Term Care

The aging of the U.S. population will be a formidable challenge to the country's systems of acute- and long-term care. Nursing homes, home care services, other adult care facilities, and rehabilitation facilities will become increasingly important components of the nation's health care system as they grow in number, size, and complexity. The creation of seamless systems of care that permit patients to move back and forth among ambulatory care offices, acute-care hospitals, subacute-care services, home care, and nursing homes within a single, integrated network of facilities and services will provide a continuum of services required for the more complex care of aging patients.

Mental Health

The mental health component of health care is often neglected in the debates on system reforms. Nevertheless, psychiatric hospitals, community mental health facilities, and community-based ambulatory services serve large segments of the population and are critically important to the effectiveness of the health care system. Mental health and physical health are contiguous conditions and should, but do not, generate the same concern and unprejudiced funding.

Voluntary Facilities and Agencies

Voluntary not-for-profit facilities and agencies provide significant amounts of health counseling, care, and follow-up and research support and should be considered major stakeholders in the health care system. It is interesting that although the voluntary sector traditionally has not received the recognition it deserves for its contribution to the nation's health care, it is now suggested as the safety net to replace the services to be eliminated in cost-cutting proposals.

Health Professions Education and Training Institutions

Schools of public health, medicine, nursing, dentistry, pharmacy, optometry, allied health, and other health care professions have a significant impact on the nature, quality, and costs of health care. As they prepare generation after generation of competent health care providers, these schools also inculcate the values, attitudes, and ethics that will govern the practices and behaviors of those providers as they function in the health care system. The influences of these schools, particularly as they contribute to the leadership of academic health care centers, are addressed in Chapter 5.

Professional Associations

National, state, and regional organizations representing health care professionals or institutions have considerable influence over legislative proposals, regulation, quality issues, and other political matters. The lobbying effectiveness of the American Medical Association, for example, is legendary. The national influence of the American Hospital Association and the regional power of its state and local affiliates are also impressive.

Other organizations of health care professionals, such as the American Public Health Association, the Group Health Association of America, American Nurses Association, and the American Dental Association, play significant roles in health policy decisions.

Other Health Industry Organizations

The size and complexity of the health care industry encourage the involvement of a great number of commercial entities. Several, such as the insurance and pharmaceutical enterprises, are major industries themselves and have significant organizational influence. The medical supplies and equipment business and the various consulting and information and management system suppliers also are important players.

Research Communities

It is difficult to separate much of health care research from the educational institutions that provide for its implementation. Nevertheless, the national research enterprise must be included in any enumeration of stakeholders in the health care industry. Government entities, such as the National Institutes of Health and the Agency for Healthcare Research and Quality, and not-for-profit foundations, such as the Robert Wood Johnson Foundation and the Pew Charitable Trusts, exert tremendous influence over health care research and practice by encouraging investigations that serve policy decision making and defining the kinds of research that will be supported.

Development of Managed Care

Managed care refers to arrangements that link health care financing and service delivery and allows payers to exercise significant economic control over how and what services are delivered. Common features in managed care arrangements are:

- *Provider panels.* Specific physicians and other providers are selected to care for plan members.
- *Limited choice.* Members must use the providers affiliated with the plan or pay an additional amount.

- *Gatekeeping.* Members must obtain a referral from a case manager for specialty or inpatient services.
- *Risk sharing.* Providers bear some of the health plan's financial risk through capitation and withholds.
- *Quality management and utilization review.* The plan monitors provider practice patterns and medical outcomes to identify deviations from quality and efficiency standards.

Health plans with these features are called MCOs. The most common MCOs are health maintenance organizations (HMOs) and preferred provider organizations. MCOs may directly employ medical staff, as in a staff model, or contract with independent providers or individual practice associations, or any combination of arrangements in between. Whatever the arrangement, however, in managed care, the provider is always economically accountable to the payer. Managed care is discussed at length in Chapter 7.

Rural Health Networks

Rural health systems are often incomplete, with shortages of various services and duplications of others. Federal and state programs have addressed this situation by promoting the development of rural health networks. Although relatively new, most of these networks strive to provide local access to primary, acute, and emergency care and to provide efficient links to more distant regional specialists and tertiary-care services. Ideally, rural health networks should assemble and coordinate a comprehensive array of services that include dental, mental health, long-term care, and other health and human services. Realistically, many of those services are lacking, and rural communities sometimes offer various incentives to attract or gain access to specific providers. When successful, however, rural health networks are a significant advantage to their communities. With sufficient structure and administrative capability, the networks can control the development of their service systems and negotiate effectively with MCOs.

With costs increasing and populations declining in many rural communities, it has been difficult for rural hospitals to continue their acute inpatient care services; nevertheless, these hospitals are often critically important to their communities. Because a hospital is usually one of the few major employers in rural communities, its closure has economic and health care consequences. Communities lacking alternative sources of health care within reasonable travel distance not only lose payroll and related business, but also lose physicians, nurses, and other health personnel and suffer higher morbidity and mortality rates among those most vulnerable, such as infants and older adults.[8]

Some rural hospitals have remained viable by participating in some form of multi-institutional arrangement that permits them to benefit from the personnel, services, purchasing power, and financial stability of larger facilities. Many rural hospitals, however, have found it necessary to shift from inpatient to outpatient or ambulatory care. The development of ambulatory care services by rural and urban hospitals is a strong health care system trend, as is the increased use of less expensive ancillary personnel. In many rural communities, the survival of a hospital depends on how quickly and effectively it can replace its inpatient services with a productive constellation of ambulatory care, and sometimes long-term care, services.

These rural hospital initiatives have been supported by federal legislation since 1991. This legislation provided funding to promote the essential-access community hospital and the rural primary care hospital. Both are limited-service hospital models developed as alternatives for hospitals too small and geographically isolated to be full-service acute-care facilities. Regulations regarding staffing and other service requirements are relaxed in keeping with the rural settings[9] and include allowing physician's assistants, nurse practitioners, and clinical nurse specialists to provide primary or inpatient care without a physician in the facility if medical consultation is available by phone.

The Balanced Budget Act of 1997 included a Rural Hospital Flexibility Program that replaced the essential-access community hospital/rural primary-care hospital model with a critical-assess hospital (CAH) model. Any state with at least one CAH may qualify for the program, which exempts CAHs from strict regulation and allows them the flexibility to meet small, rural community needs by developing criteria for establishing network relationships. Although the new program maintains many of the same features and requirements as its predecessor, it adds more flexibility to limited service hospitals by increasing the number of allowed occupied inpatient beds from 6 to 15 and the maximum length of stay before required discharge or transfer from 72 to 96 hours. The new program also allows maintenance of up to 25 total beds, with a swing bed program that allows flexibility in their use. The goal of the CAH program is to enable small, rural hospitals to maximize reimbursement and meet community needs with responsiveness and flexibility.

The Balanced Budget Act also serves rural hospitals by providing Medicare reimbursement for "telemedicine" and other video arrangements that link isolated facilities with clinical specialists at large hospitals. Advances in telemedicine technology make it possible for a specialist to be in direct visual and voice contact with a patient and provider at a remote location.

Rural health care organization networks have been formed in response to market changes. They may be formally organized as not-for-profit corporations or informally linked for a defined set of mutually beneficial purposes. Typically, they advocate at local and state levels on rural health care issues, cooperate in joint community outreach activities, and seek opportunities to negotiate with MCOs to provide services to enrolled populations.

Priorities of Health Care

Certainly, the priorities of health care—the emphasis on dramatic tertiary care, the costly and intensive efforts to fend off the death of terminal patients for a few more days or weeks, the heroic and often futile attempts to save extremely premature infants at huge expense while thousands of women go without the prenatal care that would decrease prematurity—contribute to the obvious mismatch between the rising costs of health care and the failure to improve the measures of health status in the United States. It is difficult to rationalize the goals of a system that invests in the most sophisticated and expensive neonatal services to save premature, high-risk infants while cutting back on the relatively inexpensive and effective prenatal services that would have prevented many of those poor birth outcomes in the first place.

If health care were to be governed by rational policies, the benefits to society of investing in early prenatal care that is unquestionably cost-effective would be compared with trying to salvage extremely low-weight, high-risk infants who often need prolonged care because they are inadequately developed, dysfunctional human beings. Clearly, current priorities favor heroic medicine over the more mundane, far less costly preventive care that results in measurable economic and human benefits.

The Tyranny of Technology

In many respects, the health care system has done and is doing a remarkable job. Important advances have been made in medical science that have brought measurable improvements in the length and quality of life. The paradox is, however, that as our technology gets better and more expensive, more people are being deprived of its benefits. Health care providers can be so mesmerized by their own technological ingenuity that things assume greater value than persons. For example, hospital administrations and medical staffs commonly dedicate their most competent practitioners and most sophisticated technology to the care of terminal patients while allocating far fewer resources to primary and preventive services for ambulatory clinic patients and other community populations in need of basic medical services. Some community hospitals are recognizing this disparity by conducting outreach and education programs for the medically underserved. As long as reimbursement policies continue to favor illness intervention rather than prevention, however, most institutions will find it difficult to initiate and maintain prevention initiatives and allocate staff to the potentially more productive care of ambulatory clinic populations.

No better example of the pervasive influence of technology exists than that of the continuing advances in diagnostic imaging. Although clinicians still depend on the long-established and relatively simple radiograph technology, they now have at their disposal several new and highly sophisticated computer-assisted imaging techniques that vastly expand their capability to visualize body structures and functions. The total spent on new imaging procedures in the United States is in the billions of dollars and is rising annually.

The recurring theme among health services researchers assessing the value of technologic advances is a series of generally unanswered questions, such as the following:

1. How does the new technology benefit the patient?
2. Is it worth the cost?
3. Are the new methods better than previous methods, and can they replace them?
4. Is treatment planning enhanced?
5. Is the outcome from disease better, or is the mortality rate improved?

Although many of the latest advances have gained great popularity and widespread acceptance, the rigorous assessments that address these basic questions have yet to be conducted.

Much of the philosophy underlying the values and priorities of the health care system today can be attributed to the unique culture of U.S. medicine. That philosophy owes much to the aggressive "can do" spirit of the frontier. The U.S. physicians want to do as much as possible. They order more diagnostic tests than their colleagues in other countries, pre-scribe drugs frequently and at relatively higher doses, and are more likely to resort to surgery whenever possible. Patients and their physicians regard the body as a machine, like a car, which helps explain their enthusiasm for annual checkups and devices such as pacemakers and artificial hearts. Diseases are likened to enemies to be conquered. Physicians expect their patients to be aggressive, too. Those who undergo drastic treatments in order to "beat" cancer are held in higher regard than patients who resign themselves to the disease. Some physicians and nurses feel let down when dying patients indicate that they do not want to be resuscitated or stipu-late restrictions to palliative care only.

The treatment-oriented rather than prevention-oriented health care philosophy was encouraged by an insurance system that before managed care rarely paid for any disease prevention other than immunization. It is also understandable in an era of high-technology medicine that there is much more satisfaction and remuneration from saving the lives of the injured and diseased than in preventing those occurrences from happen-ing in the first place.

The capitation concept and HMOs evolved from the expectation that health care could be improved if the financial incentives could be reversed. Rather than allowing providers to profit from treating sickness, managed care concepts reward providers for keeping patients well; how-ever, the treatment orientation so pervades U.S. health care that even the widespread development and acceptance of HMOs have yet to result in a significant and effective national effort to accomplish health maintenance and disease prevention.

Social Choices of Health Care

The emphasis on cure also has disinclined the health care professions to address those situations over which they have had little control. Acquired dependence on cigarettes, alcohol, and drugs must be counted among the significant causes of impaired health in our population. The future effects on health and medical care associated with these addictions probably will exceed all expectations. Similarly, the AIDS epidemic is as much a social and behavioral phenomenon as it is a biological one. Nevertheless, outside of the public health disciplines, the considerable influence and prestige of the health care professions has been noticeably absent in steering public opinion and governmental action toward an emphasis on health. Similarly, by comparison with resources expended on treatment after illness occurs, relatively little attention is given to changing high-risk behaviors even when the consequences are virtually certain and nearly always extreme.

The Aging Population

The aging of the U.S. population is of major significance among the health care system's emerging issues. It will increasingly affect every aspect of health care. The rate of aging is five times that of overall population growth. By the year 2050, it is estimated that 30% of the U.S. population will be over the age of 65 years. The number of persons over 85 years old will double, but the under-35 population will decline by 10%.

The growth of the population 65 years old and older presents a serious challenge to health care providers and policy makers. Those 85 years old and older are the fastest growing segment of the aging population. Projections by the U.S. Census Bureau suggest that the population 85 years old and older will grow from about 4 million in 2000 to 19 million in 2050 (Figure 1-5).[10] The size of this age group is especially demanding of the health care system because these individuals tend to be in poorer health and require more services than the younger elderly.

The sheer magnitude of the "baby boom" that followed World War II and the recent levels and composition of immigration to the United States are important factors in the growth and diversity of the aging population. Seventy-five million babies were born in the United States between 1946 and 1964, which is 70% more than during the preceding 2 decades.

Uwe Reinhardt, the James Madison Professor of Political Economy at Princeton University's Woodrow Wilson School of Public Health and International Affairs and a highly respected prognosticator of health care's economic prospects, disagrees with what he calls "the popular myth" that

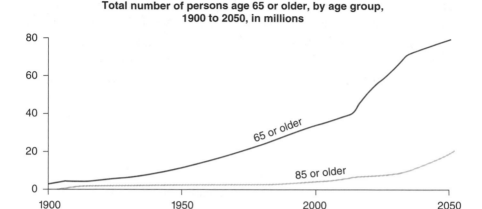

FIGURE 1-5 Total Number of Persons 65 or Older, by Age Group. *Source:* U.S. Bureau of the Census, decennial census data and population projections.

the baby boom increase in the proportion of older people in the total U.S. population will be a major contributor to the demand for health care and to total health care spending. Although he considered it "not a trivial matter in health policy," he considered the change in age distribution of the total population too gradual to have dramatic impact and other factors, such as technology development and workforce shortages, more important in contributing to health care cost increases.[11]

Although the current population of older adults is predominately white, there will be more racial diversity and more persons of Hispanic origin within U.S. older population in the coming years. There were relatively large population gains among older adults of Asian and Hispanic origin between 1980 and 1990, and those gains will increase substantially in subsequent decades.[12]

The older Hispanic population is projected to almost triple between 2000 and 2050. The older Hispanic population is growing much faster than the older black population. The number of older Hispanics was about two thirds that of the black population in 2000. In 2050, older Hispanics will exceed the number of older blacks by 25%. A similar surge in the number of non-Hispanic Asian and Pacific Islanders is also projected during the period. The proportion of the non-Hispanic white population will drop significantly from 83.5% to 64.2% (Table 1-1).[13]

Although the older adults of the future will stay more active after retiring and be better educated, the burden of incurable chronic diseases of

Table 1-1 Projected Population Age 65 and Older by Race and Hispanic Origin, 2000 and 2050

	Year 2000	Year 2050
Total	100.0	100.0
Non-Hispanic White	83.5	64.2
Non-Hispanic Black	8.1	12.2
Non-Hispanic American and Alaska Native	0.4	0.6
Non-Hispanic Asian and Pacific Islander	2.4	6.5
Hispanic	5.6	16.4

Note: Data are middle series projections of the populations. Hispanics may be of any race.

Source: U.S. Census Bureau, Population Projections of the United States by Age, Sex, Race, Hispanic Origin, and Nativity: 1999 to 2100. Published January 2000. http://www.census.gov/population/www/projections/natproj.html.

later life will be an enormous challenge to the health care system. As medical advances find more ways to maintain life, the duration of chronic illness and the number of chronically ill patients will increase. Consequently, the need for personal support will increase even more. The intensity of care required by frail older adults has the potential of affecting worker productivity. It is common for women to leave the workforce or to work part-time in order to care for frail relatives at a time when they would like to build retirement benefits for their own old age.

The increased number of older persons with chronic physical ailments and long-term cognitive disorders raises significant questions about the capability of the U.S. health care system. Much has yet to be learned by practitioners serving the aged. Health care professionals are just beginning to recognize and gradually respond to the need to focus health care for older adults away from medications or other quick-fix remedies. The system is slowly acknowledging that the traditional medical service model is inappropriate to the care of those with multiple chronic conditions. Chronically ill older patients need a multidisciplinary mix of services that must meet a broad spectrum of physical, medical, and psychosocial needs. This challenge will require a large increase in the number of health care providers trained in the special philosophies and skills of geriatric health care. The provisions of the Balanced Budget Act of 1997 that institutionalized the program of all-inclusive care for the older population in the revised Medicare reimbursement scheme symbolize growing acceptance of innovative ways to meet the needs of the older Americans.

The growing number of older adults faces serious gaps in financial coverage for long-term care needs. Unlike the broad Medicare program coverage for the acute health care problems of older Americans, the long-term care services needed to cope with the chronic disability and functional limitations of aging are largely unaddressed by either Medicare or private insurance plans. With the exception of the relatively small number of individuals with personal long-term care insurance, the major costs of long-term care services are borne by the individual older adults and their caregivers.

As a last resort, the Medicaid program has become the major public source of financing for nursing home care. Medicaid eligibility, however, requires that persons of means "spend down" their personal resources to meet the means-test criteria. For those disabled older adults who seek care in the community outside of nursing homes, Medicaid offers limited assistance. Thus, the health policy issues associated with the multidisciplinary long-term care needs of older adults mount with every year's increase in the proportion of aged Americans and every upturn in the costs of health care.

Access to Health Care

Much attention has been paid to the economic problems of health care, and considerable investments of research funds have been made to address the issues of health care quality. The third major problem, however—that of limited access to health care among the estimated 47 million uninsured or underinsured Americans—continues to confound decision makers. The issue, of course, is more a moral than economic one. Unlike most other developed nations, the United States has yet to decide on the ethical precepts that should underlie the distribution of health care. Although references frequently are made to those millions of citizens, including children, who are virtually locked out of the system, only a few professionals have had the courage to address this troublesome issue in open debate.

Polar positions have been taken by those who have addressed the question of whether society in general or governments in particular have an obligation to ensure that everyone has the right to health care and whether the health care system has a corresponding obligation to make such care available. Consider these opposing viewpoints by P. H. Elias and R. M. Sade, respectively.

Physicians who limit their office practice to insured and paying patients declare themselves openly to be merchants rather than professionals. The mercantile approach has several consequences. First, it demeans the individual physician and cheapens the profession. Second, it puts the third-party payer, as a service purchaser, in a position of greater importance than the patient. Third, it fosters the myth that physicians as a group are greedy and self-serving rather than dedicated and altruistic. And most important, it deprives a large segment of our fellow humans of care. Physicians who value their professionalism should treat office patients on the basis of need, not remuneration.[14]

The concept of medical care as the patient's right is immoral because it denies the most fundamental of all rights, that of a man to his own life and the freedom of action to support it. Medical care is neither a right nor a privilege: it is a service that is provided by doctors to others who wish to purchase it. It is the provision of this service that a doctor depends upon for his livelihood. . . . If the right to health care belongs to the patient, he starts out owning the services of a doctor without the necessity of either earning them or receiving them as a gift from the only man who has the right to give them; the doctor, himself.[15]

Although health care providers debate their individual and personal obligations to provide uncompensated care, the system itself finessed the problem for a long time by shifting the costs of care from the uninsured to the insured. This unofficial but practical approach to indigent care was ethically tolerable as long as the reimbursement system for paying patients was so open ended that the cost of treating the uninsured could easily be passed on to paying patients. The cost shifting that worked under retrospective reimbursement, however, was not feasible under prospective payment and diagnostic reimbursement guidelines. Under the current price-competitive market pressures, health care providers are in the uncomfortable position of having to apply some kind of government intervention to address the problems of health care access.

Thus, the shifting winds of health care reform only underscore the confusion of the health policy of the United States. At the same time, U.S. health policy makers would like to assure the public that the health care system provides all citizens with comparable access to health care while maintaining the freedom of the providers from government interference in decisions about service production and delivery—and add for good measure that the system exercises budgetary and cost controls in the process.

It is obvious that these goals are contradictory and that attainment of any two leaves the third uncontrolled. Thus, policy makers have been forced to choose among pairs of these goals or fail to achieve all three. In the 1990s, the government chose to let providers and insurers work out what care would be delivered and how, as long as they met government requirements for budgetary and cost controls. The third goal, equitable access, seems to have been deferred indefinitely. The achievement of some kind of universal coverage that ensures that all Americans have access to a basic level of health care will not be resolved effectively until the system's stakeholders and the supporting public can formulate and reach consensus on the fundamental values underlying the problem.

Quality of Care

Another health care system problem area relates to variations in the quality and appropriateness of medical care. The uncertainty that pervades current clinical practice is far greater than most people realize. Problems in the quality and appropriateness of many diagnostic and therapeutic procedures impact heavily on costs.

Since the November 1999 report of the Institute of Medicine that estimated that medical errors take from 44,000 to 98,000 lives per year, Congress, the president, medical institutions, and the public have been stirred to respond to a problem that has existed for years. The increasing complexity of the health care system, the potency of its pharmaceuticals, the dangers inherent in invasive surgical procedures, and the potential for error in the many information transfers that occur during hospital care combine to put patients at serious risk. The strategies proposed to cope with these problems, as well as the physician report cards, clinical guidelines, and other mechanisms designed to address inexplicable variations in the provision of medical care, are discussed in subsequent chapters.

It is important, however, to recognize the seriousness of the medical error problem. Health care errors are the leading cause of preventable deaths in the United States. Deaths resulting from medical mishaps in acute-care hospitals alone are between the fifth and eighth leading causes of all deaths in the United States. The overall burden on society is much greater when both fatal and nonfatal events are counted and when medical mishaps in medical offices, ambulatory centers, and long-term care facilities are considered.[16]

Conflicts of Interest

One of the greatest advantages of the high-technology health care systems that serve most metropolitan areas in the United States is the ability of physicians and patients to benefit from referrals to a broad range of highly specialized clinical, laboratory, rehabilitation, and other services. The array of comprehensive diagnostic and therapeutic resources available in most communities greatly enhances the clinical capability of health care providers and the care of their patients.

In recent years, however, more and more providers have begun to invest in laboratories, imaging centers, medical supply companies, and other health care businesses. In many cases, these are joint ventures with other institutions that conceal the identity of the investors. When health care providers refer patients for tests or other services to health care businesses that they own or in which they have a financial stake, there is a serious potential for conflicts of interest. In fact, for the last several years, this referral for profit has been a sensitive medical issue during congressional debates. Both federal and state governments and the American Medical Association have conducted studies that confirm that physician-owned laboratories, for example, perform more tests per patient at higher charges than those in which physicians have no investments. These conflicts of interest undermine the traditional professional role of physicians and significantly increase health care expenditures. Government attempts to limit self-serving entrepreneurial activities of physicians are driven by economic concerns. The ethical implications should be of concern to the medical profession. A major contribution would be made to the code of conduct for health care providers if the American Medical Association provided physicians with a few clear guidelines regarding the growing encroachment of commercialism on medical practice.[17]

Health Care's Ethical Dilemmas

Once almost an exclusive province of physicians and other health care providers, moral and ethical issues underlying provider/patient relationships and the difficult decisions resulting from the vast increase in treatment options are now in the domains of law, politics, journalism, health institution administrations, and the public. Since the 1970s, the list of ethical issues has expanded as discoveries in genetic identification and engineering, organ transplantation, a mounting armamentarium of highly specialized diagnostic and therapeutic interventions, and advances in technology have allowed the lives of otherwise terminal individuals to be prolonged. In addition, an energized health care consumer movement advocating more personal control over health care decisions, economic realities, and the issues of the most appropriate use of limited resources are but a few of the topics propelling values and ethics to the top of the health care agenda. There is a social dimension to health care that never existed before and that the health professions, their educational institutions, their organizations, and their philosophical leadership are just beginning to address.

Clearly, the rapid pace of change in health care and the resulting issues have outpaced U.S. society's ability to reform the thinking, values, and expectations that were more appropriate to a bygone era. Legislative initiatives are, correctly or not, filling the voids. The 1997 decision of the U.S. 9th Circuit Court of Appeals permitting physician-assisted suicide for competent, terminally ill adults in the state of Oregon is an unprecedented example. New York State's 1990 passage of health care proxy legislation that allows competent adults to appoint agents to make health care decisions on their behalf if they become incapacitated is another. Living wills that provide advance directives regarding terminal care are now recognized in all 50 states.

Issue by issue, the country is trying to come to grips with the ethical dilemmas that modern medicine has created. The pluralistic nature of this society, however, and the Judeo-Christian concepts about caring for the sick and disabled that served so well for so long make sweeping reformation of the ethical precepts on which health care has been based very unlikely.

As Americans continue to live longer and new technologies vastly improve the treatment of disease, a new generation of health plans will evolve. The basic issues of cost, quality, and access, however, will undoubtedly persist, joined by a host of new concerns. How to improve Americans' health behaviors, how to involve consumers more effectively in health care decisions, and how to determine responsibility for medical management are among the challenges of this decade.

References

1. Ginzberg E. Health care reform: why so slow? *N Engl J Med.* 1990; 32: 1464–1465.
2. Nichols LM, Ginsburg, BA, Christianson, U et al. Are market forces strong enough to deliver efficient health care systems? Confidence is waning. *Health Affairs.* 2004;23:8–21.
3. Wolinsky F. *The Sociology of Health Principles, Practitioners and Issues.* 2nd ed. Belmont, CA: Wadsworth; 1988.
4. World Health Organization. *The World Health Organization: A Report on the First Ten Years.* Geneva, Switzerland: WHO Press; 1958.
5. Blumberg DI, et al. The physician and unconventional medicine. *Alterna Ther.* 1995;1:31–35.
6. Carton B. Health insurers embrace eye-of-newt therapy. *Wall Street Journal.* January 30, 1995:B1.
7. Abelson R, Brown PL. Alternative medicine is finding its niche in nation's hospitals. *The New York Times.* April 13, 2002:B1, B3.
8. Fickenscher K, Voorman ML. An overview of rural health care. In: Shortell SM, Reinhardt UE, eds. *Improving Health Policy and Management: Nine Critical Research Issues for the 1990s.* Ann Arbor, MI: Health Administration Press; 1992:111–149.
9. Fickenscher V. An overview of rural health care. 111–149. *Annals of Internal Medicine* March 1995;Vol 122, Issue 5.
10. Federal Interagency Forum. Available from http//www.agingstats.gov/chartbook 2000/population.html (September 8, 2000). Accessed September 15, 2002.
11. Reinhardt UE. Does the aging of the population really drive the demand for health care. *Health Affairs.* 2003;22:27–39.
12. U.S. Bureau of the Census. *U.S. Population Estimates by Age, Sex, Race and Hispanic Origin: 1980–1991, Current Population Reports.* Washington, DC: Government Printing Office; 1993:15-10955, Table 1.
13. Available from http://www.census.gov/population/www/projections/natproj.html. Accessed January 24, 2004.
14. Elias PH. Letter to editor. *N Engl J Med.* 1986;314:391.
15. Sade RM. Medical care as a right: A refutation. *N Engl J Med.* 1971; 285:1281, 1289.
16. Kizer KW. Patient safety: a call to action: a consensus statement from the national quality forum. National Quality Forum for Health Care Measurement and Reporting. Available from www.qualityforum.org. Accessed September 16, 2002.
17. Relman AS. Self referral: what's at stake. *N Engl J Med.* 1992; 327:1522–1524.

CHAPTER 2

Benchmark Developments in U.S. Health Care

This chapter describes the major developments in health care in the United States and the important legislative, political, economic, organizational, and professional influences that transformed health care from a relatively simple process to one professional service and, finally, to a huge, complex, corporation-dominated industry. The effects of medical education, scientific advances, rising costs, changing population demographics, and American values and assumptions regarding health care are noted.

From its earliest history, health care, or more accurately, medical care, was dominated by physicians and their hospitals. In the 19th and early 20th centuries, participation in U.S. medicine was generally limited to two parties—patients and physicians. Diagnosis, treatment, and fees for services were considered confidential between patients and physicians. Medical practice was relatively simple and usually involved long-standing relationships with patients and, often, several generations of their families. Physicians collected their own bills and set and usually adjusted their charges to their estimates of patients' ability to pay. This was the intimate physician–patient relationship that the profession held sacred.

Free from outside scrutiny or interference, individual physicians had complete control over where, when, what, and how they practiced, and not surprisingly, they preferred to do business that way. In 1934, the American Medical Association (AMA) published this statement: "No third party must be permitted to come between the patient and his physician in any medical matter."[1] The AMA was concerned about such issues as non–physician-controlled voluntary health insurance, compulsory health insurance, and the few capitated contracts for medical services negotiated by remote lumber or mining companies and a few workers' guilds. For decades, organized medicine repeatedly battled against these and other outside influences that altered "the old relations of perfect freedom between physicians and patients, with separate compensation for each separate service."[1]

As early as the 19th century, some Americans carried insurance against sickness through an employer, fraternal order, guild, trade union, or commercial insurance company. Most of the plans, however, were simply designed to make up for lost income during sickness or injury by providing a fixed cash payment.[1] Sickness insurance, as it was originally called, was the beginning of social insurance programs against the risks of income interruption by accident, sickness, or disability. Initially, it was provided only to wage earners. Later, it was extended to workers' dependents and other people.[2]

The drive for compulsory health insurance began to build in the United States about 1915, after most European countries had initiated either compulsory programs or subsidies for voluntary programs. The underlying concern was to protect workers against a loss of income resulting from industrial accidents that were common at the time. Families with only one breadwinner, often already at the edge of poverty, were devastated by loss of income caused by sickness or injury, even without the additional costs of medical care.

At the time, life insurance companies sold "industrial" policies that provided lump-sum payments at death, which amounted to $50 or $100. The money was used to pay for final medical expenses and funerals. Both Metropolitan Life and Prudential Insurance Company rose to the top of the insurance industry by successfully marketing industrial policies that required premium payments of 10 to 25 cents per week.[2]

In 1917, World War I interrupted the campaign for compulsory health insurance in the United States. In 1919, the AMA House of Delegates officially condemned compulsory health insurance with the following resolution:[3]

The American Medical Association declares its opposition to the institution of any plan embodying the system of compulsory contributory insurance against illness or any other plan of compulsory insurance which provides for medical service to be rendered contributors or their dependents, provided, controlled, or regulated by any state or the federal government.

The majority of physician opposition to compulsory health insurance was attributed to an unfounded concern that insurance would decrease, rather than increase, physician incomes, and to their negative experience with accident insurance that paid physicians according to arbitrary fee schedules.[1]

The Great Depression and the Birth of Blue Cross

The Depression of 1929 shook the financial security of both physicians and hospitals. Physician incomes and hospital receipts and admission rates dropped precipitously. As the situation grew worse, hospitals began experimenting with insurance plans. The Baylor University Hospital plan was not the first, but it became the most influential of those insurance experiments. By enrolling 1,250 public school teachers at 50 cents a month for a guaranteed 21 days of hospital care, Baylor created the model for and is credited with the genesis of Blue Cross Hospital Insurance. Baylor started a trend that developed into multihospital plans that included all of the hospitals in a given area. By 1937, there were 26 plans with more than 600,000 members, and the American Hospital Association (AHA) started approving the plans. Physicians were pleased with the increased availability of hospital care and the cooperative manner in which their bills were paid. The AMA, however, was characteristically hostile and called the plans "economically unsound, unethical, and inimical to the public interest."[4]

The AMA contended that urging people "to save for sickness" could solve the problem of financing health care.[2] Organized medicine's consistently antagonistic reaction to the concept of health insurance, whether compulsory or voluntary, is well illustrated by medicine's response to the 1932 report of the Committee on the Costs of Medical Care. The establishment of the committee represented a shift of concern from lost wages to medical costs. Chaired by a former president of the AMA and financed by several philanthropic organizations, a group of 45 to 50 prominent Americans from the medical, public health, and the social science fields worked for 5 years to address the problem of financing medical care. After an exhaustive study, a moderate majority recommended adoption of group practice and voluntary health insurance as the best way of solving the nation's health care problems; however, even this relatively modest recommendation was too much for some physicians on the panel. They prepared a minority report denouncing voluntary health insurance as more objectionable than compulsory insurance. Health insurance, predicting or having predicted the minority, would lead to "destructive competition among professional groups, inferior medical service, loss of personal relationship of patient and physician, and demoralization of the profession."[5]

The dissenting physicians, however, did favor government intervention to alleviate the financial burden on physicians resulting from their obligation to provide free care to low-income populations. The AMA's House of Delegates reiterated its long-standing opposition to health insurance of any kind by declaring in 1933 that the minority report represented "the collective opinion of the medical profession."[6]

From the 1930s to the present, there have been many efforts to enact various forms of compulsory health insurance. It was only when the proponents of government-sponsored insurance limited their efforts to older adults and the medically indigent, however, that they were able to succeed in passing Medicaid and Medicare legislation in 1965. Voluntary insurance against hospital care costs became the predominant health insurance in the United States during those decades. Although the advocates of government-sponsored health insurance had little success in improving the access of patients to medical care, the Blue Cross plans effectively improved hospitals' access to patients.

Sensitive to the power of the health care industry to defeat health insurance proposals by raising the battle cry of "socialized medicine," almost all proposed plans emphasized accommodations to the interest of physicians and hospitals. Especially after World War II, when the federal government began to heavily subsidize hospital construction and medical research, the expansion of the health care industry, particularly physician resources, became the overriding policy objective.

The government gave a huge boost to the private health insurance industry by excluding health insurance benefits from wage and price controls and by excluding workers' contributions to health insurance from taxable income. The effect was to encourage employees to take wage increases in the form of health insurance fringe benefits rather than cash.

Because insurance companies simply raised their own premium rates rather than trying to exert pressure on physicians and hospitals to contain costs, the post–World War II health insurance system pumped an ever-increasing proportion of the national income into health care. Clearly, contributing to the inflationary spiral was preferable to incurring the wrath of physicians and hospitals by infringing on their prerogatives to set prices and control the costs of their work. Medicare and Medicaid followed the same pattern. In fact, the preamble to the original legislative proposals specifically prohibited any interpretation of the legislation that would change the way health care was practiced.

The Dominant Influence of Government

Although the health insurance industry contributed significantly to the spiraling costs of health care in the decades after World War II, it was only one of several influences. The federal government's coverage of health care for special populations played a prominent role. Over the years, the U.S. government developed, revised, and otherwise adjusted a host of categorical or disease-specific programs designed to address needs not otherwise met by state or local administrations or the private sector. Federally sponsored programs account for about 40% of this country's personal health care expenditures. Most physicians and other health professionals are trained at public expense. The government provides almost 6% of the funds available for research and development, and most not-for-profit hospitals have been built or expanded with government support. State and local governments also contribute, but in much smaller amounts.[7]

Although many of these programs are described in more detail in Chapter 7, it is important to recognize the health care policy implications of certain federal initiatives. Certainly, the Social Security Act of 1935 was the most significant social initiative passed by any Congress. The act established the principle of federal aid to the states for public health and welfare assistance, maternal and child health, and children with disabilities services. It was the legislative basis for a number of significant health and welfare programs, including the all-important Medicaid and Medicare titles.

The government increased its support of biomedical research through the National Institutes of Health, which was established in 1930, and the categorical programs that addressed heart disease, cancer, stroke, mental illness, mental retardation, maternal and infant care, and many other conditions. Programs such as direct aid to schools of medicine, dentistry, pharmacy, nursing, and other professions and their students; support of health planning, health care regulation, and consumer protections, which were incorporated in the various 1962 amendments to the 1938 Food, Drug, and Cosmetic Act, were all part of the Kennedy-Johnson presidential policy era called Creative Federalism. The aggregate annual investment in those programs made the U.S. government the major player and payer in the field of health care.

Grants-in-aid programs alone, excluding Social Security and Medicare, grew from $7 billion at the start of the Kennedy administration in 1961 to $24 billion in 1970. President Nixon expressed his intent to undo the categorical programs and shift revenues to the state and local governments. For broad general purposes, this direction was labeled New Federalism. In spite of his efforts, grants-in-aid programs grew to almost $83 billion in 1980. Congress had resisted block grants and allowed only limited revenue sharing to take place.[7]

In the meantime, federal and state governments were underwriting the skyrocketing costs of Medicare and Medicaid with no effective controls over expenditures. The planners of the Medicare legislation made several misjudgments. They underestimated the growing number of older adults in the United States, the scope and burgeoning costs of the technologic revolution, and the public's rising expectations for the latest in every diagnostic and treatment modality.

The Medicare and Medicaid programs did provide access to many desperately needed health care services for older Americans, people with disabilities, and low-income populations. Because rising Medicare reimbursement rates set the standards for most insurance companies, however, their inflationary effect was momentous. In the mid 1960s, when Medicare was passed, the United States was spending about $42 billion on health care, or approximately 8.4% of the gross national product. The cost of U.S. health care now exceeds a trillion dollars and consumes about 17% of the gross national product.

The three major health care concerns—access, cost, and quality—are particularly problematic because attempts to control one or two of those problems exacerbates the one or two remaining. It is impossible to correct all three problems simultaneously. The government attempted to improve access through the Hill-Burton Act of 1946, which increased the number and size of health care facilities substantially. In addition, President Johnson's Medicare and Medicaid legislation ensured health care payment for older Americans and low-income populations and succeeded in bringing millions of patients into a now overbuilt system. These changes, however, were made at the cost of skyrocketing expenditures and questionable quality. The health care system's excess capacity and virtually unchecked funding improved access to competent and appropriate medical care for many, but also resulted in untold numbers of clinical tests, prescriptions, surgery, and other expensive procedures that were often of questionable necessity. Almost all of the federal health legislation since the passage of Medicare and Medicaid has been aimed at reducing the costs of health care but has focused little on the reciprocal effects of reducing both the availability and quality of health care.

Efforts at Planning and Quality Control

The federal government did not ignore the issues of cost and quality; the efforts to address those concerns were essentially doomed to be ineffectual by their very designs. To get legislation passed that might alter the existing constellation of health care services or that would scrutinize how well clinicians actually practiced, the powerful medical and hospital lobbies had to be accommodated. This meant that the legislation had to be "provider friendly," allowing physicians, hospital administrators, and other health professionals to maintain control over how the legislation was interpreted and enforced.

Two legislative initiatives of the 1960s typify the circumstances surrounding federal efforts to address the problems of the health care delivery system. In 1965, the Public Health Service Act was amended to establish a nationwide network of regional medical programs to address the leading causes of death: heart disease, cancer, and stroke. Throughout the country, groups of physicians, most of whom were associated with academic medical centers, and a few nurses and other health professionals met to discuss innovative ways to bring the latest in clinical services to the bedside of the patients. As might have been predicted, representatives of each clinical specialty argued for funds to do more of what they were already doing. As a consequence, the regional medical programs improved the educational and clinical resources of their regions but did not dramatically improve the prevention or control of their target conditions.

A parallel program, the Comprehensive Health Planning Act, was passed in 1966 to promote comprehensive planning for more rational systems of health care personnel and facilities in each service region. The legislation required federal, state, and local partnerships. It also required that there be a majority of consumers on every decision-making body.[8]

Almost all of the regional medical programs and Comprehensive Health Planning Act programs across the country soon were dominated by medical–hospital establishments in their regions. Although there were many productive outcomes from the money spent through the two programs, conflicts of interest regarding the allocation of research and development funds were common, and there was general agreement that the programs were ineffective in achieving their goals. The two programs were therefore combined by the National Health Planning and Resources Development Act of 1974.

Clearly, political rather than objective assessments led Congress to presume that combining two ineffective programs would result in one successful program. Nevertheless, the legislation called for a new organization, the Health Systems Agency (HSA), to have broad representation of health care providers and consumers on governing boards and committees.

After several years, nothing had changed. Data submitted to the U.S. Department of Health, Education, and Welfare by the HSA indicated that provider board members were not representative of the overall provider work force or the consumer population. The physician/hospital administrator establishment was overrepresented, and other provider groups were underrepresented. HSA board members were predominately white males, although nonwhites and females are heavily represented in the workforce and consumer population. The HSA's function of recommending approvals of certificates of need for new or added facilities and equipment was compromised by the vested interests on the governing boards. The general ineffectiveness of HSA boards and committees in containing costs and preventing unnecessary duplication of services in their regions was recognized, and federal support ultimately was withdrawn.[9]

Several other programs beside Medicare and Medicaid were initiated during the Johnson administration to address the prevalence of mental illness and to support the education of health care professionals. The Health Professions Educational Assistance Act of 1963 provided direct federal aid to medical, dental, nursing, pharmacy, and other professional schools, as well as to their students. The Nurse Training Act supported special federal efforts for training professional nursing personnel, and during the same period, the Maternal and Child Health and Mental Retardation Planning Amendments initiated comprehensive maternal and child health projects and centers to serve people with mental retardation. The Economic Opportunity Act supported the development of neighborhood health centers to serve low-income populations.[7]

The Johnson-era programs, especially Medicare and Medicaid, put the federal government deeply into the business of financing health care. President Johnson's ambitious activation of the concept of creative federalism enriched the country's health care system and improved the access of many impoverished citizens to continually improving medical care, but it also fueled the inflationary spiral of health care costs that has yet to be constrained. It is apparent that during the last 3 decades none of the attempts to correct the unnecessary duplications of facilities and services and their excessive or inappropriate use or to contain their costs has been successful.

Managed Care Organizations

In 1973, the Health Maintenance Organization Act supported the development of health maintenance organizations (HMOs) through grants for federal demonstration projects. An HMO is an organization responsible for the financing and delivery of comprehensive health services to an enrolled population for a prepaid, fixed fee. HMOs were expected to hold down costs by changing the profit incentive from fee for service to promoting health and preventing illness.

The concept was accepted widely, and between 1992 and 1999, HMOs and other types of managed care organizations experienced phenomenal growth, accounting for the majority of all privately insured persons.[10] Subsequently, the fortunes of managed care organizations changed as both health care costs and consumer complaints increased.

Beginning in 2001, a derivative of managed care organizations, preferred provider organizations (PPOs), gained in popularity. Although PPOs encompass important managed care characteristics, they were organized by physicians and hospitals to meet the needs of private, third-party, and self-insured firms. By 2002, PPOs captured 52% of covered employees.[11]

Although the majority of Americans are now receiving their health care through some sort of prepaid managed care arrangement, the evidence that significant savings will be realized is fragmentary. Stiff increases in HMO premium rates suggest that the widespread application of HMO concepts will not provide the long-sought containment of runaway health care costs. In addition, both consumers and providers are suggesting that the HMO controls on costs are compromising the quality of care. Consumer concerns about restrictions on choice of providers, limits on availability of services, and quality of health care have evoked a managed care backlash and have generated support for government regulation of managed care organizations.

In fact, the most recent available data from a large, nationally representative sample of privately insured persons under the age of 65 years found little difference between HMOs and other types of insurance.[12] Hospital use, emergency room visits, or surgeries did not differ significantly.

The limits placed by the administrative barriers on how much health care HMO enrollees can use are considered by many patients to be an unwarranted intrusion on traditional physician/patient relationships. Public opinion polls suggest that many consumers do not trust HMOs to provide the care they need if they become sick. It is likely, therefore, that pressure by consumers for less restrictive forms of managed care will make future care management strategies and cost savings more difficult for HMOs.

The Reagan Administration

Beginning with the Reagan administration and continuing to this day are attempts, some successful, to undo or shrink the federally supported programs begun in the 1960s and 1970s. Unlike Nixon and Ford, Reagan succeeded in implementing New Federalism policies that were all but stymied in previous administrations. A significant reduction in government expenditures for social programs occurred. Decentralization of program responsibility to the states was achieved primarily through block grants. Although his attempts at deregulation to stimulate competition had little success, Reagan's implementation of prospective payment to hospitals based on diagnosis-related groups (DRGs), rather than retrospective payment based on hospital charges, signaled the new effort to contain health care costs.[13]

The DRG concept provides hospitals with a set dollar payment based on each patient's diagnosis on admission. If the hospital can discharge patients early and/or provide fewer services, it increases its profit. If patients require a longer hospital stay than the DRG allows or if more diagnostic or treatment services are needed, the hospital loses money.

The conversion of categorical and disease-specific programs to block grants, the withdrawal of federal support for professional education, and the creation of a Medicare resource-based relative value scale to adjust and contain physicians' fees are but a few examples of presidential or congressional actions to reduce the federal government's financial commitment to health care.

Biomedical Advances: Evolution of High-Technology Medicine

Health care in the United States dramatically improved during the 20th century. In the first half of the century, the greatest advances led to the prevention or cure of many infectious diseases. The development of vaccines to prevent a wide range of communicable diseases, from yellow fever to measles, and the discovery of antibiotics saved vast numbers of Americans from early death or disability.

In the second half of the 20th century, however, technological advances that characterize today's health care were developed. As so often happens with technological change, after the scientific concepts that underlie the initial breakthroughs are understood, the pace of technological development accelerates rapidly. Since the 1960s, the rate of technologic advance has increased so quickly that the announcement of new discoveries or more sophisticated equipment has become commonplace.

A few of the seminal medical advances that took place during the 1960s were the following:

- The Sabin and Salk vaccines ended the annual epidemics of poliomyelitis.
- The mild tranquilizers Librium and Valium were introduced and widely prescribed, leading Americans to turn to medicine to cure their emotional as well as physical ills.

- The birth-control pill was first prescribed and became the most widely used and effective contraceptive method.
- The heart–lung machine and major improvements in the efficacy and safety of general anesthesia techniques made possible the first successful heart bypass operation in 1964. Three years later, the first human heart transplant took place.

In 1972, the computed tomography (CT) scan was invented. The CT scan, which unlike X-rays can distinguish one soft tissue from another, is installed widely in U.S. hospitals. This valuable and profitable diagnostic imaging device started an extravagant competition among hospitals to develop lucrative patient services by making major capital investments in high-technology equipment. Later, noting the convenience and profit associated with diagnostic devices such as CT scanners and magnetic resonance imaging, medical groups purchased the device and placed them in their own offices. This practice represents one example of how hospitals, physicians, and other health service providers have come to act as isolated economic entities, rather than as members of a community of health care resources established to serve population needs. The profit-driven competition and resulting redundant capacity continue to drive up utilization and costs for hospitals, insurers, and the public.[14]

New technology, new drugs, and new and creative surgical procedures have made possible a wide variety of life-enhancing and life-extending medical accomplishments. Operations that once were complex and hazardous, requiring hospitalization and intense follow-up care, have become relatively common ambulatory surgical procedures. For example, the use of intraocular lens implants after the removal of cataracts has become one of the most popular surgical procedures (see Chapter 4). Performed on over a half-million Americans annually, the procedure takes less than an hour and has very high success rates, and complications are rare. Although the ambulatory procedure costs less than it would in an inpatient setting, the aggregate costs for eye surgery will grow as the demand for the operation escalates among the increasing number of older Americans.

Almost every medical or technological advance seems to be accompanied by new and vexing financial and ethical dilemmas. The greater ability to extend life raises questions about the quality of life and the right to die. New capabilities to use costly and limited resources to improve the quality of life for some and not others create other ethical problems.

Whatever its benefits, the increased use of new technology has contributed to higher health care costs; however, some believe that if the new technology were used properly and not overused for the sake of defensive medicine or to take advantage of its profit potential, it would actually lower health care costs.[15]

Both the AMA and the federal government have developed programs to explore these issues and to provide needed information for decision makers. The AMA has three programs to assess the ramifications of medical advancements: the Diagnostic and Therapeutic Technology Assessment Program, the Council on Scientific Affairs, and AMA Drug Evaluations.[16]

In the Technology Assessment Act of 1972, Congress recognized that "it is essential that, to the fullest extent possible, the consequences of technological applications be anticipated, understood, and considered in determination of public policy on existing and emerging national problems."[17] To address this goal, the Office of Technology Assessment, a nonpartisan support agency that works directly with and for congressional committees, was created. The Office of Technology Assessment relics on the technical and professional resources of the private sector, including universities, research organizations, industry, and public interest groups, to produce their assessments and provide congressional committees with analyses of highly technical issues. It was intended to help officials sort out the facts without advocating particular policies or actions.

The Agency for Health Care Policy and Research, created by Congress in 1989 and now called the Agency for Healthcare Policy and Quality, is intended to support research to understand better the outcomes of health care at both clinical and systems levels. It has a particularly challenging mission as technologic and scientific advances make it ever more difficult to sort out the complexities of health care and determine what works, for whom, when, and at what cost.

Roles of Medical Education and Specialization

Medical schools and teaching hospitals in the United States are the essential components of all academic health centers and are the principal architects of the medical care system. In addition to their research contributions to advancements in health care and their roles as major providers of health services, they are the principal places where physicians and other professional personnel are educated and trained. Year after year, professional schools graduate thousands of medical, nursing, and other professionals whose attitudes, values, and skills have been shaped by the educational and socialization process of their professional preparation. The annual infusion of new graduates of professional schools serves to reinforce continuously the values and policies of their teachers and role models.

During the last 30 years, medical education and policies regarding the size and nature of the physician workforce have influenced the size, structure, and operation of the American health care industry. From post–World War II to the mid-1970s, there were numerous projections of an impending shortage of physicians. The response at federal and state levels was to double the capacity of medical schools and to encourage the entry of foreign-trained physicians.[18]

The explosion of scientific knowledge in medicine and the technologic advances in diagnostic and treatment modalities encouraged specialization. In addition, the enhanced prestige and income of specialty practice attracted the majority of medical school graduates to specialty residencies. It soon became evident that specialists were being produced in numbers that would lead to an oversupply. Also, they needed to be close to their referring doctors and to associate with major hospitals, which caused graduates to concentrate in urban medical centers. At the same time, the shortage of nonspecialists among rural and inner-city populations became more serious.

Medical schools and hospitals, however, were not willing to address these related problems by giving up their high-demand, productive, and well-regarded specialist training emphases. Instead, they developed a more acceptable physician workforce policy to maintain or increase their training capacities. Schools erroneously assumed that producing an oversupply of physicians would force more physicians into primary care in underserved rural and inner-city areas. Unfortunately, this trickle-down workforce policy did little to change these problems and only added to the swelling ranks of specialists. Most new physicians still chose specialties in which the supply was already adequate and elected to practice where the surplus of physicians was increasing.

Hospitals added to the problem by developing residencies that met their own service needs without regard for oversupply. Supplemental

Medicare payments for teaching hospitals and indirect medical education adjustments for hospital-based residents were and still are strong incentives for hospitals to add residents.[19]

The failure of past physician workforce policies is evident. In 1989, despite major increases in the physician supply, rural areas in the United States had fewer than 100 physicians per 100,000 persons, compared with up to six times that many in major cities. Furthermore, increasing the number of medical graduates did not correct the imbalance between specialists and generalists.[20]

The rapid growth of managed care plans in the 1990s was expected to produce profound changes in the use of the physician workforce. The emphasis on prevention and primary care and the employment of generalist physician "gatekeepers" to control inappropriate or unnecessary use of physician specialists was expected to cause a significant oversupply of specialists by the year 2000. To stave off the surplus, many medical schools and their teaching hospitals endeavored to produce equal numbers of primary care and specialist physicians instead of the one-third/two-third ratio that had existed for years.

As soon as the effort produced a sizable increase in the number of primary care physicians, new medical workforce projections refuted the prior predictions and forecast a shortage, rather than a surplus, of specialists. Current evidence indicates that the demand for certain specialists is exceeding the supply. Quite appropriately, a majority of new medical school graduates are once again electing to prepare for practice in a medical specialty. Clearly, estimating a future physician shortage or surplus is a tenuous endeavor.

The forces of reform are exerting increasing pressures on schools of medicine and the other major health professions to change their curricula in keeping with the new emphasis on population-based thinking, prevention, and cost-effectiveness. The inflexibility of traditional departmental organization and the relatively narrow areas of expertise required of faculty, however, present formidable obstacles to needed educational reforms. Roger Bulger, president of the Association of Academic Health Centers, urged academic medical centers to "demonstrate a real commitment to multiprofessional, interdisciplinary team approaches to a patient centered system" and considers the "forces that separate various health professions" and the "devalued status of teaching within our institutions" as preventing adequate responses to the changing environment.[21]

Influence of Interest Groups

Many of the problems associated with U.S. health care result from a system shared among federal and state governments and the private health care industry. The development of fully or partially tax-funded health service proposals initiated waves of lobbying efforts by interest groups for or against the initiatives. Federal and state executives and legislators continue to receive intense pressure from supporters and opponents of health care system changes.[22] Lobbying efforts from special interest groups have become increasingly sophisticated and well financed. Since the 1970s, former congressional staffers appear on the payrolls of private interest groups, and former lobbyists assume positions on Capitol Hill. This strong connection between politicians and lobbyists is evidenced by the record number of dollars spent to defeat the Clinton Health Security Act of 1993.

Five major groups have played a key role in the debate on tax-funded health services: providers, insurers, consumers, business, and labor. Historically, physicians, the group most directly affected by reforms, developed the most powerful lobbies. Although the physician lobby is still among the best financed and most effective, it is recognized as not representing the values of large numbers of physicians detached from the AMA. In fact, several different medical lobbies exist as a result of political differences among physicians.

The American Medical Association (AMA)

The AMA, founded in 1847, is the largest medical lobby, with a membership of 287,000 individuals, yet it represents less than half of the medical professionals. The AMA was at the height of its power from the 1940s to the 1970s, opposing government-provided insurance plans by every president from Truman through Carter. Compromises gained in the final Medicare bill still affect today's program. In the 1980s, however, the AMA steadfastly opposed cuts in Medicare proposed by the Reagan-Bush administration. James S. Sammons, then AMA executive vice-president, led the opposition and alienated several congressional members through the use of highly confrontational tactics. Since 1989, when James Todd replaced Sammons, the AMA has changed its relationship with Congress.

Initially locked out of White House discussions on the Clinton plan, the AMA was later included and supported the idea of expanding health care access to all Americans. Nevertheless, cost containment, malpractice reform, and physician autonomy still remain as areas of contention.[23]

Other Physician Groups

The American College of Physicians, the American Academy of Family Physicians, the American Society of Internal Medicine, and the American College of Surgeons all make their presence known in Washington as they lobby on behalf of their members' interests.[23]

As in the case of physicians, the lobbying efforts of hospitals have also been weakened by a loss of unity. In the late 1970s, the powerful hospital lobby was able to defeat President Carter over the issue of increased cost containment; however, in 1983, President Reagan was able to pass Medicare's prospective payment system successfully, which benefited some providers but harmed others. Prospective payment set the more expensive hospitals against the less expensive ones, southern hospitals against northern ones, for-profit hospitals against not-for-profit ones, and urban hospitals against rural ones.[24]

The influence of the AHA has decreased as a result of the persistent competition in the hospital industry. Founded in 1898, the AHA is the largest hospital group, with a combined membership of approximately 42,000 facilities and individuals. Despite its large size, Reagan's Medicare victory caused disagreement within AHA's membership and lessened its leverage on the national scene. As differences have begun to subside, the power of the AHA has increased but never again has reached the level it attained in the late 1970s.

Other Hospital Groups

The Federation of American Health Systems (FAHS) has a membership of 1,400 hospitals and health systems and was founded in 1966 to represent the for-profit portion of the hospital population. When the AHA lost power in the mid-1980s, the FAHS was there to take over. The group staunchly opposes any government-imposed price controls. This stance decreased its influence after the first President Bush was defeated in 1992. After President George W. Bush reclaimed the presidency for the Republican Party, the FAHS regained some influence.

The Catholic Health Association of the United States, founded in 1915, represents the fewest members: 700 hospitals and 300 nursing homes. As such, it exercises little political power.[23] It should be noted, however, that in the current political environment, hospital associations, individually or collectively, have little influence on the legislative agenda. Although addressing the complicated problems of the U.S. health care system was one of the hottest political issues before the terror attacks of 2001, health care has dropped in political priority well below the troubled national economy and homeland security.

The American Nurses Association (ANA)

The American Nurses Association is the only major nursing interest group and serves 200,000 members. The American Nurses Association was founded in 1896; however, nurses were not very politically active until about 1980. The organization now has an elaborate network of congressional district coordinators who develop effective campaign organizations for nurses within their districts. The ANA endorsed the Clinton plan in mid-September of 1993 and earned several concessions, including elimination of state restrictions of scope of practice, direct Medicare reimbursement, and a doubling of federal support for training.[23]

Insurance Companies

Even more than physicians, nurses, or hospitals, insurers' political efforts have been viewed as completely self-serving. The efforts of insurance companies to eliminate high-risk consumers from the insurance pools and their frequent premium rate hikes have contributed significantly to the focus on cost containment and the plight of the uninsured and underinsured in the debate on health care reform. Nevertheless, the Health Insurance Association of America, founded in 1956 and representing some 300 small companies, was responsible for that seemingly endless onslaught of television commercials featuring middle-class people worrying about the limited choice of physicians and other potential dangers of cost containment in the Clinton plan.[23]

Other insurers' groups include the Group Health Association of America, founded in 1959, and the Blue Cross and Blue Shield Association, founded in 1946. The Group Health Association of America's 1,100 individual members welcomed the idea of numerous new cash-paying customers that would have been created by the Clinton plan. The 69 organizations encompassed by Blue Cross/Blue Shield have often served as insurers of last resort for Americans, resulting in a large proportion of high-risk people in its pool of nearly 70 million. The fact that enactment of reforms would change their demographic disadvantage made Blue Cross/Blue Shield an ally of Clinton and of reform in general.[23]

Consumer Groups

Although provider groups have been most effective in influencing health care legislation, the historically weak consumer movement has gained strength. Much of the impetus for health care reform on the national scene was linked to pressure on politicians from consumers concerned about rising costs and lack of security in health care coverage. Despite widespread disagreement among groups about the extent to which government involvement is needed, all are concerned about the questions of cost, access, and quality in the current health care system.

Better educated and more assertive citizens have become more cynical about the motives of leaders in both the political and health arenas and much more effective in influencing legislative decisions. A prominent example is the American Association of Retired Persons (AARP). Founded in 1958, the AARP is one of the most influential consumer groups in the health care reform movement. Because of its size and research capability, it wields considerable clout among legislators who are very aware that the AARP's 35 million older citizens are among the most determined voters.

Although a single consumer group may have some influence in shaping a legislative proposal, consumer group coalitions that rally around specific issues are much more effective in generating political pressure. For example, a political battle over revamping the Food and Drug Administration (FDA) was initiated in 1995 when conservative think tanks and drug company officials urged a receptive Congress to make major changes in the agency's operations. These changes were intended to weaken the agency's investigative powers and reduce the time required for drug companies to introduce new drugs to the consumer market. The proposed changes would require the FDA to meet deadlines for investigating and approving new drugs and allow pharmaceutical companies to submit one, rather than two, well-controlled studies as proof of effectiveness.

Consumer groups entered the debate on both sides of the issue. The biggest and best organized was the Patients' Coalition, which is made up of more than 50 national nonprofit health groups. It includes such dissimilar organizations as the American Cancer Society, National Hemophilia Foundation, Arthritis Foundation, and several AIDS organizations such as the AIDS Action Council and Gay Men's Health Crisis. The coalition rushed to the FDA's defense and urged Congress to reject the proposals that could hurt consumers. Other consumer groups support the positions of the Pharmaceutical Research and Manufacturers Association, the main industry trade group that claims that FDA reforms could be accomplished without risking safety and effectiveness.[24]

The battle continues, however, between those who think that keeping new drugs from the market while safety and effectiveness are carefully tested is denying help to those patients who might benefit from them and those who presume that drug manufacturers would take advantage of less rigorous testing to foist unproven or dangerous drugs on the market for profit. While the two sides continue to debate, administrative changes have taken place that shortened the assessment time for cancer-treating drugs in an effort to prolong life for dying patients.[25]

Business and Labor

In the 1960s and 1970s, business groups were among those that blocked health reform legislation. Today, such legislation is seen as inevitable, and employer mandates and insurance costs have become central concerns. Here, too, there is division. Small firms tended to oppose reform because they might not be able to afford to insure their workers. Large firms favored reform because their insurance coverage costs are likely to be reduced.

The National Federation of Independent Businesses, founded in 1943, has 570,000 individual members and is the largest representative of small firms. The National Association of Manufacturers has a much smaller membership of 12,500 individuals. Founded in 1895, it represents the interests of large employers. The U.S. Chamber of Commerce was founded in 1912 and represents 200,000 individuals and businesses. The Chamber and the National Association of Manufacturers have similar views on reform; they both generally welcome the equalizing effect of an employer mandate but are wary of intense government regulation.[23]

Whenever business groups are involved in an issue, labor unions are sure to make their presence felt as well. The American Federation of Labor and Congress of Industrial Organization (AFL-CIO), once over 14 million individuals strong, has had a tremendous influence on national health policy. Although job losses during the current economic downturn have reduced membership by over a million members, the influence of organized labor is significant. Intimately connected with the AFL-CIO is the Service Employees International Union, founded in 1921. It is the largest union representing health care workers, with a membership of 1 million individuals, and its president is also chairman of the AFL-CIO's health care committee.

During the mid-1940s, labor unions began to demand health care benefits as an alternative to wage increases not possible during postwar wage and price controls.[23] The two major national unions, the AFL and the CIO consolidated their power by merging in 1955. During the late 1960s, they were able to address the issues of occupational safety and health and achieved passage of the Occupational Safety and Health Act of 1970. Today, occupational safety and health hold a prominent place on the national agenda, and efforts to weaken the 1970 legislation or to reduce its enforcement are met with strong opposition from organized labor.

The Pharmaceutical Industry

In recent years, the profit-laden pharmaceutical industry increased its spending on lobbying tactics and campaign contributions to unprecedented levels. With prescription drug prices and pharmaceutical company profits at record highs, the industry correctly anticipated public and congressional pressure to legislate controls on drug prices and drug coverage for older adults on Medicare.

Between 1997 and 1999, the drug industry spent $235.7 million to lobby Congress and the executive branch. As lawmakers moved to add a prescription-drug benefit to Medicare that would include price controls, the drug industry hired 297 lobbyists—one for every two members of Congress.[26] Campaign contributions also rose to almost $14 million, a 147% increase over previous years. An industry that can spend that amount of money to block a comprehensive Medicare drug benefit that reins in sky-high drug costs is clearly costing the American public dearly. In fact, for the first time in the history of the U.S. health care system, insurers that cover prescription drug costs report that pharmaceutical costs now exceed the costs of hospital care.

More recently, the pharmaceutical industry made a calculated decision to throw its financial weight behind the Republican Party with $50 million in campaign contributions and an even larger army of lobbyists that has unlimited budgets to influence legislators. To date, it has succeeded in stifling any measure that would put a dent in its corporate earnings.[27]

In addition, the pharmaceutical industry was given a large role in crafting the 2003 Medicare Part D prescription drug benefit plan, which in 2006 began providing huge profits to drug companies. Unfortunately, those Medicare recipients who enrolled in the plan were faced with a baffling array of choices. California, for example, offers 55 prescription drug plans from which to choose, and seniors find that it is very difficult to get accurate, unbiased information. Each plan has its own premium, its own deductible, and its own co-payment for individual drugs.[28]

One of the most contentious elements in the Medicare Part D drug plan is the so-called doughnut hole. Beginning in 2006, the legislation calls for ending federal payment for a person's drug purchases after an annual spending limit is reached. Federal support resumes only after the beneficiary has spent $3,600 in out-of-pocket for prescription drugs. The "doughnut hole" directly affects the middle class and disabled retirees who do not qualify for special poverty assistance yet still live on limited fixed incomes.

Public Health Focus on Prevention

Although groups discussed in the previous section are primarily concerned with the diagnostic and treatment services that constitute over 95% of the U.S. health care system, there is an important public health lobby that speaks for health promotion and disease prevention. Often overlooked because of this country's historical emphasis on curative medicine, public health organizations have had to overcome several negative perceptions. Many health providers, politicians, and others associate public health with governmental bureaucracy or link the care of low-income populations with welfarism. Nevertheless, the American Public Health Association, founded in 1872 and having an aggregate membership of 50,000, has substantial influence on the national scene; however, because the positions of public health advocates are considered liberal in nature, the influence of the American Public Health Association wanes when the Republicans are in power and rises during Democratic administrations.

The significant contributions of both governmental and voluntary organized public health agencies to the health of the American public and the political struggles that led to those accomplishments are described in Chapter 10.

Economic Influences: Rising Costs

The single most important impetus for health care reform throughout recent history has been rising costs. Since the introduction of Medicare and Medicaid in 1965, almost all federal health law has been aimed at cost containment, but without success. Overall, health care costs have risen from 5.3% of the U.S. gross domestic product (GDP) in 1960 to over 15% in 2006. Growth in health spending has been advancing much faster than the rest of the U.S. economy. Aggregate health spending rose to over $2 trillion in 2006 or to almost $7,000 per person. In that year, health spending's share of the U.S. GDP rose to over 15%. Without major changes, government projections suggest that health spending will reach 18.7% of the GDP by 2014.[29]

Advocates of health care reform are cautiously more optimistic now that both houses of the 2007 Congress have Democratic majorities. Fundamental questions of how the complex and vested interest system should be reformed, however, remain the subjects of partisan debate.

Chapter 7 presents a comprehensive overview of the complex and interlocking systems of fiscal incentives and constraints that contribute to the rising costs of health care and the difficulties inherent in attempts to exercise control over those costs.

The Uninsured and Problems of Access to Medical Care

The problems of access to health care, exacerbated by rising costs and reductions in Medicaid coverage, are generally related to place of residence and employment status. The lack of easily accessible health care services in rural and inner city areas often presents serious problems for low-income and lower middle-income families. For the medically indigent outside of Medicaid programs, however, the absence of adequate health insurance constitutes an almost insurmountable barrier to obtaining anything other than emergency medical care. The risk of being uninsured or underinsured is greater for those who are unemployed or employed at low-level jobs that do not offer group health insurance or who are unable to work and are not covered by Medicaid.

The number of Americans without adequate or any health insurance was estimated at 37 million during the health care reform debates of 1994. In 1996, that number was estimated to have grown to 40 million. In 2004, estimates of the number of uninsured individuals were around 45 million. More recent census bureau estimates put the number of uninsured at 46.6 million Americans or 16% of the total population.[30]

Of most importance when considering the magnitude of the problem is that the composition of that uninsured population is constantly changing. When those on Medicaid or other unemployed persons find jobs that provide group health insurance, those individuals leave the ranks of the uninsured. They are replaced, however, by those who become unemployed or lose Medicaid coverage. More and more employers, upset by the ever rising costs of employee health insurance, are reducing or eliminating health insurance as a fringe benefit.

The Health Insurance Portability and Accountability Act (HIPAA)

The Health Insurance Portability and Accountability Act (HIPAA), signed into law in 1996, was intended to address the problem of the growing number of uninsured. The legislation permits individuals to continue insurance coverage after a loss or change of employment by mandating the renewability of insurance coverage except for specific reasons, such as the nonpayment of premiums. The act also regulates the circumstances in which an insurance plan may limit benefits because of preexisting conditions. It also mandates special enrollment periods for individuals who have experienced certain changes in family composition or employment status.

More sweeping in its effects is the part of the law called "Administrative Simplification." It required medical records to be computerized by October 2003. Although yet to be achieved, it is intended to reduce the costs and administrative burden of health care by standardizing the electronic transmission of many administrative and financial transactions. The standardization must also maintain the privacy of health information. As a result, the entire health care industry is involved in a costly high-tech upgrade of complex medical and financial documents to comply with the legislation.[31]

The Aging of America

The elimination or control of many infectious diseases through immunization and antibiotics; the implementation of basic public health measures that contribute to the safety of food, water, and living and working conditions; a far more nutritious food supply; and constantly improving medical care have all combined to extend the life expectancy of people in the United States. Although AIDS, accidents, and violence are causing an increasing number of deaths among young people, the vast majority of Americans live to advanced ages. The proportion of Americans aged 65 and older is projected to grow from 12.7% in 2000 to 20% in 2030. Approximately half of those older people will be over 75 years of age. The population over 85 years of age is increasing even faster. By 2050, it is expected that one in four of those over 65 years old will be 85 years or older.[32]

The increased longevity of the population, particularly those with serious or disabling chronic illness, poses serious challenges to the U.S. health care system. The problems of financing and delivering an increasingly broad array of medical and other long-term care services are already serious and will become more critical as the proportion of dependent older adults grows in relation to the number still in the workforce.

Although the medical model of curing illness, maximizing function, and preventing premature death has been beneficial to many older

Americans, it offers little to the growing number of older citizens who are not acutely or morbidly ill, but who have irreversible physical or mental limitations that require diligent care by others. Although the number and kinds of institutionally- and community-based long-term care services (described in Chapter 8) have increased, many are struggling to balance actual and perceived patient needs against their allowed benefits, rising costs, and limits imposed by third-party payers.

Of increasing importance is the need for mechanisms to support care-givers as older person care becomes the responsibility of more and more Americans. Changes in U.S. social structures have increased the stress on today's adults because they are required to provide financial, functional, or emotional support to aging family members. More women working out-side the home, a high divorce rate, the geographic dispersion of family members, an increase in the number of adults simultaneously caring for both children and aging relatives, and the rise in the proportion of older adults taking care of even older relatives make respite services, adult day care, and other strategies to reduce stress and caregiver burnout mandatory.

Values and Assumptions
that Guide Priorities

Under the leadership of the U.S. Department of Health and Human Services Public Health Service, a consortium of 300 organizations collab-orated in a process that led to the design of a decade-long national plan for reducing preventable deaths, disabilities, and diseases. The 1990 plan was called Healthy People 2000: An Overview of the National Health Promotion and Disease Prevention Objectives. Most states have devel-oped their own Healthy People 2000 objectives tailored and targeted to their own populations.

Healthy People 2000 contains the following impressive statements:[33]

The greatest opportunities for improvement and the greatest threats to the future health status of the people reside in certain subpopulations that have historically been disadvantaged economically, educationally, and politi-cally. "Healthy People 2000" calls for special attention to reducing—and finally eliminating—disparities in death, disease, and disability rates expe-rienced by these groups compared with the general population. . . . For the coming decade, perhaps no challenge is more compelling than that of equal opportunity for good health.

Unfortunately, Americans seem to hold values that shape their responses to proposals for changes in health delivery or financing that seem to put the goals of Healthy People 2000 out of reach. There is a moral commitment to the uninsured population, but much of that concern is self-serving and results from the fear of unexpected unemployment. There is a genuine desire to achieve personal peace of mind and empathy for those without it; however, there also is a lack of self-blame. As in other endeavors, there is an absence of personal accountability among both providers and consumers in the fields of health care.

Nothing illustrates the unrealistic posturing of the public health sector better than the latest set of 10-year targets for health improvement in the United States, which was assembled by a consortium of over twice as many national, professional, and voluntary organizations as produced Healthy People 2000. Healthy People 2010 essentially ignores the failure to meet 85% of the last decade's goals and establishes several hundred more equally unattainable objectives. Notably lacking in these monumental efforts to establish health improvement goals is either the organizational commitment or the strategies to make them happen.

It is indicative of a self-indulgent society that there is a limited willingness to take personal responsibility, to sacrifice for the benefit of others, and to judge each proposed change in the health service structure in terms of reasoned self-interest. The result is a basic incongruity in the U.S. system of health care. The system strives to improve an already superb ability to care for the individual patient, but it fails dismally to address the problems of the larger society.

Public Health's Lack of Preparedness

The terrorist attacks on September 11, 2001, and the 2005 Gulf Coast hurricanes revealed the lack of preparedness of this country's public health system to cope with emergency situations. Clearly, there were both "quality" and "quantity" deficits in public health preparedness. Both the number and the competencies of public health personnel available for emergency preparedness, as well as the systems in which they work, were revealed to be woefully inadequate.[34]

On the positive side, public exposure of the dwindling numbers of public health workers of highly variable competencies, employed in widely different public health organizations, was revealed as the consequences of decades of benign neglect. In Chapter 11, the extensive efforts to remedy the problems leading to the lack of emergency preparedness are discussed.

In a country facing epidemics of teenage pregnancy, sexually transmitted diseases, drug addiction, drive-by shootings, and crack-addicted infants, there seems to be a striking capacity for ignoring the truth about matters of public health and public good. Warren Bennis, author of *Why Leaders Can't Lead*, attributes this disregard in large part to the United States's historical commitment to individual freedom. He explains why the decline in societal concern for the less fortunate that started in the 1980s was so well accepted.[35]

> The conflicts between individual rights and the common good are far older than the nation, but they have never been as sharp or as mean as they are today. In fact, as the upwardly mobile person has replaced the citizen, we have less and less that is good. The founding fathers based the constitution on the assumption that there was such a thing as public virtue. James Madison wrote, "The public good . . . the real welfare of the great body of people . . . is the supreme object to be pursued." At the moment, we not only cannot agree on what the public good is, we show no inclination to pursue it.

Even the institutions in which health care providers work reflects similar values. Rosemary Stevens, author of *In Sickness and in Wealth*, writes:[36]

> By 1980 hospitals seemed obsessed with the language of management. Instead of an increased emphasis on chronic care and social services after the advent of Medicare and Medicaid—not an unreasonable expectation in programs dedicated to the older adult and low-income populations— hospital administrative training programs began to require courses in financial management. Administrators became managers, presidents, or CEOs; and the hospital journals rang with news of "product lines" (patient care), of capital financing, of diversification and innovation and of the "bottom line."

Under pressure to adjust to rapidly changing economic circumstances, many hospitals are engaging with providers in joint investments that raise serious questions about conflicts of interest. Ventures into the construction of privately owned high-technology diagnostic facilities by providers who refer patients for those services proliferate in competition with hospital facilities, apparently without concern for the ethical issues involved.

Oregon Death with Dignity Act

November 8, 1994, was a pivotal date in the U.S. social legislation. Oregon voters approved Ballot Measure 16, the Oregon Death with Dignity Act, also known as the Oregon Physician-Assisted Suicide Act. The act legalized physician-assisted suicide by allowing "an adult resident of Oregon, who is terminally ill to voluntarily request a prescription for medication to take his or her life."[37] The person must have "an incurable and irreversible disease that will, within reasonable medical judgment, produce death within six months." The Death with Dignity Act was a response to the growing concern among medical professionals and the public about the extended, painful, and demeaning nature of terminal medical care for patients with certain conditions. An additional consideration for some voters was the worry that the extraordinary costs associated with lengthy and futile medical care would exhaust their estates and leave their families with substantial debts.

A survey of Oregon physicians showed that two-thirds of those responding believe that physician-assisted suicide is ethical in appropriate cases, and almost half of the responding physicians (46%) said that they might assist in a suicide if the patient met the criteria outlined in the act.[38]

The issue of euthanasia and physician-assisted suicide has been debated for years in other countries. Although among Westernized countries, only Northern Australia has legalized physician-assisted suicide, the Netherlands has a long history of allowing euthanasia within the medical community.[39] Although technically illegal, there are specifications guiding the practice, and doctors following the guidelines are not prosecuted.[40]

Provisions of the Oregon Death with Dignity Act

A physician must meet multiple requirements before he or she can write a prescription for a lethal combination of medications. The physician must ensure that the patient is fully informed about the diagnosis, the prognosis, the risks, and likely result of the medications and the alternatives, including comfort care, pain control, and hospice care. Then a consulting physician must confirm that the patient's judgment is not impaired by a mental condition and that the decision is fully informed and voluntary. The patient will then be asked to notify next of kin. Family notification is not mandatory, however. After a 15-day waiting period, the patient must again repeat the request. If the patient does so, the physician is then permitted to write the fatal prescription.[41] Although it varies from year to year, fewer than half of the terminally ill patients who receive prescriptions actually ingests the lethal medications.[42]

The Internet and Health Care

Data collection and information transfer are critical elements of the health care system, and thus, it is not surprising that the Internet has become a major influence in U.S. health care. Eighty percent of American Internet users, or some 113 million adults have searched online for health information.[43] Consumers have access to vast resources of health and wellness information, have the ability to communicate with others sharing similar health problems, and are able to gain valuable data about medical institutions and providers that permit well-informed choices about services and procedures. Internet users are becoming more educated and participatory in clinical decision making. Physicians and other providers are now challenged by the need to deal with a more knowledgeable and involved patient population.

Health care consumers turn to the Internet, at least in part, because of dissatisfaction with the amount of information available from traditional sources. A host of websites offers everything from interactive health assessments to personalized diet and fitness programs. Internet use also provides the benefit of anonymity, convenience, and freedom from inhibitions. For those reasons, it is becoming a growing alternative to traditional in-office counseling, particularly in the field of mental health. The mental health field has initiated a variety of forms of online therapy for consumers who are more comfortable with the impersonal nature of Internet communication.

Providers also are entering the online world of health care communication. After a slow start, provider-sponsored websites are proliferating at a rapid pace. In addition to information for consumers about the provider's training, competencies, and experience, many providers encourage e-mail exchanges that invite queries and provide opportunities to respond to consumer informational needs.

A wide variety of other web-based entrepreneurial ventures have also begun to take advantage of the huge and growing market of Internet surfers. Both dependable and questionable entrepreneurs are offering consumers opportunities to cybershop for pharmaceuticals, insurance plans, medical supplies and equipment, specific physician services, and other health-related commodities. The public is well advised to be cautious in making commitments on the Internet. A listing of some of the most reliable consumer-oriented websites is in Appendix B.

The Basic Issues

The basic issues underlying efforts to improve the U.S. health care system remain, as they have for decades, concerns for costs, access, and quality. Although knowledge, technology, and resources have developed so that superb and dramatic medical care can be provided to meet even the most formidable needs of this country's population, such care is provided at unacceptable cost, with unnecessary duplications of effort, and to the exclusion of the health maintenance and preventive activities that might have reduced the incidence of the medical conditions that required those curative efforts. It is, by every assessment, a health care system focused on providing excellent care for the individuals within it, while virtually ignoring the more basic health service needs of the larger populations outside of it.

Emeritus Professor of Public Health at Yale University School of Medicine George Silver described the current health care dilemma with these observations:

> The pressures on Congress, professional groups such as the American Medical Association and the American Hospital Association, and the health care insurance companies are directed toward developing a legislative package that will ameliorate the suffering of the underserved, provide coverage for the uninsured, control costs, and satisfy doctors and hospitals without huge tax increases or intolerable additional wage assessments.

Physicians are sullen and discontented under the burden of regulations and constraints that seriously impede their flexibility and ability to use professional judgment freely. Patients are angry with inflated costs, rising insurance premiums, and various impediments and obstacles to maintaining a comfortable, friendly relationship with doctors. Other patients are unable to obtain needed medical services to the extent required, or at all. Critics and reformers attack the medical profession as greedy, uncaring, and even incompetent. Malpractice accusations proliferate, and costs and judgments soar.[44]

References

1. Numbers RL. The Third Party: Health Insurance in America. In: Vogel MJ, Rosenburg CE, eds. *The Therapeutic Revolution: Essays in the Social History of American Medicine*. Philadelphia, PA: University of Pennsylvania Press; 1979.
2. Starr P. Transformation in Defeat: The Changing Objectives of National Health Insurance, 1915–1980. In: Kindig DA, Sullivan RB, eds. *Understanding Universal Health Programs, Issues and Options*. Ann Arbor, MI: Health Administration Press; 1992.
3. Minutes of the House of Delegates. *JAMA*. 1920;74:1317–1328.
4. Leland RG. Prepayment plans for hospital care. *JAMA*. 1933;100:113–117.
5. *Medical Care for the American People: The Final Report of the Costs of Medical Care. Committee on the Costs of Medical Care*. Chicago, IL: University of Chicago Press; 1932.
6. Minutes of the Eighty-Fourth Session, 12–16 June 1933. *JAMA*, 1933; 100:44–53.
7. Lee PR, Benjamin AE. Health Policy and the Politics of Health Care. In: Lee PR, Estes CL, eds. *The Nation's Health*. 4th ed. Boston, MA: Jones & Bartlett Publishers; 1994.
8. Litman TJ, Robins LS. *Health Politics and Policy*. 2nd ed. Albany, NY: Delmar Publishers; 1991.
9. Cheekoway B, O'Rourke T, Macrima, DM. et al. Representation of providers on health planning boards. *Int J Health Serv.* 1981;11:573–581.
10. McGinley L. HMO fracas moves to who makes medical decisions. *Wall Street Journal.* February 18, 1999:A24.
11. Hurley RE, Strunk BC, White JJ, et al. The puzzling popularity of the PPO. *Health Affairs.* 2004;23:56–68.
12. Reschovsky JD, Kemper P. Do HMOs make a difference. *Inquiry.* 1999/2000; 36.
13. Lee PR, Estes CL. *The Nation's Health*. 4th ed. Boston, MA: Jones & Bartlett Publishers; 1994.
14. Ropes LB. *Health Care Crisis in America*. Santa Barbara, CA: ABC-CLIO; 1991.
15. Gallwas G. The technological explosion: Its impact on laboratory and hospital costs. *Pathologist.* 1980;31:86–91.
16. McGivney WT, Hendee WR. Technology Assessment in medicine: the role of the American Medical Association. *Arch Pathol Lab Med.* 1988; 112: 1181–1185.

17. Office of Technology Assessment. *Assessing the Efficacy and Safety of Medical Technologies.* Washington, DC: Government Printing Office; 1978.
18. Reinhardt UE. Reinhardt on reform (interview done by Donna Vavala). *Physician Executive.* 1995;21:10–12.
19. Eisenberg JM. If trickle-down physician workforce policy failed, is the choice now between the market and government regulation? *Inquiry.* 1994; 31: 241–249.
20. Schroeder SA. Academic medicine as a public trust. *JAMA.* 1989; 262: 803–812.
21. Bulger RJ. Generalism and the need for health professional educational reform, refers to the "turf-related." *Acad Med.* 1995;70:931–934.
22. Smith JP. The politics of American health care. *J Adv Nurs.* 1990; 15:187–197.
23. Sorian RM. *A New Deal for American Health Care: How Reform Will Reshape Health Care Delivery and Payment for a New Century.* New York, NY: Faulkner and Gray; 1993.
24. McGinley L. Patients' groups jump into battle over proposals to restructure FDA. *Wall Street Journal.* February 22, 1996:B5.
25. U.S. Food and Drug Administration. "Assessment Time Shortened for Cancer Drugs" Available from http:www.fda.gov/bbs/topics/news/2003/ NE00873.hymy. Accessed March 10, 2003.
26. Murray A. Trade group fight against drug review is self-defeating. *Wall Street Journal.* November 30, 2004:A4.
27 'Drug firms' political outlays skyrocket. *Wall Street Journal.* July 7, 2000: A14.
28. Time to take another look at medicare drug plans. Available from http:// www.nytimes.com/2006/11/07health/07brody.html. Accessed November 10, 2006.
29. Heffler S, Smith S, Keehan S. et al. U.S. health spending projections for 2004–2014. Available from Health Affairs Web Exclusives, http://content. healthaffairs.org/webexclusives/index.dtl?year2005. Accessed November 10, 2006.
30. U.S. Census Bureau. American fact finder. Available from http://www.census. gov/acs/www/Products/usersguide/index.htm. Accessed November 11, 2006.
31. Centers for Medicare and Medicaid Services, Health and Human Services. Available from http://cms.hhs.gov/hipaa1/default.asp. Accessed September 12, 2002.
32. U.S. Census Bureau. Projections of the total resident population by five-year age groups, and sex with special age categories: middle series, 1999–2100 (NP-T3). Available from www.census.gov/population/www/projections/ natsum-T3.html. Accessed December 8, 2004.
33. *Healthy People 2000: Midcourse Review and 1995 Revisions.* Washington, DC: Department of Health and Human Services, Public Health Service; 1995.

34. Lurie N, Wasserman J, Nelson CD. "Public health preparedness: evolution or revolution? *Health Affairs*. 2006;25:935–945.
35. Bennis W. *Why Leaders Can't Lead, The Unconscious Conspiracy Continues*. San Francisco, CA: Jossey-Bass Publishers; 1989:40.
36. Stevens R. *In Sickness and in Wealth: American Hospitals in the Twentieth Century*. New York, NY: Basic Books; 1989.
37. Emanuel EJ, Daniels E. Oregon's physician-assisted suicide law: provisions and problems. *Arch Int Med*. 1996;156:46, 50.
38. Lee MA, Nelson HD, Triden UP. et al. Legalizing assisted suicide: view of physicians in Oregon. *N Engl J Med*. 1996;334:310–315.
39. Emanuel EJ. Euthanasia: historical, ethical, and empiric perspectives. *Arch Int Med*. 1994;154:1890–1901.
40. De Wachter MAM. Active euthanasia in the Netherlands. *JAMA*. 1989; 262:3316–3319.
41. Emanuel EJ, Daniels E. Oregon's physician-assisted suicide law: provisions and problems. *Arch Int Med*. 1996;156:825–829.
42. Eighth annual report on Oregon's Death with Dignity Act, Center for Health Statistics, Oregon Department of Human Services. Available from http://www.oregon.gov/OHS/ph/pas/ar-index.shtml/. Accessed November 11, 2006.
43. Pew/Internet Reports: Health. Available from http://PPF/r/190report-display.asp. Accessed November 12, 2006.
44. Silver GA. The route to a national health policy lies through the states. *Yale J Biol Med*. 1991;64:443–453.

Hospitals: Origin, Organization, and Performance

This chapter's overview of the genesis of U.S. hospitals provides a basis for understanding their characteristics and organization. The major private and governmental insurance initiatives that contributed to the growth and centrality of hospitals in the health care system are defined. The chapter also discusses the diverse functions of hospitals, the staff who perform in them, and the management structures in which they work. Important aspects of the relationship between staff and patients are reviewed, with particular emphasis on the rights and responsibilities of patients in that often intimidating hospital environment. The chapter concludes with a discussion of the quality of care provided in hospitals and an explanation of the forces of health care system reform that made managed care an ubiquitous influence on hospital economics, service patterns, and provider relationships.

Of all the familiar institutions in U.S. society, the hospital is, at the same time, the most appreciated, most maligned, and least understood. Besides serving as a place for the treatment of the sick and injured, it may function as a research laboratory, an educational institution, and a major employer within the community.

Being a hospital patient is usually at best an unpleasant personal trial and at worst a serious, perhaps life-threatening event. Where else in the free world, outside of a prison, does an individual voluntarily submit to being confined to a room in scanty institutional garb and to being poked, prodded, jabbed with needles, questioned, fed, toileted, and alternately ignored and attended, seemingly at the whim of a legion of strangers?

Historical Perspective

The often strained relationship between patients and hospital personnel such as doctors, nurses, aides, technicians, and therapists dates back to the earliest history of health care in the United States. The indifference to patients' needs for information, comfort, and humane contact that is today a common complaint about hospital care is rooted not only in the overall history of medical care but also—and especially—in the history of hospitals.

Hospitals in early America served quite different purposes from those of today. They were founded to shelter older adults, the dying, orphans, and vagrants and to protect the inhabitants of a community from the contagiously sick and the dangerously insane.

During the 18th century, Boston was the largest city in the new democracy, with about 7,000 citizens. Philadelphia and New York each had about 4,000 people. Whatever passed for medical care in those days was provided in the home. It was necessary, however, in these and other seaport towns to provide refuge for sailors and other shipboard victims of contagious diseases who often were unceremoniously left ashore when the ships departed. The town responded by organizing pest houses, quarantine stations, or isolation hospitals to segregate the sick from the town inhabitants and to prevent the spread of disease. Because these facilities were not intended to be used by the local citizenry, they were usually located well outside the city limits.

As populations grew, mental illness became an additional problem. Individuals whose behavior offended or frightened the townspeople came to the attention of the town board. It was common in those days for the town board to order relatives or friends to build a small stronghouse, or cell, on their property to contain a person with mental illness. If the individual had no relatives or friends, the town might lease him or her at an auction to the lowest bidder, who would take responsibility for confining that individual for 1 year, usually in exchange for his or her labor.

The existence of pest houses, or isolation hospitals, also provided the towns with what seemed an ideal solution for dealing with other individuals whose presence posed a risk to or offended its inhabitants. Over time, people with mental illness or those in poor health, the homeless, and the petty criminal joined the contagious ill that occupied those facilities.

Bellevue Hospital was originally the Poor House of New York City, established in 1736 to house the "poor, aged, insane, and disreputable." In 1789 the Public Hospital of Baltimore was established for low-income populations, people with mental or physical illness, and the seafaring of Maryland. One hundred years later, in 1889, it became the now prestigious Johns Hopkins Hospital.

Eventually, almost every city of any size in early America had a pest house to isolate patients during epidemics. Most cities also had an almshouse for low-income populations, sometimes with an added infirmary. Many of today's county or municipal hospitals were originally combinations of almshouses and infirmaries.

The largest county institution, Eloise Hospital in Wayne County, Michigan, was started in 1835 to serve the "old, young, deaf, dumb, blind, insane, and destitute." It grew to 6,000 beds to care for acute and chronic illness and mental diseases and to provide domiciliary services to low-income populations. The Kings County Hospital in Brooklyn, Philadelphia General Hospital, and Cleveland City Hospital are similar examples.

Most hospitals in the United States in the 19th century were disgraceful, the antithesis of what their patients needed. They were dirty, unventilated, and contaminated with infections. They were overcrowded and offered little or no medical care. The only nurses available were former inmates or women who could get no other work. As a result, they only accelerated the spread of disease. The public, however, knew little of these conditions. Because visiting was restricted, patients were effectively cut off from the outside world. Persons with family or the means to obtain home medical or nursing care shunned hospitals.

Certain religious orders, however, saw the hospitals' clients as so helpless, so miserable with incurable disease, or so maimed by accident that they presented an opportunity for spiritual outlet for those seeking salvation through good works. Thus began the close relationships of the Protestant and Catholic religions with hospitals and hospital nursing. Religious nursing groups played a major role in the evolution of hospital care. Catholic religious orders were the first groups responsible for kindly and humane nursing performed by fairly well-educated, sincere, and devoted disciples. The American branch of St. Vincent de Paul Sisters of Charity, founded by Mother Elizabeth Seton in 1809, established hospitals that still stand in major cities across the United States.

The Protestant nursing movement began in Germany and was brought to Pennsylvania in 1850. It was based on the formal training of nurses in religion, nursing, and nursing education. The nurse teachers were called deaconesses. The Protestant church hospital, or deaconess movement, had an important influence on nursing.

Ironically, it was the Civil War of the 1860s that brought about public appreciation of the work of women in nursing. When sick or wounded soldiers were returned to their hometowns attended by obviously dedicated and capable nurses, it was the first time that relatives of those soldiers encountered women as nurses outside of their own homes. Nursing gained a much more positive image and came to be viewed as a respectable career option for women.

All of this early hospital care was focused on only the most unfortunate of the population with physical and mental illness. Although provided in the most deplorable conditions, hospital care reflected the early American concept of charity and public responsibility, which required that provision be made for low-income populations, people with physical or mental illness, vagrants, and criminals. Institutions originally classified as almshouses provided refuge for all of them. Later, physicians realized the efficacy of separating the sick population from the rest of the needy and putting them in facilities more properly called hospitals. The Pennsylvania Hospital in Philadelphia, the New York Hospital in New York City, and the Massachusetts General Hospital in Boston were founded by physicians who obtained citizen funding for charitable hospitals. Their motives, however, were not altogether in the interests of the patients. They wanted a place to practice surgery and obstetrics, to obtain patients to serve for the instruction of medical students, and to protect the well population from people with physical or mental illness.

Sources That Shaped the Hospital Industry

Health Insurance

The transformation of hospitals from simple, charitable institutions to complex, technical organizations was accompanied by a parallel growth of private hospital insurance. The percentage of the U.S. population with hospital insurance grew from 9% in 1940 to over 74% in 1986.[1]

By the 1960s, billions of dollars were flowing into hospitals from insurance companies, such as Blue Cross/Blue Shield, medical society plans, and other plans sponsored by unions, industry, physicians, and cooperatives. The availability of hospital insurance removed an important cost constraint from hospital charges. The ability of insurers to cope with ever-rising hospital costs by distributing relatively small premium increases over large numbers of subscribers opened the floodgates to hospital admissions. Expanding hospital services and relatively unrestrained reimbursement rates created an inflationary spiral that was to persist for decades.

In addition, medical advances and medical specialization encouraged hospitalization, and the hospital industry expanded to meet the demand. After World War II, the American Hospital Association (AHA) convinced Senators Lister Hill and Harold Burton to sponsor legislation that provided federal monies to the states to survey hospitals and other health care facilities and to plan and assist construction of additional facilities. The Hill-Burton Hospital Construction Act was signed as Public Law 79-75 in 1946 and became a major influence in the expansion of the hospital industry.[2] Over 4,600 projects to expand existing facilities or construct new ones were initiated within 20 years after its passage. Federal support of hospital construction was critically important to the location of hospitals in underserved rural areas.

Medicare and Medicaid

In 1966, the hospital industry was the recipient of another major legislative contribution to its fiscal well-being by the passage of Medicare, Title XVIII of the Social Security Act. The legislation provided the growing population of Americans over age 65 years with significant hospital and medical benefits. In one decisive legislative action, the large population of older Americans, the group most likely to need hospitalization, was assured of hospital care, and the hospitals were assured that they would be reimbursed on the basis of "reasonable costs."

The companion program, Medicaid, Title XIX of the Social Security Act, was established at the same time to support medical and hospital care for persons classified as medically indigent. Unlike Medicare, Medicaid required the states to establish joint federal–state programs that covered persons receiving public assistance and, if they wished, others of low income. Because the states had broad discretion over eligibility, benefits, and reimbursement rates, the programs that developed differed widely among the 50 states.

Medicare, and to a lesser extent Medicaid, had enormous impact on hospitalization rates in the United States. In a little over 10 years after the implementation of Medicare, persons over 65 years old were spending well over twice as many days in the hospital as those 45 to 64 years old.[3] Because the rising Medicare rates became the standards for establishing hospital reimbursement rates in general, Medicare probably did more to fuel the rising costs of hospital care than any other factor.

The Medicare and Medicaid programs also had another effect. Because these programs provided government funding for the hospital care of low-income population and older adults, they altered the long-standing nature or mission of hospitals by diminishing the traditional charitable or social role of those voluntary institutions. It was not long after the implementation of those programs that hospitals became increasingly focused on profit, maximizing the more lucrative activities, and closing or reducing services that operated at a loss. In the 1980s, hospitals, along with most of U.S. industry, became market oriented and aggressively enterprising. The monetary incentives built into the Medicare system favored entrepreneurial, short-term financial interests.

Rosemary Stevens, author of *In Sickness and in Wealth: American Hospitals in the Twentieth Century*, wrote this: "One effect was to bring hospitals into prominence as enterprises motivated by organizational self-interest, by the excitement of the game, by greed."[4] She concluded with this:[5]

> Medicare and Medicaid, supposedly designed to promote egalitarianism, fostered sharp inequities in the health-care system while disarming criticism from low-paid American workers and the poverty population. The stage was set for today's struggles to rethink, once again, the American health-care system—and to redefine the relative roles of voluntarism, government, and business for the last few years of the twentieth century.

Growth and Decline in Numbers of Hospitals

The number of hospitals in the United States increased from 178 in 1873 to 4,300 in 1909. In 1946, at the close of World War II, there were 6,000

American hospitals, with 3.2 beds available for every 1,000 persons. That year, Congress passed the Hill-Burton Hospital Construction Act to fund expansion of the hospital system to achieve the goal of 4.5 beds per 1,000 persons.[6] The system grew thereafter to reach a high of approximately 7,200 acute-care hospitals.

During the 1980s, however, medical advances and cost-containment measures caused many procedures that once required inpatient hospitalization to be performed on an outpatient basis. Outpatient hospital visits increased by 40% with a resultant decrease in hospital admissions. Fewer admissions and shortened lengths of stay for patients resulted in a significant reduction in the number of hospitals and hospital beds. Health care reform efforts and the acceptance of managed care as the major medical practice style of U.S. health care resulted in enough hospital closings and mergers to reduce the number of governmental and community-based hospitals in the United States to approximately 5,700.

Types of Hospitals

Acute-care hospitals are distinguished from long-term care facilities such as nursing homes, rehabilitation centers, and psychiatric hospitals by the fact that the average stay of their patients is less than 30 days. Such hospitals have one of three basic sponsorships:

1. They may be operated as voluntary not-for-profit entities.
2. They may be owned and managed by profit-making corporations.
3. They may be public facilities, supported and managed by governmental jurisdictions.

Hospitals may also be divided into teaching and nonteaching hospitals. Teaching hospitals are affiliated with medical schools and provide clinical education for medical students and medical and dental residents. They, and many hospitals not affiliated with medical schools, also provide clinical education for nurses, allied health personnel, and a wide variety of technical specialists.

Only about one-fifth of hospitals are teaching facilities affiliated with one or more of the allopathic and osteopathic medical schools in the United States. Most teaching hospitals are voluntary not-for-profit institutions or government-sponsored public hospitals. The last survey of this country's hospitals conducted by the AHA concluded that there were

2,958 voluntary not-for-profit hospitals sponsored by religious groups or other community-based organizations. They constitute over 80% of the 5,756 registered hospitals in the United States.[7]

They include large numbers of small community general hospitals and smaller numbers of large tertiary-care facilities. These large tertiary-care facilities are usually affiliated with medical schools. The presence of medical school faculty with strong research interests and the availability of medical residents to assist in the collection of clinical data put teaching hospitals in the forefront of clinical research on medical conditions and treatments.

The federal government, through the U.S. Department of Veterans Affairs (VA), or the U.S. Public Health Service, operates 226 public hospitals. In addition, state and local governments maintain over 1,100 public hospitals. These public hospitals are usually large and well staffed with full-time attending physicians and residents. Such hospitals are usually teaching hospitals, with a heavy preponderance of economically disadvantaged patients.

Public hospitals in many localities deliver the fiscally problematic, but essential, community services that other hospitals are reluctant to provide. These high-cost, low-return services include sophisticated trauma centers, psychiatric emergency services, alcohol detoxification services, other substance abuse treatment, and burn treatment. In addition, there are 456 nonfederal psychiatric hospitals.

Investor-owned for-profit hospitals grew from a few physician-owned facilities before the 1965 Medicare and Medicaid legislation to 868 in 2005.[7] Most for-profit hospitals belong to one of the large hospital management companies that dominate the for-profit hospital network. An increasing number, however, are physician-owned specialty hospitals. Such hospitals usually limit their services to treatments in one of three major specialty categories: orthopedics, surgery, or cardiology.

Although these new specialty hospitals are typically upscale facilities with many patient luxuries, they usually operate with greater efficiency and provide excellent care in their few targeted services. Nevertheless, they have raised a series of concerns about their performance and their effect on community hospitals.

First, it is clear that specialty hospitals treat the less complex, more profitable cases, leaving the more difficult, less profitable, or uninsured patients to be served by community hospitals. Second, because physician-owners of specialty hospitals profit directly by the value of services provided by their hospitals, there are concerns that clinical decisions may be influenced by financial incentives.[8]

Supporters of physician-owned specialty hospitals point out that the physician-owners take great pride in the quality of care provided in their hospitals, that they also work in community hospitals, and that their facilities enhance their communities by paying taxes as for-profit agencies.[9]

The number of beds in not-for-profit, state and local government, and federal hospitals decreased in the last decade, whereas the much smaller number of beds in for-profit facilities increased slightly. The last annual survey of the AHA counted about 947,000 staffed beds among all U.S. registered hospitals in the United States.[10]

Financial Condition of Hospitals

The fierce competition among hospitals to survive potentially catastrophic economic challenges caused many to rethink their attitudes toward their patients. Hospitals now face the almost impossible task of making their facilities and services more user friendly while implementing organizational changes and staffing reductions designed to keep them economically viable in a highly aggressive marketplace.

At least one third of U.S. hospitals are failing financially, and another third are in precarious condition. Caught between rising costs and falling revenues, hospitals have been desperately seeking ways to cope with deteriorating market conditions.

Beginning in the mid-1990s, thousands of hospitals were involved in mergers, acquisitions, and other multihospital deals in an effort to capture and solidify market shares and gain economies of scale. In 1996 alone, 235 deals involved 768 hospitals.[11] Although the service and financial outcomes of the mergers and other deals vary from location to location, there is little evidence that the multihospital strategies are meeting expectations. In fact, some of the mergers that combined facilities with differing administrative and clinical cultures have only added to their economic problems.

Those economic problems result from a combination of factors over which the hospitals have little control. The Balanced Budget Act of 1997, which reduced payments for Medicare patients below the costs of treating them, wrecked havoc on U.S. hospitals. At the same time, hospital changes were held in check by hard-bargaining managed-care organizations.

In contrast to the restraints on revenues, costs were rising at an unprecedented pace. Costly new technology, pharmaceuticals, and services, as well as significant inflationary increases, combined with declining occupancy to significantly reduce operating margins.

The federal government, realizing that the Balanced Budget Act cuts to hospital revenues were too deep, passed a Balanced Budget Relief Act to restore a small portion of those cuts. The financial damage, however, was significant, and additional cuts in Medicare payments to providers proposed in the Medicare budgets of succeeding years have kept many hospitals teetering on the edge of insolvency and bankruptcy.

The more recent development of private specialty hospitals and diagnostic centers owned by physicians introduced competition with community hospitals for their most profitable services. The continuing losses to the community hospitals that also provide those services are significant.

Academic Health Centers, Medical Education, and Specialization

Medical, dental, nursing, pharmacy, and allied health schools and their teaching hospitals are the principal sources of education and training for most health care providers. Major universities with several or all of those different schools join them in organizational entities called academic medical centers or academic health centers. Much of the basic and clinical research in medicine and other health care disciplines are conducted in these health centers and their related hospitals. The teaching hospitals usually provide the most technologically advanced care in their communities and also offer inpatient and ambulatory care for economically disadvantaged populations. Thus, the three objectives of academic health centers—education, research, and service—are fulfilled most adequately by teaching hospitals.

The influence of these medical centers on health care during the last few decades has been extraordinary. The advances that occurred in the medical sciences and technology that resulted in the introduction of life-saving drugs, anesthetics, surgical procedures, and other therapies and the development and use of sophisticated computerized diagnostic techniques increased both the use and the costs of hospital services. Physicians could intervene more successfully in the course of an ever-increasing array of conditions of disease and injury, and they enthusiastically exercised those capabilities. This increased intervention resulted in increases in both the life expectancy of most Americans and the proportion of the gross national product devoted to health care; however, these advances also significantly expanded the knowledge base and performance skills required of physicians to practice up-to-date clinical medicine.

Medical education and training, led by the academic medical centers, responded by increasing the number of physicians with in-depth expertise in increasingly narrow fields of clinical practice. Specialization and subspecialization grew, subdivided, and grew more. More and more physicians limited their activities to narrower and narrower fields of practice. In doing so, they greatly increased the overall technological sophistication of hospital practice along with the number of costly consultations that take place among specialist hospital physicians; the amount of expensive equipment, supplies, and space maintained by hospitals to serve specialist needs; and, in general, the complexity of patient care. The contributions of highly specialized clinical practice to the quality of hospital care have been both extraordinarily beneficial and regrettably negative. Although the superspecialists of U.S. medicine have given the profession its justified reputation for heroic medical and surgical achievements, specialization also has fragmented and depersonalized patient care and produced a plethora of often questionable tests, procedures, and clinical interventions.

Although academic medical centers have contributed admirably to the advancement of medicine, and especially hospital-delivered medical and surgical care, they have not brought their impressive expertise to bear effectively on solving the delivery system problems that have plagued their industry. Rather, the commitments of academic medicine to high-technology research and patient care and its adherence to traditional organizational structures and professional roles have prevented it from taking the lead in correcting health care system problems. As a result, medical education and medical organizations in general are reacting to, rather than guiding, the changes taking place.

The Hospital System of the Department of Veterans Affairs

The tax-supported, centrally directed Veterans Health Administration of the VA is the country's largest health care system and a significant component of America's medical education system. In 2006, the VA owned and operated 156 hospitals, most of which are affiliated with medical schools. The VA also operates 136 nursing homes, 43 residential rehabilitation facilities, and over 800 outpatient clinics. With its large number of hospitals and other facilities, over 12,000 full-time salaried physicians, over 900 dentists, and 33,000 nurses, the medical care program of the VA would be expected to be a prime target for the congressional cost cutters of large and expensive federal programs. With the current conflicts in Iraq and Afghanistan, however, the VA has regularly escaped the competitive pressures of the rest of the system. Instead, with broad bipartisan political support, the VA has received an annual congressional appropriation consistently higher each year than requested in the president's budget. Apparently, the strong political advocacy for veterans in the United States restrains any congressional initiative to give up VA hospitals in favor of subsidizing the care of veterans in the private sector.[12]

Like the rest of the hospital industry, the VA is reorganizing its facilities to lower costs, improve the quality of its care, and better integrate its patients throughout the system. Its major change has been the creation of 22 networks called Veterans Integrated Service Networks, each of which functions as a vertically integrated delivery system.[13]

An important part of the VA's organizational transition is its Health Services Research and Development Service. It works to improve the quality of health care for veterans by examining the impact of the organization, financing, and management of health services on their quality, cost, access, and outcomes. Health Services Research and Development Service programs span the continuum of health care research and delivery—from clinical research to dissemination of research results to the application of the findings to clinical, managerial, and policy decisions. The latter activities are especially important because the VA is facing rising costs and an aging and sicker patient population.

For over 8 years, the VA has operated a Quality Enhancement Research Initiative, which incorporated the findings of evidence-based research into improvements in patient care. The developed and tested interventions resulted in significant improvements in the quality of care received by veterans.[14]

In April 2007, however, the previously well-earned reputation for excellent care provided by the VA system was undone by public exposure of the dreadful circumstances of care at Walter Reed Army Medical Center in Washington, DC. An independent panel, headed by two former secretaries of the Army, issued a sweeping indictment of the leadership, training, staffing, and physical facilities. The conditions they reported included filthy physical facilities and a bureaucratic maze that left severely injured soldiers in limbo for months.[15]

Apparently, the hospital was unprepared, understaffed, and overwhelmed by the numbers, severity, and patterns of blast-related injuries to the military in Iraq. Such individuals require extremely complex and lengthy rehabilitation services to assure maximum functional and psychosocial outcomes.[16] Neither the staff nor the physical facilities of the hospital were judged adequate to meet the challenge.

Structure and Organization of Hospitals

The organizational structure of today's hospital is a complex maze of committees, departments, personnel, and services. In addition to being a caring, people-oriented institution, it is at the same time a many-faceted, high-tech business. It operates just like any other large business, with a hierarchy of personnel, channels of authority and responsibility, and constant concern about its bottom line. Likewise, the people who work in hospitals exhibit the same range of human characteristics as their counterparts in other businesses. Patients and their families trying to obtain the best possible results from the services of a hospital, therefore, should base their approach on the same principles that they use in dealing with other service entities. They need to determine who is in charge, what services to expect from whom and when, with what results, and at what cost to them.

The following general description of hospital structure and organization uses the voluntary not-for-profit community hospital as the example because this type of institution has historically provided the model for hospital organization. The direction, control, and governance of the hospital are divided among three influential entities: the medical staff, the administration, and the board of directors or trustees. The major operating divisions of a hospital represent areas of the hospital's functions. Although they may use different names, the usual units are medical, nursing, patient therapy, diagnosis, fiscal, human resources, hotel services, and community relations.

Medical Division

The medical staff is a formally organized unit within the larger hospital organization. The president or chief of staff is the liaison between the hospital administration and members of the medical staff. Typically, the medical staff consists primarily of medical physicians, but it also may include other doctoral-level professionals, such as dentists and psychologists.

A major role of the medical staff organization is to recommend to the hospital board of directors the appointment of physicians to the medical staff. The board of directors approves and grants various levels of hospital privileges to physicians. Such privileges commonly include the right to admit patients to the hospital, to perform surgery, and to provide consultation to other physicians on the hospital staff. Another medical staff function is to provide oversight and peer review of the quality of medical care in the hospital. It performs this function through a number of medical staff committees, which coordinate their efforts closely with the hospital's administration and committees of the hospital's board of directors.

Members of the medical staff who have completed their training and are in practice are referred to as attending physicians. In addition, the hospital usually has a house staff of physicians who are engaged in postmedical school training programs under the supervision of attending staff members. These members of the house staff are referred to as residents. They rotate shifts to provide 24-hour coverage for the attending medical staff's patients in the specialty departments to which they are assigned.

There is no universal rule as to how a hospital's medical departments or divisions are organized. Most often, the types of practice of the hospital's medical staff determine the specialty components within the medical division. Medicine, surgery, obstetrics and gynecology, and pediatrics are usually major departments. In larger hospitals and in most teaching hospitals, the subspecialty areas of medical practice are represented by departments as well. In the internal medicine specialty, subspecialty departments might include cardiology or cardiac care, ophthalmology, urology, oncology, gastroenterology, pulmonary medicine, endocrinology, otolaryngology, and a variety of others. In the surgical area, subspecialties might include orthopaedics, thoracic, neurosurgery, cardiac surgery, and plastic and reconstructive surgery. Each medical department or division in a hospital is headed by a physician department head or chairman, who is charged with overseeing the practice and quality of medical services delivered in the department. In a teaching hospital, either the department head or another designated attending physician is responsible for coordinating the required educational experiences of medical students and residents.

Nursing Division

The nursing division usually comprises the single largest component of the hospital's organization. It is subdivided by the type of patient care delivered in the various medical specialties. These nursing units are composed of a number of patient beds grouped within a certain area to allow centralization of the special facilities, supplies, equipment, and personnel pertinent to the needs of patients with particular conditions. For example, the kinds of equipment and skills and the level of patient care needs vary considerably between an orthopedic unit and a medical intensive care unit.

A head nurse, often carrying the title of "nurse manager," has overall responsibility for all nursing care in his or her unit. Such care includes carrying out the attending physician's and house staff physician's orders for medications, diet, and various types of therapy. In addition, the nurse manager supervises the unit's staff, which may include nurses' aides and orderlies. The nurse manager is also responsible for coordinating all aspects of patient care, which may include services provided by other hospital units, such as the dietary department, physical therapy department, pharmacy, and laboratories. The nurse manager also has the responsibility for coordinating the services of departments such as social work, discharge planning, and pastoral care for the patients in the unit.

Because nursing services are required in the hospital at all times, staff is usually employed in three 8-hour shifts. Normally, the nurse manager of a unit will work during the day shift, and two other members of the nursing staff will assume what is referred to as charge duty on the other two shifts of the day. Charge nurses report to the nurse manager.

A nursing supervisor may have management responsibility for a number of nursing units. These nursing supervisors in turn report to a member of the hospital's administration, who is usually a vice-president for nursing or an assistant administrator.

It is also common to find an individual with the title of ward clerk or unit secretary on each nursing unit. The ward clerk assists the head nurse with paperwork and helps to coordinate the other hospital services related to patient care.

Allied Health Professionals

Not as well known as the physicians and nurses who are central to the care and treatment of patients in hospitals is the wide array of personnel who provide other hospital services that support the work of the physicians and nurses and the others who operate behind the scenes to make the facility run smoothly.

Staff members in an increasingly diverse array of health care disciplines are now classified as allied health personnel, and their roles in the complex health care system are often not recognized or well understood by the public. Allied health personnel support, complement, or supplement the functions of physicians, dentists, nurses, and other professionals in delivering health care to patients. They contribute to environmental management, health promotion, and disease prevention.

There are now over 200 allied health occupations and specialties, and advancing medical technology is likely to create the need for even more personnel with highly specialized training and relatively unique skills. Those who are responsible for highly specialized or technical services that have a significant impact on health care are prepared for practice through a wide variety of educational programs offered at colleges and universities.

The range of allied health professions may be best understood by classifying them by the functions they serve in the delivery of health care. Some disciplines may serve more than one of these functions:

1. *Laboratory technologists and technicians* play a major role in the diagnosis of disease, the monitoring of physiologic function, and the effectiveness of medical interventions. Medical technologists, nuclear medical technologists, radiologic technologists, and cytotechnologists are but a few of the specialists on whom hospitals depend.

2. *Allied health practitioners of the therapeutic sciences* are essential to the treatment and rehabilitation of patients with a wide variety of

injuries and medical conditions. Examples include physical, occupational, and speech therapists and physician assistants.

3. *Behavioral scientists* are crucial to the social, psychological, and
patient education activities related to health maintenance, disease
prevention, and accommodation to disability. Professionals in this
category include social workers, health educators, and rehabilitation counselors in mental health, alcoholism, and drug abuse.

4. *Specialist support service personnel* include those who perform
administrative and management functions and others with special
expertise that often work closely with the actual providers of
patient care. Health information administrators, formerly called
medical record administrators, food service administrators, dietitians, and nutritionists are examples of personnel in this category.

The following descriptions of some of the key hospital services reflect
the close functional relationships among the various kinds of highly specialized individuals required to staff hospital services.

Diagnostic Services

Every hospital either maintains or contracts with laboratories to perform
a wide array of tests to help physicians diagnose illness or injury and monitor the progress of treatment. One such laboratory is the pathology laboratory, which examines and analyzes specimens of body tissues, fluids, and
excretions to aid in diagnosis and treatment. These laboratories are usually supervised by the hospital's pathologist, who is a physician specialist.

The radiology department, directed by a physician specialist called a
radiologist, provides radiographs for a variety of diagnostic purposes and
may also provide radiation therapy for the treatment of certain disorders.
Grouped under the rubric "diagnostic imaging services," a wide array of
more sophisticated imaging equipment has been developed that incorporates computer technology. This includes computed tomography (CT),
magnetic resonance imaging (MRI), and positron emission tomography
(PET). Unlike radiograph technology, which is limited to providing
images of the body's anatomical structures, these imaging advances have
unique abilities to visualize structures in several planes, and with PET,
even quantify complex physiologic processes occurring in the human
body. Thus, they add immeasurably to the understanding and treatment

of major ailments, including heart disease, stroke, cancer, epilepsy, and Alzheimer's disease.

A variety of other diagnostic services also may be available through specific medical specialty or subspecialty departments, such as cardiology and neurology. For example, a noninvasive cardiac laboratory administers cardiac stress testing to assess a patient's heart function during exercise. Obstetricians commonly use an imaging capability called ultrasonography to visualize the unborn fetus.

Rehabilitation Services

Rehabilitation or patient support departments provide specialized care to assist patients in achieving optimal physical, mental, and social functioning after resolution of an illness or injury. One such department is physical medicine, where diagnosis and treatment of patients with physical injuries or disabilities are conducted. This department is headed by a specialist physician called a physiatrist, who usually works with a team of physical therapists, occupational therapists, and speech therapists. Other health-related specialists, such as social workers, may provide additional services to support the rehabilitation of patients with complex problems.

Other Patient Support Services

The hospital pharmacy purchases and dispenses all drugs used to treat hospitalized patients. The department is headed by a licensed pharmacist, who is also responsible for pharmacy technicians and others who work under his or her supervision.

Among other functions, the social services department helps patients about to be discharged to arrange financial support and coordinate needed community-based services. Generally, the social services department assists patients and their families achieve the best possible social and domestic environment for the patients' care and recovery. Such services are available to all hospital patients and their families.

Discharge planning services (discussed in more detail later in this chapter) may or may not be a part of the social services department. Frequently, staffing includes both nurses and social workers who are responsible for planning posthospital patient care in conjunction with the patients and their families. The discharge planning department becomes involved when the patient requires referral for one or more community services or placement in a special care facility after discharge.

Nutritional Services

The nutritional services department includes food preparation facilities and personnel for the provision of inpatient meals, food storage, and purchasing and catering for hospital events. It may also operate a cafeteria for employees and, in larger hospitals, may sponsor educational programs for student dietitians. An important function of this department's staff is educating patients on dietary needs and restrictions. This department usually is headed by a chief dietitian who has a degree in nutritional science, and it may be staffed by any number of other dietitians and clinical nutrition specialists with specific expertise in dietary assessment and food preparation.

Administrative Departments

Hospitals contain other professional units that provide a wide variety of nonmedical services essential to the management of the hospital's physical plant and business services. Patients are certainly aware of two of them: the admissions department, through which a hospital stay is initiated, and the business office, through which a hospital stay is terminated. These units are two of the many components of the hospital's complex management structure.

The general administrative services of the hospital are headed by a chief executive officer or president who has the day-to-day responsibility for managing all hospital business. He or she is the highest ranking administrative officer and oversees an array of administrative departments concerned with financial operations, public relations, and personnel. Most larger hospitals have a chief operating officer, who oversees the operation of specific departments, and a chief financial officer, who directs the many and varied fiscal activities of the hospital. Those key administrative officers are commonly positioned as corporate vice presidents. The large number of employees and the wide array of individual skills required to staff a hospital competently call for a personnel or human resources department with highly specialized labor expertise. That department is also usually headed by a vice president for human resources. Because nursing is such a large component of the hospital's service operations, the larger facilities also maintain a chief nursing executive at the vice-president level.

During the past 20 years, as the information needs of hospitals have increased in volume and complexity, new departments, often referred to as management information systems, have evolved. These departments are usually directed by computer science professionals and are responsible for managing hospitals' extensive computer systems. Those systems extend from office word processing to medical record transcription to transmittal of clinical laboratory findings to financial data processing. Increasingly, hospitals' management information systems departments are engaged in the computer management of patient care data necessary to evaluate the quality and cost-effectiveness of hospital services.

Hotel Services

Hotel services are generally associated with the hospitality functions common to hotels. They include building maintenance, security, laundry, television, and telephone services.

Complexity of the System

Unlike the nonhospital health services, over half of which employ fewer than five persons, almost two-thirds of hospital employees work in facilities with more than 1,000 workers.[17] Major hospital systems may have thousands of employees, significant turnover of personnel requiring training and indoctrination of new employees to the complicated procedures of the organization, and a maze of information transmission requirements with high potential for miscommunication. The newer diagnostic and therapeutic methods that are increasingly effective are also increasingly complex.

Thus, even this very limited description of the hospital's complex structure and organization should make it clear that with so many different kinds of employees and so many interrelated systems and functions, it is a small wonder that hospitals work at all, much less as well as they do. With the multitude of tasks that are performed every day by the hundreds of employees in a busy hospital, misunderstandings and information breakdowns in patient care are inevitable. In acknowledgment of the fact that their organizations are too complex and their employees too compartmentalized in their responsibilities to solve system problems, the majority of this country's hospitals have patient representatives, sometimes called patient advocates, to serve as ombudsmen for the patients. They are prepared to intervene on behalf of the patients in a wide variety of situations. The phone numbers of those patient representatives are usually provided to patients in the material given them during the admission process or left conspicuously in their rooms.

Types and Roles of Patients

Nowhere in the early development of hospitals was the patient considered as anything other than an unavoidable burden to society. In its mercy, society provided the hospital as a refuge—and incidentally, a workplace for the physician and his disciple, the medical student. Patients receiving this charity were expected to be grateful for the shelter and nursing care and even for the opportunity to lend their bodies and illnesses for medical practice. On the other hand, patients who could afford to pay for their medical and nursing care continued to receive it in the comfort and dignity of their homes.

By 1900, proper training in nursing, effective anesthetic agents, modern methods of antisepsis and sterilization, and other medical advances had revolutionized hospital practices. Hospitals changed from merely supplying food, shelter, and meager medical care to the unfortunate needy and contagious to providing skilled medical, surgical, and nursing care to everyone; however, the belief persisted that patients in the hospital, removed from their usual social environment, were in a dependent relationship with charitable authorities. Remnants of the idea that these professionals have the knowledge and authority to decide what is best for grateful and uncomplaining patients persist to this day, regardless of the expense to the patient or the merit of the services.

Unfortunately, the behavior of many patients and their families has been conditioned to reinforce this philosophy. In the hospital, otherwise assertive, independent individuals tend to assume a passive and dependent "sick role." Numerous sociological studies of patient behavior have concluded that the patients who behave in the traditional submissive sick role help to preserve the authoritarian attitude of health care providers that most consumers now consider patronizing and inappropriate.[18]

Rights and Responsibilities of Hospitalized Patients

Patients in hospitals have individual rights, many of which are protected by state statutes and regulations. The constitution of the United States and, in particular, its Bill of Rights are not suspended when a citizen enters a hospital. In fact, since 1972, the AHA has published a "Statement on a Patient's Bill of Rights" that is displayed prominently in every hospital in the country. In addition, hospitals are required by their accrediting body to make this information known to every patient admitted. Very importantly, the statement recognizes that the hospital, in addition to the physician, has a responsibility for the patient's welfare. In fact, the ultimate responsibility for everything that happens within the hospital, including the medical care provided, lies with the hospital institution and its board of directors.

Many hospitals, other institutions, and government agencies have modified the language of the original AHA Statement on a Patient's Bill of Rights to represent more accurately their individual interpretations of their responsibilities or to communicate better with special populations. In addition to posting these statements on the walls of the facility, hospitals also distribute their modified versions under their own organization title with the admission documents provided to patients.

The following description of major patients' rights is a synthesis of the statements posted by several hospitals. Patients have the right to:

1. Receive respectful and considerate treatment, including respect for their personal privacy, during examinations, tests, and all forms of interaction with their physicians, staff members, and others involved in their care.
2. Know the names and titles of all individuals providing their care and the name of the physician responsible.
3. Complete and understandable explanations of their diagnosis, treatment, and prognosis. They also have the right to designate another individual to receive such explanations on their behalf.
4. Receive from the physician all of the information necessary to give informed consent before any procedure or treatment. Such information should include a description of the procedure or treatment, the estimated period of convalescence, the risks involved, the risk

of not accepting the treatment or procedure, and any alternative options.

5. Request and receive consultation on their diagnosis and treatment or obtain a second opinion.
6. Set limits on the scope of treatment that they will permit or refuse treatment and be informed of the consequences of such refusal.
7. Leave the hospital, unless unlawful, even against the advice of their physicians and receive an explanation of their responsibilities in exercising that right.
8. Request and receive information and assistance in discharging financial obligations to the hospital, and review a complete bill, regardless of the source of payment.
9. Since April 2004, the federal HIPAA law requires hospitals as well as physicians and clinics to provide patients with access to their own records on demand, as well as someone capable of explaining anything that is confusing or difficult to understand.
10. Receive assistance in planning and obtaining necessary support services after their discharge.

Those endowed with individual rights are always expected to assume certain reciprocal individual responsibilities. Patients are obligated to act responsibly toward physicians and hospitals by cooperating with all reasonable requests for personal and family information. It is to their own benefit that patients inform medical or hospital personnel if they do not understand or do not wish to follow instructions. If a patient would like a family member or other advocate to be involved in treatment decisions, that individual should be identified to the physician, and the hospital and contact information should be provided.

It is also incumbent on patients to recognize that hospitals are highly stressful institutional settings and that other patients, as well as the hospital personnel, deserve consideration and respect. Courtesy to others in the close confines of hospital quarters is most appreciated.

In no other institutional setting are individual rights at greater risk of being compromised than in a hospital; however, the risks do not arise from a purposeful disregard for patients by physicians or the hospital staff or from their individual or collective determination to subject patients to treatment against their will. The personal integrity of patients may be unintentionally violated as a result of certain institutional circumstances and factors unique to the hospital setting. These institutional circumstances arise from the fact that the hospital, like most large complex organizations, has a life of its own, which pulses with an infinite array of daily scheduled events that pervade every aspect of its functioning. There are schedules for changing beds, bathing patients, serving meals, administering medications, obtaining specimens, providing therapy, checking vital signs, performing surgery, housekeeping, admitting, discharging, doing rounds, receiving visitors, performing examinations, and finally, preparing patients for the night.

The vast number of tasks that evolve from the care needs of up to several hundred people who are ill each day requires the planning and scheduling of every activity if they are all to be accomplished within a 24-hour period. The pressure of the daily schedule often makes it difficult for hospital personnel to pay attention to the special needs of individual patients. Even though a patient's particular schedule of tests, procedures, treatments, and examinations is uniquely related to his or her condition and the physician's orders, it also is influenced by the needs of fellow patients and the schedules of the physicians, technicians, technologists, nurses, nurses' aides, therapists, students, and numerous others involved directly or indirectly in the patient's care.

A patient's treatment may also be modified by the schedule of those daily institutional events, which although unrelated to his or her treatment can have an impact on what happens or does not happen on any given day. Such institutional events include inspections, grand rounds, nursing in-services, unplanned staffing shortages, and an array of technical problems with any of the hundreds of the pieces of medical equipment used to perform the daily functions of a sophisticated hospital.

As it becomes clearer that the schedule, rather than the patients' needs, drives the caregivers, the second major reason why patient rights may be in jeopardy in the hospital setting emerges. Physicians may not be aware of the many aspects of daily care in the hospital that determine whether patients will be comfortable and reasonably satisfied during their hospital stay. Physicians are likely to spend only a few minutes a day with each patient. That means that patients nearly always depend on the nursing staff and other support personnel for the medical and personal care they should receive. Very importantly, nurses are supposed to be continuously monitoring each patient's condition and alerting the physician to any change in a patient's status; however, the number of patients for whom a nurse is responsible and the number of tasks that the nurse is required to perform during the course of a single work shift make it extremely difficult, or sometimes impossible, to fulfill that obligation. In addition, the increasing number of caregivers involved with each patient provides additional opportunities for failures of communication and subsequent mistakes in the treatment programs for individual patients. Although hospitals do their best to develop fail-safe systems to protect patients against the possibility of human error in the delivery of their care, mistakes can happen. One patient can receive a medication intended for another. The report of a laboratory test can get lost and require the repeat of an uncomfortable procedure. A physician's instructions can be overlooked, and the patient may be deprived of something that he or she was supposed to receive. The patient may continue receiving something that was supposed to be stopped. A nurse's note alerting the physician to a change in the patient's condition may be missed, and the patient may fail to receive something that he or she requires.

Progressive hospital systems encourage patients to recognize their vulnerability during hospitalization and urge them or their family members to function as active participants in, rather than passive recipients or observers of, hospital care. In addition, state health departments, which certify hospitals to operate, ensure the right of patients to press complaints about hospital care and services. Hospitals are required by law to investigate patient complaints and respond to them. In fact, a hospital must provide a written response if a patient so requests.

Important Decisions, Informed Consent, and Second Opinions

No description of the structure and processes of hospitals would be complete without mention of the very important personal decisions regarding medical care that patients are asked to make, often, unfortunately, under circumstances that are stressful if not intimidating. A cornerstone of the personal rights of hospitalized patients is the right to know:

- What is being done to them and why
- What the procedure entails
- How the procedure can be expected to benefit them

- What risks or consequences are associated with a procedure
- What the probability of risks and consequences is

In short, in almost all cases, the doctrine of informed consent ensures that patients have ultimate control over their own bodies. This doctrine, first recognized legally in 1914, has been reaffirmed repeatedly over the years and is now generally recognized to encompass not only all of the previously mentioned elements, but also the right to receive information about alternative forms of treatment to the one being recommended.

A physician has no legal right to substitute his or her judgment for the patient's in matters of consent. This principle means that even though a physician may believe a certain intervention is in the patient's best interest, the patient has the absolute right to reject that recommendation. The right of patients to refuse a certain procedure or treatment until they are satisfied that it is in their best interest allows them to stay in control of their health care.

That is why it is considered appropriate for patients to obtain second opinions to satisfy concerns about the necessity for various tests and other procedures. Because there is evidence that seeking the opinion of a second physician regarding the need for surgical and other invasive procedures often results in a decision to reject the original advice, many insurers now require a confirming second opinion before agreeing to pay for surgical procedures.

In many medical situations, the wisest course of action is uncertain or debatable. The need for certain surgical procedures is one good example. Few people realize that the medical needs for some common operations have never been clearly defined by scientific studies. When such studies have been performed, many procedures, even those that surgeons once favored, have turned out to offer no real benefit or improvement over alternative treatments. Unlike the introduction of new drugs, which must be extensively tested to document safety and benefits before they can be marketed, new operations have been introduced and become popular based on clinical impressions, rather than the systematically collected information necessary to determine in what circumstances the benefits justify the risks. Because the best estimates are that only 20% of the more than 20 million operations performed in the United States each year involve critical, life-threatening emergencies in which the physician must operate immediately, patients usually have time to deliberate carefully over the need for surgery and its potential risks and benefits.

Diagnosis-Related Group Hospital Reimbursement System

Until 1983, a patient stayed in the hospital until the physician decided that he or she was well enough to leave. If the patient was going to a nursing home or some other institution, sometimes that patient had to remain in the hospital until a bed became available in the other institution. In most cases, however, physicians had a considerable amount of leeway in making decisions about the length of a patient's stay in the hospital, and they usually tried to balance the best interests of the patients with those of the hospital.

For this and other reasons, the length of time patients stayed in the hospital varied, even among those being treated for the same condition. In fact, the patterns of medical care varied considerably from one geographic location to another. For many years, physicians on the West Coast of the United States have discharged patients from hospitals 2 or more days earlier than their counterparts in the Northeast for patients with the same conditions. Apparently, differing regional medical practice patterns guide physician behaviors.

In any case, each hospital monitored its own situation. Each had a utilization review committee made up of physicians and administrators who were required to review the lengths of stay of hospitalized patients and to ensure that neither the quality of care nor the efficiency of the hospital was being compromised by physicians' decisions.

During the 1970s and early 1980s, however, the cost of hospital care rose so fast that health insurance companies and big corporations that paid huge insurance premiums to cover the hospitalization costs of their workers dramatically increased the pressure on federal agencies to find a way to stem the rising tide of hospital expenses.

Two factors made change imperative. Hospitals were paid a set amount for each day that a patient stayed in the facility. That amount was determined retrospectively by determining what it cost per day per bed to operate the hospital the year before. Under that arrangement, the hospital had no incentive to keep costs down. In fact, if it did, it would receive a smaller daily reimbursement rate the next year than if it spent freely. Furthermore, it became clear to the government and the insurance companies that they were paying not only for uncontrolled costs per hospital day, but also for hospital days that were not necessary. On a national scale, hundreds of thousands of hospital days that did not benefit the patients, at a cost of several hundred dollars per day, amounted to a huge and valueless financial burden. Hospital costs were forcing the federal Medicare program, which served older Americans, to exceed all financial projections.

There was another worry as well. Not only are unnecessarily long hospital stays expensive, but they also can be dangerous to the patients' health. Older patients are especially vulnerable. Patients are exposed to infections and diseases in hospitals that they would not face at home. In addition, many older patients lose the ability to do some of the basic activities of daily living, such as dress, feed, or toilet themselves during a long stay in a hospital. Those patients come out of the hospital less able to function than when they went in. Shortened stays in hospitals, especially for older patients, can often be beneficial as well as less expensive.

In 1983, the federal government radically changed the way hospitals would be reimbursed for the costs of treating Medicare patients. The new payment system is referred to as diagnosis-related groups (DRGs) and is designed to provide hospitals with a financial incentive to discharge patients as soon as possible. It is a prospective payment system, which means that the patient's diagnosis determines how much the hospital will be paid, and the hospital knows that amount in advance. The payment is a set amount based on the average cost of treating that particular illness or condition. If the patient requires less care or fewer days in the hospital than the DRG average, the hospital is paid the average cost regardless, and the hospital makes money. If the patient requires a longer stay or more care than the DRG average, the hospital loses money.

This carrot-and-stick system was adopted quickly by almost all states and hospital insurance companies and now affects all hospital patients, not just Medicare patients. It quickly changed hospital behavior. The built-in system of financial rewards and punishments caused hospitals to discharge patients more quickly and sometimes before they were completely recovered, a practice that has increased the need for home-delivered health care services. In addition, medical staff is much more conservative about ordering tests and procedures that are of marginal value in diagnosis and treatment. Now hospitals do everything they can to ensure that their average cost in a particular DRG category stays within the reimbursement limit. In most cases, the incentive to discharge patients as soon as possible does not cause problems. In some cases, however, it does, and patients have to be readmitted for further treatment. A more detailed discussion of the impact of this reimbursement method on the financial viability of hospitals is provided in Chapter 7, which deals with the financing of health care.

Discharge Planning

The hospital is responsible for employing discharge planners to help patients arrange for safe and appropriate accommodations after a hospital stay. Using information provided by the patient or the patient's family, a discharge planner must see to it that the patient who needs follow-up services, such as home care, will obtain them. The planner must then help make the specific arrangements that are necessary. If the patient requires a transfer to another level of institutional care, such as a nursing home, it is the responsibility of the discharge planner to arrange that transfer before the patient can be discharged from the hospital.

The hospital's financial incentive to discharge patients as soon as possible should never cause patients to be discharged before they are medically ready to leave and before arrangements have been made to ensure that they will receive the necessary posthospital care. Patients who feel that either of these two conditions will not have been met by their anticipated discharge date have the right to appeal that date. If they cannot persuade their physician or discharge planner to reconsider the discharge decision, they can ask the hospital for a written notice of discharge. For those receiving Medicare, the written notice will allow 2 free Medicare-covered days in the hospital, whether or not they decide to appeal.

The hospital's discharge notice must include instructions on how the patient can have the hospital's decision reviewed by the peer review organization (PRO). The PRO is an organization under contract with the federal government to ensure that hospitals and physicians follow Medicare rules. Every geographic area in the United States is covered by a federally designated PRO. Patients have 3 calendar days after receiving written notice to ask the hospital to refer their case to the PRO. The PRO then has 3 working days to return its decision.

The PRO will reverse the decision to discharge and require Medicare to cover the costs of the additional days if it is convinced that the patient is in need of continuing hospital care. If the PRO does not reverse the decision, the hospital can bill the patient directly for any stay after 2 days following its written notice to the patient. There is also a mechanism to appeal the PRO's decision and a further process for a Medicare appeal.

Subacute Care

It was inevitable under recent economic pressures that hospitals would find ways to increase utilization, fill empty beds, and increase revenues. Subacute care, a level of care that falls between inpatient hospitalization and long-term or nursing home care, provided one such opportunity.

Subacute care is a mix of rehabilitation and convalescent services that requires 10 to 100 days of care. It is a level and duration of care inappropriate to either acute-care hospitals or most skilled nursing facilities. Nevertheless, both hospitals and nursing homes have created special units within their facilities to provide for subacute care. Because that care level falls between well-established reimbursement formulas, setting up acute-care facilities has allowed hospitals and nursing homes to find different ways to capture the highest reimbursement rates.

Some hospitals have licensed their subacute-care facilities separately from the rest of the hospital to exempt them from the prospective payment system. Others have converted a hospital-based skilled nursing facility to subacute care. Still others have transformed an entire acute-care facility to a long-term care facility. Unlike acute-care facilities, these long-term care hospitals receive higher cost-based reimbursement from Medicare.[19]

In any case, subacute care, viewed as a new financial opportunity for health care institutions, has become one of the fastest growing developments in the hospital and nursing home industries. Managed care providers welcome the opportunity to direct patients to subacute-care facilities that can treat them effectively for a fraction of the cost of traditional hospital care.

The rapid development of subacute care and the accompanying switch from prospective payment to cost-based reimbursement, however, has prompted the federal government's Health Care Financing Administration and agencies in several states to take steps to halt the spread of subacute-care units within both hospitals and nursing homes until the value of subacute care can be determined. Questions about whether hospitals or nursing homes are more suitable to administer subacute care have been raised. In addition, because the focus of subacute care is more on new forms of reimbursement than on a new type of service, studies are under way to determine the cost-effectiveness and usefulness to patients of this type of care. Clearly, it is a high-stakes development in the hospital industry.

Market-Driven Reforms Affecting Hospitals

Although the American public and Congress resisted the health care system reforms proposed by President Clinton in the failed Health Security Act of 1993, market forces continued to alter the health care environment with remarkable rapidity. With consumers, employers, government, and commercial payers intensifying their demands for lower costs, higher quality, better access, and more information about outcomes, most hospitals undertook a series of competitive efforts to retain and, if possible, improve their market positions. Many engaged in mergers and consolidations intended to effect economies of scale and place them in a better position to negotiate with managed care organizations and other payers. Others, in communities with excess hospital capacity, either closed or converted to other uses, such as ambulatory or long-term care facilities.

Since 1980, approximately 2,000 hospitals closed in the United States, and hospital inpatient days declined by one third. Furthermore, with an increasing number of medical services occurring in ambulatory settings, hospitals are facing the need to reduce inpatient capacity and refocus their service efforts on intensive care and other inpatient essentials.[20]

New Insurer Pressures

The almost total penetration of managed health care in communities across the United States continues to have a profound impact on the hospital industry. Managed care organizations, striving to provide cost-effective care to increasingly large populations of enrollees, exert significant influence over both the use and the cost of hospital services. Additionally, managed care organizations obtain and pay serious attention to measures of performance among hospitals so that they can ensure that their enrollees have timely access to high-quality care. Negotiating with managed care organizations and competing with other hospitals in an open market on the basis of documented performance and cost-effectiveness continue as formidable challenges to most hospitals.

Controlling costs without decreasing the quality of the product, the essential principle of successful commercial ventures, presents a dilemma to many hospitals. In many instances, voluntary hospitals remained financially viable for reasons unrelated to the efficiency and quality of their performance. Now, with health care purchasers increasingly relying on revealing measures of service cost and quality, their continued viability will depend on accountability for every aspect of performance with zero tolerance for waste of effort and resources. Those hospitals that cannot compete successfully for major patient populations under the oversight of managed care organizations are unlikely to survive the reformation of the hospital industry.

Patient-Focused Care

One of the consequences of high-technology hospital care was the industrialization of patient care activities. The corporate thinking that swept the hospital industry in the 1970s and 1980s brought production-line concepts to what formerly had been very personal, high-touch, rather than high-tech, relationships between patients and caregivers, primarily nurses.

Rather than being patient oriented, the care became task oriented, with every chore identified and delegated to the person at the lowest skill level who was capable of carrying it out. Thus, a nurse might be assigned the task of going from patient to patient just taking vital signs, temperatures, blood pressures, and pulses. Another individual, not necessarily a nurse, might be only bathing those same patients, another drawing blood, another handing out medications, and so forth. The end result for patients was a succession of relatively anonymous caregivers, none of whom had a knowledgeable relationship with the patients they served. Responsibility and accountability for the total care of patients became increasingly diffuse. Opportunities for patients to fall into the cracks between the many caregivers increased, and more midlevel managers were necessary to oversee operations. Any questionable gains in efficiency were achieved at the costs of patient satisfaction, communication, and personal care.

Patient satisfaction studies reflected an increase in patient complaints about the loss of identity, dignity, and respect for them as individuals that characterized their hospital stay. Particularly frustrating to many hospital patients and their families was the difficulty that they experienced in obtaining information or even identifying someone capable of answering questions. For most, the lack of communication between hospital staff, including physicians, and the patients and their families was the most irritating aspect of the hospital experience.

After an extensive survey of over 6,000 hospital patients and 2,000 individuals who accompanied patients during their hospital stays, as well as research drawn from field visits and focus groups, the Picker/Commonwealth Program for Patient-Centered Care, established in 1987, was able to identify a series of patient care failings common among hospitals. Unquestionably, the diffusion of clinical responsibility that complicates communication among caregivers and the flow of information between caregivers and patients affect the quality of clinical care. In addition to making patient experiences unpleasant and stressful, communication and coordination breakdowns make for needless duplications of effort and the delay or omission of important procedures and tasks. One devastating finding was that as many as 20% of patients concluded that no one was in charge of their hospital care.

It is significant in the Picker/Commonwealth findings that the most technologically sophisticated teaching hospitals with the most specialized medical staffs also are viewed as the least sensitive to the personal and cultural values, concerns, and perceptions of their patient populations. Conversely, the cultural homogeneity of staff and patients and the relative simplicity of small community hospitals are viewed as more conducive to patient-sensitive care. Clearly, the advances in medical care and the industrialization of many, if not most, hospitals has caused the medical system to lose touch with its essential constituency—its patients—and its essential mission to serve their needs.[21]

Of course, some very large and sophisticated hospitals did not follow the crowd, and they stand out as highly mission oriented, innovative, and sensitive to patient needs and wants. They reshaped their patient care systems on the strengths of their highly skilled nursing personnel to be extremely responsive to patient concerns and to measure precisely how patients experience the process and outcomes of the care they receive.

Beth Israel Hospital in Boston and Cedars-Sinai Medical Center in Los Angeles are two excellent examples of patient-focused hospital care. The quality of nursing care is deemed as important to the safety and well-being of patients in those hospitals as it is to the progress of their medical care. Excellent hospitals give nurses a meaningful role in the care and treatment of patients, and Beth Israel Hospital has been cited many times as the model for other hospitals. Its primary care nursing program, developed in 1974, has one of the most successful histories of patient-centered care. Each patient is assigned a registered nurse (RN) who is responsible for designing a coordinated individual plan of care. The primary care nurse assumes 24-hour responsibility for maintaining continuity of care from admission to discharge and coordinates all other caregivers in the process.[22]

Similarly, Cedars-Sinai Medical Center pioneered the concept of patient-focused care with organizational redesigns, clinical practice guidelines, and firm accountability for the quality of patient care. The dedication and effectiveness of the nursing staff are reflected in its reputation as one of the world's most diversified and sophisticated medical centers and its repeated 95% patient satisfaction ratings.[22]

Clearly, the trend is moving away from the industrial model of hospital care that eroded public trust and confidence in hospital care and toward small team responsibility for the quality of patient services. To lure patients who now have more options, hospitals are focusing on friendlier staff, better food, and more amenities. Many hospitals have done away with visiting hours and invite patients' family members to stay as long as they like. Hospitals will even accommodate visitors who stay the night with reclining chairs and delivered breakfasts.[23]

Integrated Health Systems

The forces of cost containment, the rise of purchaser influence, declining trends in inpatient utilization, and demands of managed care organizations for higher levels of service organization and accountability converged in the 1980s to compel hospitals to rethink their strategic market positioning. In contrast to the 2 previous decades, which were marked by service expansion and diversification, the business environment now suggested that future viability would depend on removing excess capacity through consolidation and improved coordination of services.

The demands of managed care organizations for efficiency, cost controls, coordination of services, and accountability for service outcomes necessitated radical shifts in hospital strategic planning. McManus et al.[24] characterizes the impacts of these changes: "Providers will not just treat episodes of illness or injury, but will focus on wellness, prevention and primary care, and truly manage the total health and well-being of patients. Success will no longer be measured by census, admissions and profits, but by the health and well being of communities served."

As major players in the health care delivery system, hospitals were forced to respond to the new imperatives of managed care by leading efforts at reorganizing and reconfiguring service delivery components within their communities. Both horizontal and vertical system integration strategies began to emerge as hospitals sought to make their organizations attractive to the managed care industry.

Horizontal Integration

Under the general business definition, horizontally integrated organizations are aggregations that produce the same goods or services. They may be separately or jointly owned and governed, operated as subsidiary corporations of a parent organization, or exist in a variety of other legal or quasilegal relationships. According to Roger Kropf:[25]

> In the hospital industry, horizontal integration was viewed as potentially advantageous because a chain of hospitals might be able to purchase supplies and services at a volume discount, would be able to hire specialized staff at the corporate level to increase expertise, would be able to raise capital less expensively on the securities markets, and would be able to market hospital services under a single brand name in a number of communities.

Both for-profit and not-for-profit hospitals engaged in horizontal integration in an effort to meet the economic imperatives of the changing industry climate. The horizontal integration strategy spawned large numbers of hospital mergers and acquisitions and significant growth in the number of multihospital systems during the 1980s. As the trend in inpatient utilization and lengths of stay continued their declines throughout the 1980s, managed care organizations and other large purchasers of health care were increasing demands for the availability of comprehensive, continuous care housed within discrete, accountable systems. For this and other reasons, horizontal integration as a primary strategic initiative declined in favor.

Mergers and acquisitions have continued to the present, but often for reasons different from the advantages initially identified. Now, in communities across the United States, with managed care saturating markets more than penetrating them, consolidation of facilities, staff, and other resources of previously separate organizations has become critical to the survival of a rational health care delivery system.

Vertical Integration

Vertically integrated organizations are ones that operate a variety of business entities, each of which is related to the other. In health care, a vertically integrated system includes several service components, each of which addresses some dimension of a population's health care needs. The system may be fully comprehensive, with a complete continuum of services ranging from prenatal to terminal care. Other systems may contain some, but not all, of the services required by a population. A fully comprehensive vertically integrated system in its ideal form would include all facilities, personnel, and technologic resources to render the complete continuum of care, which comprises (1) all outpatient primary care and specialty diagnostic and therapeutic services, (2) inpatient medical and surgical services, (3) short- and long-term rehabilitative services, (4) long-term chronic institutional and in-home care, and (5) terminal care. Such a system also would include all required support services such as social work and health education. In theory, vertically integrated systems offer attractive benefits to their sponsoring organizations, patients, physicians, and other providers, as well as payers.

Sponsors of vertically integrated organizations gain the advantage of an increased market share across a mixture of high-profit, loss-generating, and break-even revenue sources. They benefit from an increased likelihood of retaining patients for many or all of their service needs. In addition, they are advantageously positioned to negotiate with managed care organizations by ensuring the availability of comprehensive, continuous care for an insured population at competitive prices. For patients, the most obvious benefit is continuity of care throughout the various system components and improved case management. Physicians and other providers benefit both from greater certainty about the flow of patients to their practices and improved ease of referrals. Managed care organizations and other large purchasers view integrated organizations favorably because of the relative ease of negotiating pricing with one organization instead of several. In addition, quality monitoring, patient case management, and physician and other provider activity can be managed and monitored more efficiently when they are all part of the same organization.

The Quality of Hospital Care

It has always been easier to evaluate the quality of the medical care provided in hospitals than that provided in medical offices or other delivery sites because of the availability of comprehensive medical records and other sources of clinical information, systematically collected and stored for later recovery. The definition of quality, however, derives from both various operational factors and the measures or indicators of quality selected and the value judgments attached to them. For many years, quality was defined as "the degree of conformity with preset standards" and encompassed all of the elements, procedures, and consequences of individual patient–provider encounters. Most often, however, the standards against which care was judged were implicit rather than explicit and existed only in the minds of peer evaluators.

The peer-review technique had both benefits and failings. A common peer-review quality-assurance process used in hospitals until the 1970s was the chart audit. Periodically, an audit committee made up of several providers appointed by the hospital medical staff would review a small sample of patient records and make judgments as to the quality of care provided.

Such audits were ineffective for several reasons. First, the evaluators used internalized or implicit standards to make qualitative judgments. Second, there was no rational basis for chart selection that would permit the evaluators to extrapolate the sample findings to the broader patient population. Third, even if deficiencies were identified, the auditors were reluctant to take corrective action because their deficient colleagues might be on the next audit committee reviewing their patient care.

Avedis Donabedian of the University of Michigan made an important contribution to quality-of-care studies by defining the three basic components of medical care—structure, process, and outcome. Structural components are the qualifications of the providers, the physical facility, equipment, and other resources and the characteristics of the organization and its financing.[26] Until the 1960s, the contribution of structure to quality was the primary, if not the only, quality-assurance mechanism in health care. Traditionally, the health care system relied on credentialing mechanisms, such as licensure, registration, and certification by professional societies and specialty boards, to ensure the quality of clinical care.

Hospital reviews for accreditation by the then Joint Commission on Accreditation of Hospitals were also based almost exclusively on structural criteria. Judgments were made about physical facilities, the equipment, the ratios of professional staff to patients, and the qualifications of the various personnel. The underlying assumption of structural quality reviews was that the better the facilities and the qualifications of the providers, the better the quality of the care rendered.

The past focus on structural criteria assumed quite erroneously that enough was known about the relationship of the structural aspects of care to its processes and outcomes to identify the critical or appropriate structural indicators. It was much later that hospital accreditation involved process criteria and more recently outcomes.

The process components are what occur during the encounters between patients and providers. Process judgments include what was done, how appropriate it was, and how well performed, as well as what was omitted that should have been done. The assumption underlying the use of process criteria is that the quality of the actions taken during patient encounters determines or influences the outcomes.

The outcomes of care are all of the things that do or do not happen as a result of the medical intervention. Only recently has quality assurance in the hospital field focused on the relationships among structure, process, and outcomes. In the past, it had always been argued by providers that so many different variables influence the outcomes of medical care that it is inappropriate and unfair to providers to attribute patient outcomes solely to medical interventions. That argument was dismissed, however, with the introduction of computerized information systems and sophisticated analytical techniques that permit the collection and analysis of data on most or all of the potential intervening influences and allow the findings to be adjusted for patient differences. Now, quality-of-care data are routinely standardized to account for age, gender, severity of illness, accompanying conditions, and other variables that might influence outcomes.

Landmark Studies of Quality of Hospital Care

In the early 1960s, the Columbia University School of Public Health and Administrative Medicine, with M. A. Morehead as director, conducted a study of the quality of hospital care provided to members of the Teamsters Union in New York City. The union was investing heavily in hospital services for their members and families and wanted to determine whether the quality of those services justified that large expenditure. Teams of medical experts in a variety of specialties were asked to review large samples of patient records and decide whether the care was justified, appropriate, and acceptably provided. The standards of care on which the decisions were based were not explicit and agreed on beforehand but left to personal judgments of the medical experts reviewing the records.[27]

As might be expected from academically based, board-certified specialists using internalized standards for judging the quality of care, they found that medical care provided by physicians, most like themselves, those who were fellows of specialty boards, was more likely to be optimal. They also concluded, after assembling the findings for all of the individual medical and surgical specialties, that the care provided in hospitals closely affiliated with medical schools was better than that provided in other hospitals.

In spite of the bias introduced into the study by the use of implicit standards that reflected the evaluators' personal values, beliefs, and practice styles, the report, for the first time, documented unquestionably the proportion of hospital admissions that were deemed unnecessary or questionable; the amount of care that was considered inappropriate, poor, or questionable; and a finding, which the public has yet to fully appreciate, that there are significant differences among hospitals and medical staffs in the quality of care they provide.

A host of parallel studies followed that was more rigorously designed and that used consensually derived, explicit performance criteria that reached essentially the same conclusions. Quality-of-care research repeatedly finds that the quality of hospital care is highly variable and is related to the influence of medical school affiliations and to the specialty training of the medical staff.

Variations in Medical Care

In 1973, two researchers, John Wennberg and Alan Gittlesohn, published what would be the first of a series of papers documenting the variations in the amounts and types of medical care provided to patients with the same diagnoses living in different geographic areas.[28]

Those publications emphasized that the amount and cost of hospital treatment in a community had more to do with the number, specialties, and individual preferences of the physicians than the medical conditions of the patients.

At the same time, concerns about the variability of hospital care and the conclusions from studies on its quality prompted federal action. The Social Security Act was amended to create a national network of local professional standards review organizations, which were charged with ensuring that health care services purchased in whole or in part by the Medicare, Medicaid, or maternal and child health programs conform to appropriate professional standards and are delivered effectively and efficiently.

With persistent concerns about improving the quality of hospital care and containing soaring costs, various groups have formed to survey and report on the quality of hospital care. Chief among them has been the Leapfrog Group. It was founded in November 2000 by the Business Roundtable with support from The Robert Wood Johnson Foundation. Members include more than 160 Fortune 500 corporations and other large private and public sector health benefits purchasers that represent more than 36 million enrollees. The Leapfrog Group fields the Leapfrog Hospital Quality and Safety Survey, a voluntary online survey that tracks hospitals' progress toward implementing all 30 of the safety practices endorsed by the National Quality Forum. The Leapfrog website, www.leapfroggroup.org, displays each hospital's results and is updated each month with data from additional hospitals; anyone can review the results at no charge. Leapfrog has compiled the first free online database of programs across the country that offer financial or nonfinancial rewards and incentives for improved performance. The Leapfrog Incentive and Reward Compendium is also available at www.leapfroggroup.org.[29]

Hazards of Hospitalization

Medical errors have been a serious problem in hospitals for years, but improving patient safety did not become a serious national concern until recently. Although those in the health professions and more knowledgeable members of the public have long been aware of the error-prone nature of hospital care, it was not until the November 1999 release of a report prepared by the prestigious National Academy of Science's Institute of Medicine (IOM) on medical mistakes that the magnitude of the risks to patients receiving hospital care became common public knowledge.

By extrapolating the findings of several well-conducted studies of adverse events occurring in hospitals to the 33.5 million hospital admissions in the United States during 1997, the IOM report concluded that as few as 44,000 and as many as 98,000 deaths occur annually because of medical errors.[30] The report put the magnitude of the problem in the context of other comparable concerns by noting that more people die from medical errors in a year than motor vehicle accidents or breast cancer and that medication errors alone kill more people than workplace injuries.

Errors are defined as "the failure to complete a planned action as intended or the use of a wrong to achieve an aim."[29] Those errors may be attributed to failures in diagnostic, treatment, or surgical procedures, selection or doses of medication, delays in diagnosis or treatment, and a host of other procedural lapses, including communication or equipment failures.

There is general agreement that system deficiencies are the most important factor in the problem and not incompetent or negligent physicians and other caregivers. Modern medicine with its highly effective but extremely complex diagnostic and therapeutic methods can be formidably risky. Extensive surgical procedures are error prone, as are increasingly powerful therapeutic drugs. Miscommunication among overstressed employees is common in busy hospitals. With so many steps and so many people involved in the care of hospital patients, the potential for error grows with every patient day, and small lapses develop into large tragedies.[31]

The IOM report presents a series of recommendations to improve the quality of care during the next 10 years. The report lays out a comprehensive strategy for reducing medical errors through a combination of technologic, policy, regulatory, and financial strategies intended to make health care safer. Better use of information technology such as bedside computers, avoidance of similar-sounding and look-alike names and packages of medications, and standardization of treatment policies and protocols would help to avoid confusion and reliance on memory and handwritten communications. The most controversial of the recommendations, however, is the call for a nationwide mandatory reporting system that would require states to report all "adverse events that result in death or serious harm."[32]

The health care system and its practicing physicians will have to make radical changes in cultural attitudes and individual prerogatives, however, before the necessary system changes and reporting requirements can be institutionalized. The IOM report, which moved awareness of the magnitude of medical errors from the anonymity of the hospitals to the nation's media and subsequently to the halls of Congress, has already produced vociferous debate over issues of mandatory or voluntary reporting. Questions of liability, confidentiality, and avoidance of punishment must be settled before any reporting legislation can be passed. In the meantime, other recommendations for more focus on patient safety by professional groups, medical societies, health care licensing organizations, and hospital administrations could be followed with more immediate benefits.

Shortage of Nurses Creating Staffing Crisis

Three factors have combined to drive a hospital nursing shortage to crisis proportions. First, increasing dissatisfaction with staffing reductions, overwork, and too little time to maintain the quality of patient care is driving nurses out of hospitals into early retirement or into home or ambulatory care. Second, with the heavy work responsibilities of nursing as a career and many other more attractive options, fewer young people were entering that clinical field. Last, aging of the current nurse workforce will accelerate staffing losses. With one third of the currently employed nurses over 50 years of age, only an increasing pool of new nurses entering the pipeline will rescue hospital nursing from its critical shortage.[33]

The consequences are serious. There is increasing evidence that nurse staffing is related to patient outcomes in both medical and surgical cases. Studies indicate a direct link between the number of RNs and the time they spend with patients and the number of serious complications and patient deaths. Low nurse staffing increases the likelihood that some patients will suffer pneumonia, shock and cardiac arrest, and gastrointestinal bleeding, and some patients will die as a result.[34]

Although the nursing shortage is far from over, the situation has improved. In the last few years, pay increases, relatively high national unemployment rates, and private initiatives aimed at encouraging men and women to become nurses have resulted in employment growth among RNs. The influx of foreign-born RNs and the return to nursing of older women accounted for a large share of the increase in nurse employment. Unfortunately, faculty shortages in schools of nursing have limited class size even when applications have increased. Thus, the nurse shortage will continue for some time.[35]

Current Research Efforts in Quality Improvement

After the Joint Commission on Accreditation of Hospitals recognized the development of multi-institutional hospital networks and changed its name to the Joint Commission on Accreditation of Healthcare Organizations, it produced a new and quantitatively measurable definition of quality with a results focus. The new definition characterizes the quality of a provider's care as the degree to which the care delivered increases the likelihood of desired patient outcomes and reduces the likelihood of undesired outcomes, given the current state of medical knowledge.

This objective and quantitative definition of quality contrasted sharply with the previous subjective and qualitative definition that required estimates of adherence to somewhat nebulous performance standards. It also left room for nonclinical outcomes, such as accessibility (the ease with which patients can avail themselves of services) and acceptability (the degree to which health care satisfies patients).

Hospitals now conduct regular patient satisfaction studies to obtain patients' views about the services they receive. Such studies encompass several aspects of care, including access, convenience, information received, financial coverage, and perceived quality. It is particularly important for hospital executives to monitor how well their patients' comfort and communication needs were met. Patient satisfaction studies add a new dimension to the definition of quality. "Quality" becomes what the patient receives as judged by the patient, rather than what the facility provides as judged by the providers.

During the decade of the 1980s, when the focus on health care costs caused insurance companies, businesses, and government regulators to become more interested in what was going on in health care, the appropriateness of care became an increasingly important issue. Closely related to the cost and quality dilemma associated with high technology was the problem that some patients received too many procedures, tests, and/or medications that were inappropriate, useless, or even harmful. Although some of the tests and procedures were probably performed to protect the physician or hospital from potential malpractice litigation, some reflected unexplainable regional variations in medical practice, and some were clearly driven by the reimbursement system at the time that rewarded physicians for doing more, not less.

A large number of studies have examined the appropriateness of the use of various medical tests and procedures. Using similar methods, researchers compared medical records against well-established criteria for performing specific medical procedures. Those procedures were then rated as performed for "appropriate," "inappropriate," or "equivocal" reasons. The RAND Corporation summarized the findings of a number of RAND-supported research studies, as shown in Figure 3-1.[36]

Overall, it appears that a significant proportion of hospital procedures is performed for inappropriate reasons. The proportion of all procedures judged to be questionable or equivocal also shows wide-ranging variation. "On average, it appears that one-third or more of all procedures performed in the United States are of questionable benefit."[36]

Hospitals That Join Newest Quality Initiative Save Lives

For several years after the IOM's shocking report about the number of deaths caused by hospital errors, Dr. Donald Berwick, a Harvard professor and president of the nonprofit Institute for Healthcare Improvement, challenged hospitals to improve their quality of care and save lives. By June 2006, over 3,100 hospitals had signed on to his "100,000 Lives Campaign." They agreed to implement six types of changes designed to prevent lethal mistakes. The changes were aimed at preventing medication errors, preventing hospital-acquired infections, deploying rapid-response teams to cope with emergency situations, and the like. Although all participating hospitals did not initiate all six changes, after 18 months, Dr. Berwick estimated that about 122,300 patient lives were saved.[37]

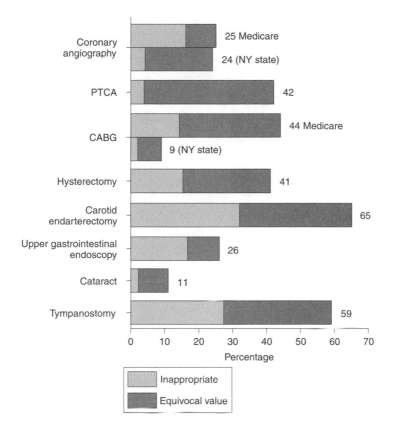

Notes: PTCA, percutaneous transluminal coronary angioplasty; CABG, coronary artery bypass grafting.

FIGURE 3-1 Proportion of Procedures Judged Either "Clinically Inappropriate" or "Of Equivocal Value": Summary of Selected Studies. *Source:* Reprinted with permission from: Rand Health Research Highlights, "Assessing the Appropriateness of Care: How Much is Too Much?" RB-4522, © RAND.

Responsibility of Governing Boards for Quality of Care

Although the medical staffs and other professional providers of patient care in hospitals make the decisions and carry out the procedures that lead to the patient care outcomes, it is the governing boards of hospitals that are ultimately responsible for the quality of the care provided. The board is responsible for the hospital's quality-assurance and risk-management programs, all of the quality-improvement programs, and the oversight of the medical staff. The latter responsibility is discharged primarily through its oversight of and final decisions regarding appointments and privilege delineations of medical staff members. Otherwise, oversight of the medical staff is delegated to the various committees of the medical staff organization.

The board oversees the hospital's quality assurance programs and related functions by monitoring specific information regarding program effectiveness in the identification and resolution of patient care problems and of the medical staff in quality assurance. Some of the indicators that hospital boards regularly review are as follows:

• Mortality rates by department or service
• Hospital-acquired infections
• Patient complaints
• Patient falls
• Adverse drug reactions
• Unplanned returns to surgery
• Hospital-incurred traumas

Needless to say, only the most diligent and dedicated lay board members are capable of interpreting these data and then formulating clear and understandable explanations for their occurrence. Health care reforms are intended to address these problems specifically.

Hospitalists: A Rapidly Growing Innovation

As discussed in more detail in Chapter 5, physicians, called "hospitalists," are rapidly taking over the care of inpatients in U.S. hospitals. Hospitalists, usually internists by training, assume responsibility for the care of inpatients from admission to discharge. They substitute for the patient's primary physician for the period of the hospital stay and provide and/or coordinate all patient care by staff and specialists. Because hospitalists are based in the hospitals, they are able to provide more responsive and continuous care than patients' primary physicians, whose hospital visits are brief and less frequent.

Because it is generally accepted that the presence of hospitalists shortens lengths of stay, improves the continuity and quality of hospital care, and has economic advantages to hospitals, hospitalist medicine is rapidly becoming the preferred model of inpatient care.[38]

Forces of Reform: Cost, Quality, and Access

The performance benchmarks of cost, quality, and access that, with few exceptions, hospitals addressed for decades with moderate enthusiasm and little, if any, effect have now become the survival criteria for the future. Because the scientific breakthroughs and technology advancements that made hospitals the complex institutions they have become, hospital care has been both admired for its diagnostic and therapeutic accomplishments and criticized for its costly inefficiencies, duplications, and its inequities in access and quality. Ironically, the same high technology that contributed so much to hospitals' medical achievements also has been used to reveal their performance shortcomings in uncompromising detail. The sophisticated computerized clinical information systems that supported the research that focused on the cost-effectiveness or outcomes of expensive medical interventions have increasingly documented and given public recognition of system deficiencies. Studies similar to that of the IOM,[39] which took 2 years of reviewing scientific articles, conducting hearings, and making site visits at health care institutions, came to the conclusion that the poor quality of health care is a major problem in the United States. Citing widespread overuse of expensive technologies, underuse of inexpensive "caring" services, and error-prone application of health care services, these studies concluded that the system deficiencies not only wasted money, but also actually harmed patients.[40]

The continuing public debate over the escalating costs of health care and the increasing number of major employer/employee disputes over sharing the costs of insurance premiums have raised the level of health cost awareness of most Americans. In addition, the disruptions in long-standing relationships between specialist physicians and patients in managed care arrangements and the position promulgated by managed care organizations that some medical care is wasteful and unproductive have focused patients' attention on the possibility that in some cases there may be inverse relationships between costs and quality.

Clearly, there is an increasing interest in major changes in the health care system, and hospitals, as a major component of the system would be seriously affected. Unfortunately, no consensus has emerged as to how to change it. Whether reform is to be incremental or comprehensive, whether it should focus on the economic problems or the organizational and delivery problems, or both are still open questions.[41]

Whatever the final form of U.S. health care after the industry-wide reformation takes place, there is general agreement that hospitals will no longer be the axis on which the rest of the system turns. Reduced in both capacity and importance, hospitals will simply be essential components of community-based and integrated systems of primary, tertiary, long-term, and home health care with significant public health and disease prevention functions.

Stephen Shortell of Northwestern University has encapsulated in seven steps the changes that hospitals will have to make to reposition themselves to function effectively in the future. Those steps are as follows:[42]

1. Becoming part of an integrated health system
2. Developing new management structures
3. Building capacity for population-based needs assessment
4. Forging new relationships with physicians
5. Re-engineering clinical processes
6. Implementing total quality management
7. Focusing on outcomes

There will be great variation in the capability of America's thousands of hospitals to adjust to what they will interpret as radical reversals of form and function. In the new hospital market economy, however, it appears likely that the Darwinian law of nature, survival of the fittest, will determine which hospitals will remain to serve the American public in the 21st century.

References

1. Stevens R. *In Sickness and in Wealth: American Hospitals in the Twentieth Century.* New York, NY: Basic Books; 1989.

2. Stevens R. *In Sickness and in Wealth: American Hospitals in the Twentieth Century.* New York, NY: Basic Books; 1989:399.

3. Stevens R. *In Sickness and in Wealth: American Hospitals in the Twentieth Century.* New York, NY: Basic Books; 1989:293.

4. Stevens R. *In Sickness and in Wealth: American Hospitals in the Twentieth Century.* New York, NY: Basic Books; 1989:319.

5. Stevens R. *In Sickness and in Wealth: American Hospitals in the Twentieth Century.* New York, NY: Basic Books; 1989:320.

6. Teisberg EO, Vayle EJ. *The Hospital Sector in 1992.* Boston, MA: Harvard Business School; 1991.

7. Fast Facts on US Hospitals. Available from http://www.aha.org/aha/resource-center/statistics-and-studies/fast-facts,ht. Accessed July 3, 2007.

8. Gutman S. Specialty hospitals: a problem or a symptom? *Health Affairs.* 2006;25:95–105.

9. Greenwald L, Cromwell J, Adamache W. et al. Specialty versus community hospitals: referrals, quality, and community benefits. *Health Affairs* 2006; 25:106–118.

10. Fast Facts on US Hospitals. Available from http://www.aha.org/aha/resource-center/statistics-and-studies/fast-facts,ht. Accessed October 23, 2006.

11. Bellandi D. Spinoffs, big deals dominate in '99. *Modern Healthcare.* 2000; 30:36.

12. Facts About the Department of Veterans Affairs. Available from http://www.va.gov/about-va/. Accessed October 25, 2006.

13. Gilles RR, Shortell SM, Young GJ, et al. Best practices in managed organized delivery systems. *Hospitals Health Services Admin.* 1997;42:299–321.

14. Francis J, Perlin J. Improving performance through knowledge translation in the Veterans Health Administration. *J Continuing Educ Health Professions.* 2006;26:67.

15. Panel on problems at Walter Reed issues strong rebuke. *New York Times.* April 12, 2007:A-11.

16. Peake JB. Beyond the Purple Heart: continuity of care for the wounded in Iraq. *N Engl J Med.* 2005;352:219–222.

17. U.S. Department of Commerce. *County Business Patterns, 1997.* Washington, DC: U.S. Government Printing Office.

18. Bachmeyr AC. *Hospital Care in the United States: A Study by the Commission on Hospital Care.* Cambridge, MA: Harvard University Press by Commonwealth Fund; 1947.

19. Anders G. Hospitals rush to remodel to offer subacute care—and get paid twice. *Wall Street Journal.* October 3, 1996:A1, A8.

20. Shortell SM. *The Future of Hospitals and Health Care Management.* Washington, DC: VA Office of Research and Development, n.d.

21. Gerteis M, Leviton SE, Daily J, et al. *Through the Patient's Eyes: Understanding and Promoting Patient-Centered Care.* San Francisco, CA: Jossey-Bass, Publishers; 1993.

22. Sunshine L, Wright JW. *The Best Hospitals in America.* New York, NY: Henry Holt and Company; 1987.

23. Rundle RL. We hope you enjoy your stay. *Wall Street Journal.* November 22, 2004:R5.

24. McManus GL, Dong C, Wilson JE. et al. The integrator of care: a coordinated health care system. *Health Care Strategic Manage.* 1993;10:17–19.

25. Kropf R. Planning for health services. In: Kovner AR, ed. *Health Care Delivery in the United States.* New York, NY: Springer Publishing Co. 1995:353.

26. Donabedian A. Evaluating the quality of medical care. *Millbank Memorial Fund Q.* 1966;44:166–206.

27. Columbia University. *A Study of the Quality of Hospital Care Secured by a Sample of Teamster Family Members in New York City.* New York, NY: Columbia University School of Public Health and Administrative Medicine; 1964.

28. Wennberg JE, Gittlesohn A. Small area variation in health care delivery. *Science.* 1973;182:1102–1108.

29. The Leapfrog Group. the Leapfrog Incentive and Reward Compendium. Available from http://www.leapfroggroup.org/. Accessed January 5, 2005.

30. Kohn LT, Corrigan JM, Donaldson MS, et al. *To Err is Human: Building a Safer Health System.* Washington, DC: Institute of Medicine; 1999:1–4.

31. Kohn LT, Corrigan JM, Donaldson MS, et al. *To Err is Human: Building a Safer Health System.* Washington, DC: Institute of Medicine; 1999: 3.

32. Kohn LT, Corrigan JM, Donaldson MS, et al. *To Err is Human: Building a Safer Health System.* Washington, DC: Institute of Medicine; 1999:75.

33. Dworkin RW. Where have all the nurses gone? *Public Interest.* 2002:23–36.

34. Needleman J, Buerhaus PI, Stewart M, et al. Nurse staffing in hospitals: is there a business case for quality. *Health Affairs.* 2006;25:204–211.

35. Buerhaus PI, Staiger DO, Averbach DI, et al. Trends: New signs of a strengthening U.S. nurse labor market? *Health Affairs, Web Exclusives.* 2004:W4.526.

36. RAND Health Research Highlights. *Assessing the Appropriateness of Care: How Much Is Too Much?* Santa Monica, CA: Rand Corporation; 1998.

37. Hospital initiative to cut errors finds about 122,300 lives were saved. *Wall Street Journal.* June 15, 2006:D6.

38. Glabman M. *Hospitalists: The Next Big Thing.* American Hospital Association, Center for Healthcare Governance, Trustee; Chicago, Ill: Health Forum, Inc. May 2005:7–11.

39. Lohr KN. *Medicare: A Strategy for Quality Assurance.* Vol I. Washington, DC: National Academy Press; 1990.

40. Palmer RH, Adams ME. Quality improvement/quality assurance taxonomy: a framework. In: Grady ML, Bernstein J, Robinson S., eds. *Putting Research To Work in Quality Improvement and Quality Assurance.* Washington, DC: U.S. Department of Health and Human Services; 1993:13–37.

41. Fuchs VR, Emanuel EJ. Health care reform: why, what, when. *Health Affairs.* 2005;24:1399–1414.
42. Shortell SM, Reinhardt UE. Creating and executing health policy in the 1990s. *Improving Health Policy and Management: Nine Critical Research Issues.* Health Administration Press, Baltimore, MD: Academy of Health Services; 1992:5–6.

CHAPTER 4

Ambulatory Care

This chapter reviews the major elements of ambulatory (outpatient) care. Ambulatory care encompasses a diverse and growing sector of the health care delivery system. Physician services are the chief component; however, hospital outpatient and emergency departments, community health centers, departments of health, and voluntary agencies also contribute important services, particularly for the uninsured and vulnerable populations. Ambulatory surgery is a continuously expanding component of ambulatory care, as new technology allows an increasing number of procedures to be performed safely and economically outside the hospital.

Overview and Trends

Ambulatory care comprises health care services that do not require overnight hospitalization. Ambulatory care is the predominant mode of health care delivery in the United States. Once largely consisting of visits to private physicians' offices and hospital outpatient clinics and emergency departments, ambulatory care today encompasses a broad and expanding array of services.

New medical and diagnostic procedures and technological advancements allow procedures previously requiring hospitalization to be performed on an outpatient basis. As early as a decade ago, many surgical procedures commonly warranted a few, and often several, days of stay in the hospital. Now, the majority of all surgical procedures are performed on an ambulatory basis.

In addition to the numerous new diagnostic and treatment tools available in the outpatient setting and the advanced technology that makes outpatient treatment safe and effective, financial mandates also have driven services into the ambulatory arena. Beginning in the 1980s, prospective hospital reimbursement replaced retrospective payment on a national scale through Medicare's initiation of the diagnosis-related group (DRG) payment system. The new payment system provided financial incentives to decrease the duration of inpatient stays and to increase service delivery efficiency. Hospitals responded to the new payment system by shifting procedures and services amenable to outpatient delivery from the more expensive inpatient environment to less expensive and more efficient ambulatory delivery systems.

Both DRGs and increasing pressures from health care purchasers to control costs contributed to the rapid expansion of health maintenance organizations and other forms of managed care. With an emphasis on providing services in the least expensive, most effective manner possible, managed care organizations exerted a powerful influence that compelled a shift toward the appropriate use of ambulatory services to replace more expensive inpatient care.

Ambulatory care capacity has expanded in both the hospital-based and non–hospital-based, or "freestanding," settings. Historically, hospitals operated virtually all ambulatory or outpatient clinics within the hospital's main facilities or in contiguous facilities on the hospital campuses. Most larger hospitals still operate clinic services on site, and many have retained ambulatory surgical services within the main facility in response to community need, physician demand, and teaching activity. The conversion of underused inpatient units also provided a cost-effective means for hospitals to accommodate the shift to ambulatory surgical services and other ambulatory procedures within the hospital.

Beginning in the 1980s, hospitals expanded their service networks to include geographically distributed freestanding facilities throughout their service areas, both for routine diagnosis and treatment and for ambulatory surgical services. In addition to cost considerations, two other factors have influenced this trend for hospitals. First, the 1980s and 1990s saw a rising consumer demand for conveniently located, easily accessible facilities and services, two factors frequently lacking on hospital campuses and the large building complexes associated with them. This is particularly true for large teaching hospitals, which are often located in congested urban centers and are perceived as inconvenient to increasing numbers of suburban dwellers. Second, with the growing concerns of inner-city hospitals about competition with other institutions for market share of profitable outpatient services and referrals for inpatient care, hospitals recognized the need to expand their service distribution network to larger segments of the community by establishing conveniently located facilities. Hospitals also recognized that some ambulatory services, such as surgery, could be operated most efficiently off site and be removed from the scheduling complexities and other requirements of a system that must accommodate a vast array of physician and patient needs.

Independent of hospital organizations, for-profit corporations' freestanding facilities providing ambulatory, primary, specialty, and surgical services have proliferated. In addition to profitability and cost-control features attractive to insurers, responsiveness to consumer preferences has also been a primary driver in these developments.

The decade of the 1990s saw a continuing upward trend in the total number of ambulatory care facilities owned and operated by hospitals, physicians, and independent chains. Services provided by these facilities are diverse and represent a response to population demographics in their respective service areas as well as reimbursement opportunities. A partial listing of the array of ambulatory care facilities includes cancer treatment, diagnostic imaging of many different types, renal dialysis, pain management, physical therapy, cardiac rehabilitation, outpatient surgery, occupational health, women's health, and wound care.

A significant corollary to developments in ambulatory care delivery for hospital-operated and independent organizations has been the entry of physicians into the business of outpatient diagnostic, treatment, and surgical services previously available to their practices in only the hospital setting. The same factors operative in the larger industry—technological advances making the purchase, maintenance, and operation of the required equipment feasible and cost-effective in freestanding facilities; consumer demand for convenient, user-friendly environments; and profitability—have compelled this development.

Physician involvement in this arena has paralleled that of hospitals in practice areas, such as ophthalmologic surgery for lens replacement and laser therapy, certain types of gynecologic surgery, fiber-optic gastrointestinal diagnosis, chemotherapy, renal dialysis, computed tomography (CT) scanning, magnetic resonance imaging (MRI), and more. The implications of this trend for hospitals' business volume and revenue have been significant as physicians and hospitals emerge as competitors engaged in the same lines of business. These developments are permanently, and in the view of some, negatively altering the long-standing relationships between physicians and their affiliated hospitals and are discussed in more detail later in this chapter.[1]

The ambulatory care delivery system is changing and growing rapidly as its various organization models evolve, including new efforts to measure quality relative to costs. The service constellation also is growing rapidly and becoming more diverse. As the reimbursement system continues to evolve and new treatment modalities are developed, ambulatory service provider roles continue refinement. Although we cannot expect to address every hybrid of the evolving ambulatory care delivery system, this chapter provides a framework for understanding the origins, development, and future direction of this important sector of the health care delivery system.

Private Medical Office Practice

It is common to think of ambulatory services organized and delivered under some institutional aegis, such as a hospital or the community-based clinics of public health departments; however, private physician office practices constitute the predominant mode of ambulatory care in the United States. In 2005, the most recent year for which data are available, the National Center for Health Statistics estimates that patients made 963 million visits to physician offices: 573 million to primary care physicians, 200 million to surgical specialists, and 190 million to medical specialists.[2] Since 1995, primary care and surgical care office visits increased by approximately 20%; visits to medical specialist offices increased by 37%. Figure 4-1 compares visit rates among physician offices, hospital outpatient departments, and emergency departments.

The way that physicians organize and operate their private practices has evolved from a variety of factors. The single most significant development has been a continuing increase in the number of group practice arrangements and their size. An increasing number of physicians are partners or salaried employees of group practices.[3]

The origins of group practice can be traced to the Mayo Clinic in the late 19th century. The Mayo Clinic group practice generated considerable controversy among physicians. A 1932 report by the Committee on the Costs of Medical Care endorsed organized group practices and the use of insurance payments. The American Medical Association (AMA) condemned

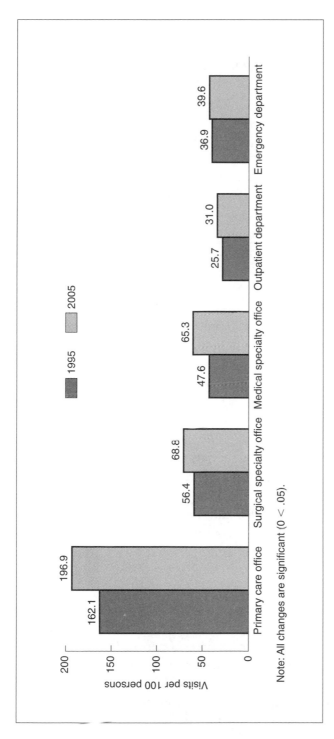

FIGURE 4-1 Ambulatory patient visit rates by setting type: United States, 1995 and 2005.
Sources: National Ambulatory Medical Care Survey and National Hospital Ambulatory Medical Care Survey.

the report, declaring that group and salaried physicians were unethical. The controversy erupted into a legal battle when Group Health Insurance was organized in Washington, DC in 1937. The AMA informed physicians that the plan was unethical and expelled all Group Health Insurance–salaried physicians. Hospitals received lists of "reputable physicians." "The Washington, DC Medical Society and the AMA were subsequently indicted, found guilty, and fined for having conspired to monopolize medical practice."[4] Around the country, local medical societies lost attempts to obstruct the formation of group practices. For the next few decades, negative confrontations occurred as physicians sought participation in developing group health plans. Participating physicians were socially ostracized and denied hospital privileges. By the 1950s, because of effective legal challenges against organized medicine and a physician shortage, opposition to group practice subsided.

Before 1950, most physicians had solo practices. Since then, rising specialization, changing economics, and the desire for more control over their lifestyles caused physicians to group together, either in single fields, such as primary care, or into multispecialty groups. Group practice involves several physicians practicing together in some type of coordinated arrangement. In contrast to an individual physician, fee-for-service payment basis, most groups pay their members a salary augmented with a percentage of practice net profits.

The old solo-practice model made the physician responsible for his or her entire patient caseload 24 hours a day, every day of the year. Before the proliferation of specialties, these physicians normally provided all of the medical care required by their patients, with the exception of surgery or occasional consultation. The demands on their time and stamina were enormous. Aside from occasional coverage arrangements with a colleague to allow for brief time off, their schedules were relentless and unpredictable.

Beginning in the 1960s, several factors influenced a major shift from the solo mode of private practice to group practice. Social movements in the United States produced a heightened awareness of lifestyle adaptations that allowed healthy accommodation for personal growth and balance between professional and personal responsibilities. In the same period, medical specialization burgeoned as the growth in medical knowledge and technological advances increased exponentially. Rapidly advancing knowledge in every field of medicine and the resulting specialization created new challenges for the solo generalist and the specialist. Most obvious were increasing demands on physicians to maintain a command of a body of knowledge that was continuously yielding new diagnostic and therapeutic breakthroughs in virtually every field of practice.

The introduction of Medicare reimbursement in 1966 dramatically altered the private medical office and its financial, billing, and reimbursement processes. Before the government's entry into financing private practice services, physician reimbursement came from largely two sources: personal patient payments or third-party private insurance. Blue Cross/Blue Shield and a relatively small number of other private indemnity carriers comprised most of the third-party payments. Billing and collection were relatively simple. When Medicare began providing primary coverage for everyone over the age of 65 years, private physicians' offices found themselves dealing with a new insurance carrier and a vast array of new government regulations and fee schedules. In addition, many Medicare recipients also carried supplemental private insurance contracts to reimburse the balance that Medicare did not cover. For the private physician's office, the regulation, complexity, and volume of billing requirements burgeoned. Solo-practice office administration, once the province of the physicians themselves, with possibly a receptionist and a part-time bookkeeper, now required an increased level of sophistication and a great deal more time.

Other factors also influenced the shift to group practice. Malpractice insurance costs began to rise dramatically in the 1970s. Inflation fueled rising office lease and rental expenses. The need for more sophisticated administrative support services increased with advancing technology and more complex billing and record-keeping requirements. As technology advanced and diagnostic equipment became available for in-office use, groups could benefit from sharing equipment acquisition costs and ensuring the volume necessary to justify ongoing staffing and maintenance. Physicians recognized that group practice could provide other economies of scale through shared administrative overhead.

Group practice evolved in two forms. One consisted of groups of physicians in the same discipline, usually primary care, surgery, obstetrics, or pediatrics. The other form was multidisciplinary specialty practices, usually including primary care physicians in collaboration with several major specialties or subspecialties. There were important features that both generalist and specialist physicians found more attractive in group practice than solo practice. First, although typically each physician carried his or her own caseload of patients, physicians could arrange a routine, preplanned schedule of after-hours call and weekend and vacation coverage. Another attractive dimension of group practice was that it provided a professionally supportive environment.

With the continuing growth of medical information and knowledge required to maintain state-of-the-art competencies and an ever-expanding range of diagnostic and therapeutic alternatives available, group practice enables physicians to access each other's knowledge and experience in an informal consultative environment. This interchange of information not only provided professional support but also introduced an informal system of peer review to each physician's practice, which, in theory, could contribute to patient care quality. Group practice also enabled patient orientation to alternative coverage arrangements, and thus, their expectation of seeing or contacting another physician in the absence of their own could be established in advance. Today, approximately 20% of medical practices with three or more physicians comprises over one half of all office-based physicians.[5]

Multispecialty group practices evolved for many of the same reasons as single-specialty groups. For specialists, a major benefit was that group membership reduced reliance on patient referrals from other community physicians because economic incentives made keeping the business inside the group beneficial to all members. Patients also benefited by having diagnosis, treatment, and consultation services available at one location. The arrangement also facilitated communication and coordination of results and findings and speeded the turnaround of information.

Surgical group practices evolved similarly to those in the general and other specialty medical fields for similar reasons; however, surgeons have tended to avoid multispecialty grouping. Instead, most are either general surgeons or specialists in such areas as gastrointestinal, cardiothoracic, vascular, or orthopedic surgery. Economies of scale afford the same advantages in these practices as those in general medical and multispecialty practices with respect to sharing operating costs.

Growth in managed care also caused changes in the characteristics of physician practices. A 2006 report from The Center for Studying Health System Change found that 89% of physicians contract with managed care organizations.[6]

Other Ambulatory Care Practitioners

In addition to physicians, a number of other licensed health care professionals conduct practices in ambulatory settings. Among the most common are dentists, podiatrists, social workers, psychologists, physical therapists, and optometrists. Like physicians, they may practice singly or in single-specialty or multispecialty groups. For example, there are general solo-practice dentists and multispecialty dental groups who provide general preventive and curative services, as well as services in specialties such as periodontics and orthodontics. Likewise, psychologists in a group may include both generalists and specialists in forensic, child, and other types of psychological interventions. Chapter 6 discusses physicians, nurses, and other health professions in detail.

Ambulatory Care Services of Hospitals: History and Trends

Acute care voluntary hospitals have operated outpatient clinics since the 19th century. The early ones were located predominantly in urban centers whose indigent populations lacked access to private medical care. At that time, the provision of outpatient services was largely a function of government-sponsored public hospitals. With the proliferation of the voluntary not-for-profit hospitals beginning in the early 20th century, outpatient clinics provided a means for those hospitals to fulfill part of their charitable mission by serving low-income populations who had little, if any, access to private physicians. Hospital outpatient clinics also provided a teaching setting for university-affiliated hospitals, which trained physicians as part of their community mission.

Historically, hospital outpatient clinics were a low-status component of the constellation of hospital care. J. H. Knowles, who was then director of the Massachusetts General Hospital, wrote in 1965, "Turning to the outpatient department of the urban hospital, we find the stepchild of the institution. Traditionally, this has been the least popular area in which to work, and as a result, few advances in medical care and teaching have been harvested here for the benefit of the community."[7]

Because they cared for a low-income population, hospital outpatient clinics addressed complex medical and social problems, poor compliance with treatment regimens, and discontinuity in care. Hospitals did not support the outpatient clinics with equipment and staff. Medical students and hospital-affiliated physicians of lowest tenure or rank, who agreed to see clinic patients in return for admitting privileges, staffed the clinics.

Today, hospital outpatient clinics, particularly those in urban centers, still function as the community's safety net for the medically indigent population; however, the status of those services within the hospital and the roles and positions of physicians working in them have changed radically. The change has been most dramatic since the early 1980s, when an array of factors converged to increase both the volume and scope of available hospital outpatient services. Far from the stepchild image characterized by Knowles, hospitals view outpatient clinical services as helping to ensure a source of inpatient admissions and generating revenue from the use of hospital ancillary services.

No longer the repository for reluctant physicians and students obligated to work there, now hospital outpatient clinics are organized along the lines of private physician group practices and are aesthetically pleasant, well equipped, and customer oriented. With respect to the hospitals' financial picture, the direction is clear. In 1980, outpatient services revenue constituted only 13% of total voluntary hospital revenues in the United States.[8] The figure rose dramatically throughout the 1980s and 1990s and continues to increase. The outpatient share of total hospital revenue currently stands at 35.2%.[9]

Because clinic services traditionally were organized both for the social goal of caring for the needy and for providing teaching and research opportunities, they have tended to be organized by human organ systems and the diseases that affect them. For example, medical clinics, in addition to general medicine, might include clinics for dermatology (skin), cardiology (heart), gastroenterology (digestive tract), rheumatology (bone and connective tissue), and other specialties. In addition to general surgery, surgical clinics might include such specialties as orthopedics (bone), vascular (circulatory system), and others. This type of organization was attractive to attending specialists, researchers, and educators because it allowed narrowly focused concentration on particular patient complaints and illnesses. Beyond this benefit, however, the complex interactions among physicians and patients inherent in this anatomic organization of services have a broad range of both positive and negative implications for both.

For the patient, specialty clinics provide a sophisticated approach to diagnosis and treatment by physicians with special interests and training in their conditions. Also, the teaching functions of clinics often result in thorough and exhaustive examination and case review for the students' benefit that might not otherwise occur in a nonteaching setting.

Treatment in hospital specialty clinics also has drawbacks for patients. Often, specialty clinics treat patients only on certain days each week or on 2 or 3 days per month, depending on the demand for the service. Patients with multiple conditions may have to visit several specialty clinics, necessitating many return visits at which different physicians see them. Because communication among physicians in different specialty clinics can be uncertain, patients may receive conflicting advice or instruction, may be medicated inappropriately with drugs prescribed by several different specialists, and may "fall through the cracks" when a complaint arises that does not seem to fit the specialty area of one of their providers. Similarly, for the physician, this type of categorical treatment environment requires a high degree of initiative to maintain accurate, current information on patients treated by multiple specialists. Beginning in the 1950s, as medical specialization continued, additional subdivision of the teaching hospitals' outpatient clinic services was required to support medical training needs, further exacerbating these problems of continuity and coordination of care. The training requirements of medical students and residents, who could be required to rotate through different specialty clinics as often as monthly, created still more rifts in continuity for patients who, in the course of one illness, might be seen by several different practitioners in the same clinic.

Beginning in the early 1980s, several influences began to have an impact on how hospital outpatient clinic services were organized and delivered. One major influence was the adoption of the DRG hospital reimbursement method, which emphasized decreased lengths of stay. For hospitals, an anticipated result would be declining inpatient revenues. Another major factor was the growing importance of managed care organizations and their emphasis on the role of primary medical care. These issues also brought a heightened realism to several years of growing concern on the part of medical educators. The uncontrolled proliferation of specialists at the expense of maintaining a balanced supply of general physicians would have to be addressed to respond to payer and rising consumer demands for more cost-effective, efficient, and coordinated care.

Facing declining inpatient revenue, increasing influences of managed care, and shifting medical education emphasis to primary medicine, hospitals initiated reorganization and expansion plans for outpatient clinic services that focused heavily on primary care areas. Teaching hospitals planned jointly with their affiliated medical schools, and non-teaching facilities followed suit to pursue expansion of both the volume and array of outpatient services with primary care as the core. Teaching hospitals also undertook outpatient clinic reorganizations, creating primary care centers under the direction of paid, full-time "geographic" faculty department heads with administrative, clinical, and teaching oversight responsibility.

Hospitals hired full-time and part-time physicians as employees who, with medical school faculty appointments, undertook ongoing responsibility for day-to-day patient care, teaching, and supervision of students and residents. Primary care physician employees were organized into practice group models along the lines of private group practices. This primary care model provided a rational structure for the general medical care of clinic patients and helped ensure appropriate referrals and coordination of patient care within and among outpatient clinic specialty units.

The group model of outpatient primary care also more adequately supported the hospitals' teaching mission by alleviating reliance on voluntary physician staffing of clinic sessions and student supervision responsibilities. Medical students and residents were provided a more supportive and consistent learning environment by interacting with members of the practice group continuously instead of with different mentors over the course of their rotation. Patients benefited from improved coordination of their care and the opportunity to develop a relationship with an individual provider, who functioned as their private attending physician. Although the distribution and organization of most specialty clinic services have not changed appreciably in teaching hospitals, developments in the organization of primary care in hospital-based clinics have made a major contribution to the coordination and appropriate delivery of services to hospital-based outpatient clinic consumers.

Outpatient business continued to expand, and although hospital admissions and lengths of stay decreased, similar reorganizations were undertaken in certain consumer-sensitive service areas. As one example, during the 1980s, the upscale, childbearing-age female population began spinning off into a major consumer group. Hospitals saw an opportunity to attract new business by reorganizing obstetrics and gynecology services. The old, hospital-based clinics were relabeled with attractive titles such as "Women's Center," and facilities were renovated, decorated, and equipped to mimic state-of-the-art private medical offices. The purely clinical services were augmented by free or low-cost health information and education services, with emphasis on prevention, wellness, and personal service. Hospitals undertook extensive public relations and media campaigns to attract the privately insured and self-paying population. Hospitals undertook many other similar initiatives in outpatient clinical areas that appeared to hold promise for new business and enhanced revenue streams.

Although major changes have occurred in the organization and delivery of hospital outpatient clinics over the past 20 years, fiscal and operational challenges remain for the urban-based teaching hospitals' outpatient clinics. Some have enjoyed considerable success in attracting new patients with private insurance and self-pay capability and have succeeded in achieving a healthier balance in their previously predominant caseload of Medicaid or charity-care patients; however, as long as our health care system leaves millions of individuals with inadequate or no insurance concentrated heavily in urban areas, it can be expected that the caseloads of hospital-based outpatient clinics will remain heavily dominated by the medically indigent population.

Hospital Emergency Services

U.S. hospitals operate 3,795 hospital emergency departments, representing a 10% decrease in the number of emergency departments since 1995.[10] In 2005, there were an estimated 115.3 million visits to hospital emergency departments, about 219 visits to emergency departments every minute. Overall, emergency department visits have increased by 20% since 1995.[10] The increase in emergency department visits is attributed to overall population growth, a decrease in the number of available emergency departments, increases in the numbers of older Americans, constrained capacity in other outpatient settings, and increasing numbers of uninsured (Figure 4-2).[11]

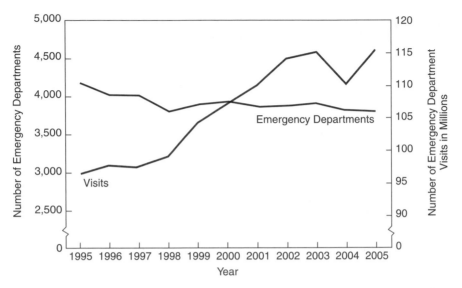

FIGURE 4-2 Trends in number of emergency department visits: United States, 1995–2005.
Sources: CDC/NCHS National Hospital Ambulatory Medical Care Survey, American Hospital Association.

Approximately 15.5% of patients arrive at emergency departments by ambulance, and about 12% of visits result in hospitalization.[10] Emergency department use is heaviest for persons 75 years of age and older, infants, Medicaid beneficiaries, Asian or Pacific Islanders, and African Americans.[10] The visit rate by uninsured individuals is about twice the rate of persons with private insurance, reflecting the safety net function of emergency departments.[2,11] The reasons for emergency department visits encompass a broad spectrum, ranging from life-threatening conditions to those treatable in primary care settings. The Centers for Disease Control reports that almost half of metropolitan center hospitals routinely experience emergency department crowding and that one third of hospitals report the need to divert ambulances to other emergency departments because of a lack of capacity.[12] Today, emergency departments in most hospitals are highly sophisticated facilities equipped with advanced technology and specialty staff, available 24 hours a day, 365 days a year. Although designed to care for life-threatening illness or injury, the public increasingly looks to them for medical care that ranges from the unnecessary to the routine. A high proportion of emergency department visits is

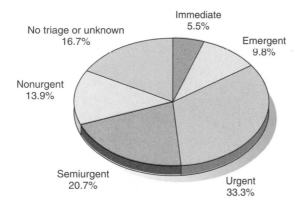

Notes: Immediate is a visit in which the patient should be seen immediately. Emergent is a visit in which the patient should be seen in 1–14 minutes. Urgent is a visit in which the patient should be seen within 15–60 minutes. Semiurgent is a visit in which the patient should be seen within 61–120 minutes. Nonurgent is a visit in which the patient should be seen within 121minutes to 24 hours. No triage or unknown is a visit in which there is no mention of an immediacy rating or triage level in the medical record, the hospital did not perform triage, or the patient was dead on arrival.

FIGURE 4-3 Percent distribution of emergency department visits by immediacy with which patient should be seen.
Source: CDC/NCHS National Hospital Ambulatory Medical Care Survey.

deemed to be nonurgent (Figure 4-3).[10] Medicaid patients represent the highest emergency department visit rate and privately insured persons the lowest rate (Figure 4-4).[10]

Over one-third of annual emergency room visits (41.6 million visits) are for injuries, poisoning and adverse effects of prior medical treatment.[10] The latter include complications of medical and surgical procedures and adverse effects of medication. About 1.9% of visits are made by individuals discharged from the hospital in the previous 7 days.[10] Many primary emergency department diagnoses are related to chronic conditions such as asthma, cancer, cerebrovascular disease, congestive heart failure, chronic obstructive pulmonary disease, depression, hypertension and heart disease resulting from obstruction of arterial blood flow.[10] One contributing factor to inappropriate emergency department use is patients' self-interpretation of symptoms. Also, when physicians receive after-hours calls or calls regarding potentially serious complaints and it is neither practical nor seems appropriate for the patient to be seen in the private office, physicians may direct patients to the emergency department for

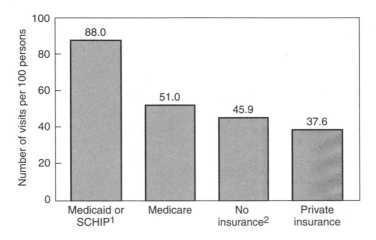

¹SCHIP is State Children's Health Insurance Program.
²Includes self-pay, no charge, and charity.
NOTES: The denominator for each rate is the population total for each type of insurance obtained from the 2005 National Health Interview Survey. More than one source of payment may be recorded per visit.

FIGURE 4-4 Emergency department visits per 100 persons by payment source.
Sources: CDC/NCHS National Hospital Ambulatory Medical Care Survey, CDC/NCHS, National Health Interview Survey.

immediate care. Physicians may also use the emergency departments of hospitals to perform certain tests or examinations requiring equipment not available in their offices. Because state and federal regulations require that hospitals turn no one away, patients know that the emergency department is a guaranteed resource regardless of their ability to pay or the nature of their complaint.

Emergency departments immediately treat discrete episodes of serious illness and injury; however, they are a poor consumer choice for routine care. First, care is much more expensive than in an appropriate ambulatory setting because it consumes the time of specialist personnel for conditions in which that level of personnel is unnecessary. Second, waiting times are often long because true life-threatening cases appropriately have priority. Third, the emergency department, by its nature, is not organized or staffed to provide follow-up care for routine illnesses. To promote appropriate care for patients who inappropriately present at the emergency department, staff will refer them, when possible, to ambulatory primary care services. Initially, managed care organizations attempted to curb inappropriate emergency department use by requiring their members to obtain telephone preauthorization before going to the emergency department and by imposing financial disincentives through copays of emergency department fees when the visit did not result in hospitalization; however, the consumer backlash against such restrictions resulted in most states passing "prudent layperson" legislation, which requires insurance companies to reimburse costs based on care that a reasonable person would consider necessary.[13]

Despite the recognition that inappropriate emergency department use drives up costs and results in inadequate continuity of care, many individuals who lack resources to pay for care, are unaware of other sources of care, or find the emergency department the most accessible source of care when private physicians are unavailable. Until the health care system successfully reduces financial barriers to care and achieves a universal, basic level of access to routine medical care, a large volume of inappropriate emergency department use can be expected to persist.

In the past, like other teaching hospital outpatient clinics, the emergency department was a place of indenture for medical interns or residents who were required to provide coverage as a component of their training. Often, to earn extra income, residents would contract to "moonlight" extra hours for their assigned hospital or for other hospital emergency departments. Nonteaching hospitals also often hired residents on a contracted basis to cover the emergency department or required attending staff to provide rotating coverage.

From both the physicians' and patients' perspective, this staffing configuration was less than ideal. Physicians working in emergency departments under these arrangements often had little training or experience with the illnesses and injuries encountered there. Over the past 20 years, the greatly expanded knowledge, techniques, and equipment available for the care of critically ill and injured patients and concerns about liability resulting from deploying physicians without specific training and experience in emergency care have resulted in dramatic changes in how emergency departments are staffed and organized and services are delivered.

Since 1979, emergency medicine has been recognized as a medical specialty with accompanying requirements for extended specialty training and experience to attain board-certified status, as in the other medical specialty fields. Now, physicians qualified by training and experience in emergency medicine staff most hospital emergency departments. Several corporations employ groups of board-qualified or board-certified emergency medicine physicians and contract their services to hospitals. Medical schools with accredited training programs in emergency medicine may staff their affiliated hospitals' emergency departments as a faculty practice group and provide clinical training there for department residents, similar to the organization of other outpatient clinics.

In addition to physicians, emergency departments are staffed by nurses with advanced education and training in the triage and care of critically ill or injured patients. Emergency departments also employ an array of other personnel who provide clerical support and medical and nursing assistance. Depending on the needs of the population served by the hospital, emergency department staff may also include mental health professionals and social workers. On-call arrangements with hospital staff members of other departments or with contracted professionals typically meet other needs of patients presenting at the emergency department.

Freestanding Services

Non–hospital-based, or freestanding, ambulatory care facilities may be owned and operated by hospitals, hospital systems, or physician groups or by independent, for-profit, or not-for-profit single entities or chains. Many hospital systems, independent entities, and chains operate multiple ambulatory care facilities that provide a wide array of services, including ambulatory surgery, occupational health services, physical rehabilitation, substance abuse treatment, renal dialysis, cancer treatment, diagnostic imaging, cardiovascular diagnosis, sports medicine, and urgent/emergent care. Technology advances, entrepreneurial business opportunity, the drive to reduce costs and consumer preferences for convenient services continue advancing freestanding services as major components of the health care delivery system.

The diversity of services available in freestanding facilities prevents a comprehensive discussion of their organizational features in this text; however, the following provides an overview of the major types of freestanding facilities that are playing roles in the rapid expansion of ambulatory care services.

Primary Care Centers

As an outgrowth of many of the same factors that fueled the reorganization, expansion, and enhancement of hospital-based clinic services, freestanding primary care centers have proliferated rapidly since the 1980s. For hospitals, the desire to capture new market share, to ensure the flow of inpatient admissions, to bring new volume to ancillary departments such as laboratory and radiology, to enhance revenues, and to improve service delivery efficiency to meet the demands of managed care have all contributed to the move toward off-site facility development. For teaching hospitals, these facilities, like hospital-based clinics, continue to play important roles in providing a teaching environment for students and residents in internal medicine, family medicine, obstetrics and gynecology, and pediatrics. Depending on state licensure requirements, they may be operated as extension clinics of the hospital or as hospital-affiliated corporate entities. Increasingly, physicians are investing in development and ownership of freestanding facilities as business opportunities that provide high-quality, practitioner- and patient-friendly sites in which to carry on their practices.

Typically, freestanding primary care facilities approximate the appearance and organization of a private physician's office. Staff physicians may themselves be the owners, or they may be employees of the owner entity. In hospital-operated facilities, staff physicians are commonly employees of the owner hospital, or in the case of a teaching facility, physicians may be jointly compensated through a medical school–affiliated faculty practice group and the hospital.

In addition to primary care physicians, staff may include registered nurses, nurse practitioners, physician assistants, medical office assistants, laboratory personnel, receptionists and clerical support, information technology personnel, social workers, and case management staff. In many ambulatory care facilities, nurse practitioners and physician assistants are the mainstays of the day-to-day operation, providing a broad range of services, including physical assessments, diagnosis, patient histories, education, and counseling. Nurse practitioners, often with specialized training in specific areas such as pediatrics, women's health, geriatrics, and adult medicine, are generally acknowledged as highly effective in carrying out their responsibilities and are well accepted by patients. Registered nurses, nurse practitioners, and physician assistants also triage patients and counsel and educate patients via phone contact.

Urgent Care Centers

The first urgent care centers opened in the 1970s. There are now estimated to be more than 15,000 such facilities in the United States, with about 200 more opening each year.[14] Ownership is diverse, including for-profit corporate chains, single entities, hospitals, private physician groups, and managed care organizations. These facilities meet consumer needs for convenient care of non–life-threatening, episodic illness. They operate for extended hours, including evenings, weekends, and holidays, and accept patients on a walk-in basis. Some centers enable patients to register online with a brief medical history in advance to expedite their visit. Physician staff members are usually specialists in internal, family, or emergency medicine, and the urgent care practice setting is gaining recognition as a specialty area of practice in itself. The American Academy of Urgent Care Medicine established in 1997 is dedicated to the standardization and advancement of the practice of urgent care medicine and is presently working toward formal recognition of this new specialty and development of residency training programs.[14]

Urgent care centers may employ registered nurses, nurse practitioners, physician assistants, and reception or other support staff and may provide radiology and basic laboratory services. Acceptable payment typically includes all forms of insurance, cash, and credit cards.

From the consumer standpoint, urgent care centers fill gaps in the delivery system created by the rigidity of private physician appointment scheduling and unavailability during nonbusiness hours. The centers provide a much more convenient and user-friendly alternative to a hospital emergency department during hours when private physicians are not available. In addition, for individuals who are new to a community and have not had the opportunity to establish a physician relationship, the centers can meet immediate needs in a convenient, economical manner without incurring the long waits and expense of the hospital emergency department. Typically located in highly visible facilities, such as storefronts in commercial areas, they offer valued convenience and ease of accessibility to their consumers. Because they are a less expensive alternative to the hospital emergency department, managed care organizations will usually fully reimburse members' use of urgent care facilities when their physicians are not available. Urgent care facilities may also take the form of "fast-track" sections within hospital emergency departments that are open extended hours.

Urgent care centers make clear to patients that they do not provide ongoing care for chronic conditions, although they may be the site where a chronic condition such as diabetes or hypertension is initially diagnosed. If patients do not have a routine source of care, center personnel may encourage them to obtain one and may provide information about area physicians or primary care centers that are accepting new patients to encourage continuity. To maintain positive relationships with area physicians whose patients they have treated, the centers may forward records of treatment to the patients' physicians.

Hospitals have expressed concern that urgent centers may succeed in culling significant numbers of paying patients, leaving to their emergency departments a disproportionate share of the most ill and expensive-to-treat patients. In areas where the centers have proliferated, the private physician community also has voiced concerns about the availability of such facilities affecting patients' motivation to develop a relationship with a primary physician. Nonetheless, the growth in numbers of urgent care centers is a clear indication that consumers perceive them as a positive alternative to the hospital emergency department, and for those without a primary physician, they can truly be a safety net provider.

Retail Clinics

Clinics operated at retail sites such as pharmacies and supermarkets are a rapidly emerging form of ambulatory care. The first ones opened in 2000 in the Minneapolis-St. Paul area in grocery stores.[15] There are currently about 12 retail clinic corporations in the United States. Known by consumer-friendly names, such as "MinuteClinic" and "TakeCare," the operations are appearing in CVS pharmacies, Walgreen's, Wal-Mart and Target stores, and many other locations throughout the country. They represent an entrepreneurial response to consumer demand for fast, affordable treatment of easy-to-diagnose, acute conditions. Typically staffed by nurse practitioners or physician assistants, a physician is not required on site, although many clinics have physician consultation available by phone. MinuteClinic, which uses the slogan "You're Sick, We're

Quick," is one of the most aggressively expanding chains, headed by the former CEO of Arby's. Since 2005, MinuteClinic expanded from 22 clinics in 2 states to 81 clinics in 10 states. It declared plans for 300 clinics by the end of 2006.[16] TakeCare has identified plans for 1,400 clinics by the end of 2008.[16] Patient polls to date indicate a high degree of satisfaction with the availability and use of the clinics. The clinics' lower cost has captured insurers' attention, particularly as employers require workers to pay larger premium shares and increased co-payments and deductibles. Many insurance companies are contracting with retail clinics to allow patients to pay only co-pays. Some employers are encouraging retail clinic use by waiving the co-pay entirely.[16]

The clinics' scope of practice is narrower than that of urgent care centers. A 2006 report for the California HealthCare Foundation, "HealthCare in the Express Lane: The Emergence of Retail Clinics," notes that there are strategic, practical and regulatory reasons for the narrow scope.[15] The report cites the strategic importance of maintaining low prices, minimal staffing, rapid patient turnaround, and the use of software to manage a predetermined range of potential diagnoses. Practically, the practice scope is limited to conditions that do not require private spaces, such as for disrobing, and that can be diagnosed with simple laboratory procedures that do not fall under state or federal regulatory requirements.

Reactions to the clinics from the organized medical community vary from acceptance of this development as a consumer choice to strong opposition. Primary care physicians have many concerns about quality and continuity of care as well as competition. The American Academy of Family Physicians has the retail clinic phenomenon under study and in 2006 issued a list of desirable clinic attributes that include the definition of service scope, evidence-based medicine, a team approach with primary physicians, referral arrangements, and electronic health records. Some physicians concede that retail clinics are filling a need for rapid access that their offices do not offer. A past president of a state medical society noted, "MinuteClinic has exposed an Achilles' heel of office-based practice. There is an access problem. If there were not, care options such as MinuteClinic or similar counterparts would not be venturing in for-profit medicine."[16] The American Medical Association at its 2007 annual meeting petitioned federal and state regulators to investigate retail clinics for possible conflicts of interest, noting that its petitions are prompted by stores' claims that the clinics increase prescription drug sales and help increase other sales. The AMA alleges potential conflicts of interest on the basis that clinics are not independent of the stores selling the drugs and prescriptions that retail clinics recommend or prescribe. Among other misgivings, "The AMA says retail clinics undermine and disrupt the relationship between patients and their doctors, and make it much harder to decide who is responsible when things go wrong."[17] The AMA also takes issue with health insurers allowing retail clinics to waive or lower patient co-payments while continuing to require physicians to collect the fees, arguing that this practice may actively influence patients to choose the clinic over a physician visit on the basis of cost rather than quality.[16] As retail clinics continue proliferating, much more will be learned about the quality, profitability, and impacts on the health care delivery system. For the present, this growing ambulatory care business is under close observation by employers, insurers, retailers, investors, and the medical and consumer communities.

Ambulatory Surgery Centers

Ambulatory or outpatient surgery accounts for 70% of all surgeries performed.[18] The National Center for Health Statistics defines ambulatory surgery as "surgical and non-surgical procedures performed on an ambulatory (outpatient) basis in a hospital or free-standing center's general operating rooms, dedicated ambulatory surgery rooms, and other specialized rooms such as endoscopy units and cardiac catheterization labs."[19] Outpatient surgery continues to be a major contributor to the overall growth trend in ambulatory care.

In the 1970s, physicians led the development of freestanding ambulatory surgery centers, as they saw opportunities created by advancing technology to establish quality and cost-effective alternatives to inpatient surgery. Ambulatory surgery centers were physicians' solutions to frustration with in-hospital bureaucracy, operating room schedule difficulties, and patient inconvenience.[20] Today, physicians have ownership of approximately 90% of freestanding ambulatory surgery centers.[20]

Hospitals also responded to the demand for outpatient surgery, faced with competition from physician-run freestanding facilities and insurer demands for lower costs. Between 1982 and 1992, outpatient surgeries in community hospitals increased over 200%, while inpatient procedures declined by more than 32%.[21] Between 1999 and 2005, the number of Medicare-certified ambulatory surgery centers grew from 2,786 to 4,506, with an average annual growth rate of 8.3%.[20]

Several factors promoted the increase in ambulatory surgical procedures as alternatives to inpatient surgery. One of the most significant factors was the development of general anesthetics that resolved safely and quickly, enabling patients to return to normal functioning within a few hours. Advancements in surgical equipment, techniques, and materials reduced or eliminated the invasive nature of many procedures and their complications and risks. With these and other technologic advances making outpatient surgery increasingly feasible and safe, mounting financial pressures resulted in Medicare, insurance companies, and managed care organizations requiring that certain procedures be performed in the less costly ambulatory setting unless physicians are able to demonstrate undue medical risks to the patient, requiring an inpatient stay.

The initial years of the shift from inpatient to ambulatory surgery provided opportunities for hospitals to convert space into efficient, cost-effective care delivery areas, encouraging the development of separate surgical management systems for ambulatory and complicated cases. Although initially this conversion entailed capital expenditures and staffing additions, well-managed ambulatory surgical centers quickly became profitable.

Freestanding ambulatory surgical facilities, owned and operated by hospitals, physicians, or independent entities, offer several advantages over the in-hospital services, including enhanced aesthetics, ease of accessibility, and the opportunity to customize the scheduling and organization of service delivery independent of hospital bureaucracy. It is not surprising that they were embraced rapidly by physicians who were freed from the rigors of operating room scheduling, staff, and equipment availability typical in the hospital setting. Patients view freestanding facilities as far more user friendly and responsive to their needs than their hospital-based counterparts.

The majority of ambulatory surgery centers comply with state licensure, certification, and accreditation requirements. Ambulatory surgery centers that furnish services to Medicare beneficiaries must be certified by Medicare on important parameters related to patient safety and care quality. Many ambulatory surgery centers also voluntarily submit to accreditation reviews by the Joint Commission on Accreditation of Healthcare

Organizations, the Accreditation Association for Ambulatory Health Care, or the American Association for the Accreditation of Ambulatory Surgery Facilities.[22]

Patient care quality has benefited significantly from improved technology and advanced, less traumatic surgical techniques applied in the ambulatory setting. Patients experience fewer complications, much faster recovery, and less disruption to normal activity from ambulatory than from hospital inpatient surgery. Continuing advances in surgical and anesthetic procedures and technology will provide opportunities to move even more types of inpatient surgery into the ambulatory setting. Recent developments include applications for laser surgery, laparoscopic surgery, and endoscopy.

The National Center for Health Statistics first conducted the only national study of hospital-based and freestanding ambulatory surgery centers from 1994 to 1996. After the 1996 study, tracking was discontinued because of a lack of resources, but was reinitiated in 2006. New data will be solicited from a nationally representative sample of approximately 60,000 ambulatory surgery cases in hospital-based and freestanding ambulatory surgery centers and will provide data for planning, evaluation, and administrative activities by government, professional, scientific, academic and proprietary institutions as well as private citizens. Survey reports are expected by late 2008.[23]

Community Health Centers

Federally funded, community-based primary care centers originated during Lyndon Johnson's presidency in the mid-1960s and represented a facet of that administration's social reform movement labeled the "war on poverty." Originally authorized by the Office of Economic Opportunity, coordinating responsibility was transferred to the Public Health Service in the mid-1970s. Funded under Section 330 of the Public Health Service Act, the organization and staffing patterns of these facilities draw from earlier models of public health services oriented toward the needs of underserved communities.[24] Centers were initially established in cities and in rural communities across the country, and although they differed from each other with respect to size and the scope of available services, they had common characteristics rooted in federal funding requirements, including focus on needs of the underserved, comprehensive primary care, professional staffing, community involvement, and partnerships between the public and private sectors. Subsequent amendments to Section 330 established specialized primary care programs for migrant workers, the homeless, and residents of public housing.

Community health centers are typically staffed by multidisciplinary teams that include physicians, nurses, social workers, nutrition science professionals, and support personnel. The staffing pattern reflects a commitment to a comprehensive service approach to address the multidimensional nature of health and health-related needs of underserved populations. Target patients are minorities, childbearing-age women, infants, persons with HIV/AIDS, substance abusers, and individuals and families who experience health service access barriers for any reason. In addition to primary care, preventive care, and dental services, community health centers assist patients to link with other supportive programs and services such as public assistance, Medicaid, the Women, Infant and Children supplemental nutrition program, and the Children's Health Insurance Program. Many community health centers also offer onsite laboratory testing, pharmacy services, and radiology services and may provide transportation, translation, and health education services as specific needs dictate. To facilitate access to services, community health centers may also employ outreach workers drawn from the centers' service areas. These workers receive training in health and social service needs assessment and advocacy for early intervention and continuity of care.

Today, community health center grants are administered by the Bureau of Primary Care, Health Resources and Services Administration of the Department of Health and Human Services. Fees for services are based on income and may be offered without charge to the neediest patients. The program has grown substantially over the years from 104 centers in the early 1970s to over 1,000 centers with multiple delivery sites. In recognition of health centers' safety net functions, a 6-year initiative was launched in 2002 to expand access to health centers' access points and medical capacity. To date, through additional grants, the initiative has created over 500 new access points, and 300 more are planned between 2007 and 2008, focusing on high poverty rate counties. With a 2007 federal appropriation of $1.9 billion, the centers will serve over 14 million people, over 40% of whom are uninsured. Other revenue sources include state and local governments, Medicare and Medicaid, and private insurance. Medicaid reimbursement provides the largest share of the centers' patient revenue (Figure 4-5).[25]

Community health centers may be organized under the aegis of local health departments, as part of larger human service organizations, or as stand-alone, not-for-profit corporations.

Public Health Ambulatory Services

The delivery of ambulatory health services by state or municipally supported sources has its roots in the early American ethic of community responsibility for care of needy members. Since the colonial period, altruistic citizens sought the charity of the community to provide for the less fortunate by supporting the development of almshouses or "poor houses" to care for the needy and orphaned children. Many of these institutions became the precursors of community hospitals.

With the evolution of state and local governments' roles in providing welfare services and the development of the public health discipline in the late 19th and early 20th centuries, tax-supported state and local departments of health began providing ambulatory services. As the provision of personal health services evolved under health department auspices, so did the opposition of organized medicine, based on the contention that government was competing with private practice medicine for patients. The influence of organized medicine's opposition was largely successful in

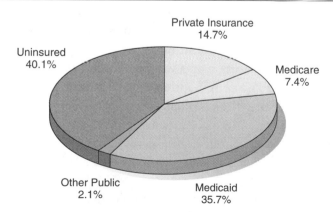

FIGURE 4-5 Health center patients by payment source.
Source: Health Resources and Services Administration, Bureau of Primary Health Care.

limiting the health departments' personal health services to providing care for patients in only the lowest income population groups and to offering other types of care in which private physicians had little interest.

Services that became the domain of health departments included the administration of preventive public health measures, such as disease screening, immunization programs, and communicable disease case finding and treatment. Also, for population groups lacking the means to pay or with only Medicaid coverage, health department services often filled gaps for family planning, obstetrical care, well-baby care, and pediatric and adult medicine. All levels of government carry out public health activities and services, but "the most visible activity occurs in the 3,000 county, city and other municipal health departments throughout the country."[26]

Today, the scope of patient care services available from the local health departments varies widely. These services can range from purely prevention-oriented programs, such as immunizations and well-baby care, to complete personal health services offered through freestanding ambulatory care centers. Many health departments also provide home care services, usually through a public health nursing division. Home care services may include communicable disease case finding, infant and child health assessments, and follow-up visits for ambulatory care patients to ensure compliance. Some health departments operate certified home health agencies under the auspices of Medicare to provide home-based services for older adults. In many municipalities, the local health department has responsibility for providing school-based, preventive services, such as vision screening and other types of screening services, general physical examinations, and immunizations. Most health departments provide community education on a variety of health-related topics such as sexually transmitted disease prevention, nutrition, cancer prevention and screening, smoking cessation, avoidance or control of environmental hazards, maternal and child health, and aspects of healthy lifestyles. Historically, support for public health services has included combinations of city, county, and state funding, plus federal or state disease-specific or block grant funds.

Public health ambulatory services staff may include physicians, nurses, aides, social workers, public health educators, and clerical and administrative staff, who function under the overall administrative direction of a local health officer. This health officer may or may not be a physician, depending on the population size of the jurisdiction and individual state or municipal requirements. Depending on the area, the governmental aegis may be state, county, or city.

Beginning with the Reagan era in the 1980s and its philosophy of advocating private enterprise over government sponsorship as a means to promote more efficient and effective public service, there has been a decided movement of local health departments to privatize personal health services. Federal and state subsidies for public health services declined, accompanied by decreased grant funding for disease-specific programs. During the same period, community penetration of hospital and other organization-sponsored ambulatory care programs increased markedly. With the enactment of the State Children's Health Insurance Program through the Balanced Budget Act of 1997, every state and many local health departments were activated in a massive outreach effort to identify and enroll uninsured children. Programs vary widely among the states; however, in many instances, departments of health are actively involved at the state and local levels in planning and implementing the activities of this initiative.

The September 11 attacks and threats of bioterrorism have brought a renewed focus to the role of the federal, state, and local public health organizations in providing public protection and supporting national security. With acknowledgment that "over the past two decades, the infrastructure has greatly deteriorated," the Centers for Disease Control and Prevention continues to be awarded new grants to focus on interventions that will respond to community public health threats.[27]

Voluntary Agencies

Not-for-profit agencies operate a variety of ambulatory health care services throughout the United States. Services have evolved from a variety of sources, often cause related, to address needs of population groups afflicted by specific diseases or types of conditions. Asthma, diabetes, multiple sclerosis, and cerebral palsy are but a few of the conditions addressed. As not-for-profit organizations, many are chartered by states as charitable organizations and maintain tax-exempt status with the Internal Revenue Service. These designations allow them to collect charitable contributions for which their donors may receive tax deductions. Governed by boards of directors who receive no compensation for their services, these organizations may be operated by a totally volunteer staff or employ numerous paid professionals and have annual operating budgets of several million dollars.

Characteristically, voluntary ambulatory health care agencies were established through the advocacy of special interest groups that desired to address the health care or health-related needs of a population group whose needs were not being adequately met by existing community services. Some operate as single entities, others as independent affiliated agencies of national organizations. Planned Parenthood Federation of America is an example of one such organization. Its clinics provide preventive care, education, and direct services for gynecologic care and contraception in numerous locations throughout the United States. Another example is the United Cerebral Palsy Association, which provides or arranges for specialized medical, social service, rehabilitative, and other services for individuals with cerebral palsy and their families. Frequently, legislative advocacy related to the organization's interests at the federal, state, and local levels is a major component of not-for-profit organization activity.

Financial support for voluntary ambulatory health care agencies is diverse. Sources may include charitable contributions, private payment, third-party insurance reimbursement (including Medicare and Medicaid), and federal, state, or local government grants. In many agencies, a large proportion of clients are uninsured or underinsured and lack personal resources, making financial subsidies crucial to continued viability. Agencies with missions to serve the neediest members of the community continue meeting challenges posed by the ebb and flow of government grant dollars and community economic conditions that affect philanthropic support through efficient business practices and a variety of private fundraising activities. The penetration of managed care also challenged voluntary agencies that serve populations with special needs. To position better their organizations for managed care contracting, they formed coalitions and networks to capture larger segments of the service population, instituting new quality and efficiency monitoring systems to aid in contract negotiations and working through their professional advocacy groups to ensure protection of their client interests.

Although voluntary agencies provide only a small fraction of the ambulatory care services, as compared with hospitals and other ambulatory care organizations, they are important as repositories of community values, as symbols of community charity and volunteerism, and as advocates for populations with special needs.

Continued Future Expansion

The focus of the U.S. health care delivery system has shifted from the hospital to expanded use of ambulatory care services. Major, continuing forces driving this shift will be advances in medical technology and diagnostic and treatment modalities that allow more services to be provided safely and effectively in the outpatient setting, cost-reduction initiatives by government payers, private insurers, and managed care organizations, and consumer demands for more convenient, accessible services. A determination of the ultimate role of retail clinics in the ambulatory care landscape awaits acquisition of experience with and accumulation of evidence regarding patient outcomes, satisfaction, costs and profitability. Formal challenges from the organized medical community may also bear on the clinics' future.

References

1. Goldsmith J. Hospitals and physicians: not a pretty picture. *Health Affairs.* 2007;26:w72–w75. Available from http://content.healthaffairs.org/cgi/content/full/26/1/w72. Accessed March 19, 2007.
2. Burt CW, McCaig LF, et al. *Ambulatory Medical Care Utilization Estimates for 2005. Advance Data From Vital and Health Statistics*, no. 388. Hyattsville, MD: National Center for Health Statistics; 2007. Available from http://www.cdc.gov/nchs/data/ad/ad388.pdf. Accessed July 1, 2007.
3. U.S. Department of Labor, Bureau of Labor Statistics. Physicians and surgeons: occupational outlook handbook: 2006–2007 edition, 1, Bulletin 2600. Available from http://www.bls.gov/oco/print/ocos074.htm. Accessed March 19, 2007.
4. Raffel MW, Raffel NK. The U.S. health system: origins and functions. 4th ed. Albany, NY: Delmar Publishers; 1994:36–44.
5. Hing E, Burt CW. Office-based medical practices: methods and estimates from the National Ambulatory Medical Care Survey: advance data, No. 383 (March 12, 2007). Available from http://www.cdc.gov/nchs/data/ad/ad383.pdf. Accessed March 24, 2007.

6. Center for Studying Health System Change. Proportion of U.S. physicians without any managed care contracts ticks up. Available from http://www.hschange.com/content/839/. Accessed March 26, 2007.

7. Knowles JH. The role of the hospital: the ambulatory clinic. *Bull NY Acad Med.* 1965;41:68–70.

8. Fraser I, Lane L, Linne E. Ambulatory care: a decade of change in health care delivery. *J Ambulatory Care Manage.* 1993;16:1–8.

9. Health Industry Distributors Association. Trends and forecasts, September 2005. Available from http://hidanetwork.com/document.asp?document_id=10160. Accessed April 4, 2007.

10. Nawar EW, Niska RW, Xu J, et al. National hospital ambulatory medical care survey: 2005, emergency department summary. Advance Data no. 386, Hyattsville, MD: National Center for Health Statistics. Available from http://www.cdc.gov/nchs/data/ad/ad386.pdf. Accessed July 7, 2007.

11. Cunningham PJ. What accounts for differences in the use of hospital emergency departments across U.S. communities? *Health Affairs.* 2006; 25: w324–w336.

12. Centers for Disease Control, Media Brief. Almost half of hospitals experience crowded emergency departments. Available from http://www.cdc.gov/media/pressrel/r060927.htm?s_cid=mediarel_r060927_x. Accessed March 11, 2007.

13. American College of Emergency Physicians. What is the status of the prudent layperson legislation? Available from www.acep.org/NR/rdonlyres/39822026-4FFF-44C2-AFB5-2D6E1482F2BD/0/issue_pl_status.pdf. Accessed March 19, 2007.

14. American Academy of Urgent Care Medicine. The trend toward urgent care medicine. Available from http://www.aaucm.org/viewpoints.asp. Accessed March 24, 2007.

15. California HealthCare Foundation (prepared by Mary Kate Scott, Scott & Company). Health care in the express lane: the emergence of retail clinics. Available from http://www.mcms.org/downloads/Healthcareintheexpresslaneretailclinics.pdf. Accessed July 7, 2007.

16. American Academy of Family Physicians. Retail health clinics are rolling your way. Available from http://www.aafp.org/fpm/20060500/65reta.html. Accessed July 8, 2007.

17. Medical News Today. AMA calls for investigation of retail health clinics. Available from http://www.medicalnewstoday.com/healthnews.php?newsid=75308&nfid=crss. Accessed July 8, 2007.

18. Jackson C. Cutting into the market: rise of ambulatory surgery centers. Available from http://www.ama-assn.org/amednews/2002/04/15/bisa0415.htm. Accessed July 7, 2007.

19. Hall MJ, Lawrence L. Ambulatory surgery in the United States, 1996. Hyattsville, MD: National Center for Health Statistics Advance Data, No. 300; August 12, 1998:3.

20. American Association of Ambulatory Surgery Centers. Ambulatory surgery centers: a positive trend in health care. Available from http://www.aaasc.org/features/documents/ASCTrendReport118061.pdf. Accessed July 3, 2007.
21. Casalino LP, Devers KJ, Brewster LR, et al. Focused factories? Physician-owned specialty facilities. *Health Affairs.* 2003;22:56–67.
22. American Association of Ambulatory Surgery Centers. Ambulatory Surgery Center Fact Sheet. Available from http://www.aaasc.org/advocacy/ASCFact Sheet.htm. Accessed July 5, 2007.
23. National Center for Health Statistics. National survey of ambulatory surgery. Available from http://www.cdc.gov/nchs/nsas.htm. Accessed March 4, 2007.
24. Health Resources and Services Administration. Bureau of Primary Health Care, health center history. Available from http://bphc.hrsa.gov. Accessed March 25, 2007.
25. Health Resources and Services Administration. HRSA's FY 2007 budget will complete president's health center initiative. Available from http://newsroom.hrsa.gov/inside-hrsa/mar2007.htm. Accessed March 30, 2007.
26. Wall S. Transformation in public health systems. *Health Affairs.* 1998;17:65.
27. Frist B. Public health and national security: the critical role of increased federal support. *Health Affairs.* 2002;21:119.

CHAPTER 5

Medical Education and the Changing Practice of Medicine

This chapter provides an overview of the growth and change in medical education from the colonial apprentice system to today's high-technology, specialty-oriented instruction in the basic sciences and clinical fields. The evolution of specialty and subspecialty practice is discussed, as is the funding of graduate medical education. The changes in the practice of medicine and physician relationships with hospitals and insurers after the introduction of managed care are also reviewed. More recent developments such as clinical practice guidelines, physician report cards, Internet use, and new ethical issues are defined. The chapter concludes with a discussion of the future of medical practice.

There were no medical schools in colonial America. Women treated the sick at home with the help of medicinal herbs, the advice of friends, and some self-help publications of questionable credibility. There were a few university-trained physicians in Europe, but not many came to the colonies. Those European physicians trained other physicians in an apprentice relationship. Because there was no formal method of testing or licensing new physicians after they concluded their apprenticeship, they were free to practice with no outside control.

The first medical school in America was established in 1756 at the College of Philadelphia (later the University of Pennsylvania). Shortly after that, a second was founded at King's College (later Columbia University) in 1768. Both schools remained very small, graduating only a handful of students each year.

Training under a single physician remained the most common method of physician education until the founding of hospitals in the mid-18th century. Physicians not only brought their own apprentices to the hospital, but they encouraged other students to observe patient treatment. This practice became so popular that the Philadelphia Hospital began to charge students who were not apprenticed to physicians on the staff. By 1773, the hospital decided to regulate this system so that an aspiring physician could pay a fee to the hospital and be formally apprenticed to the institution for 5 years.[1] Physicians were granted a certificate on the completion of their apprenticeship.

By 1800, there were still only four medical schools in the United States. In addition to the ones in Pennsylvania and New York, Harvard University had opened one in 1783 and Dartmouth College in 1797. The schools were small, with three or four faculty members teaching all of the courses. At the time, there were still very few restrictions on who could practice medicine. Regulatory procedures were almost nonexistent. The first law concerning medicine in the colonies was enacted in Virginia in 1639 to control physician fees.[2] Various states attempted to enact medical licensing legislation during the 18th and early 19th centuries, but "by the time of the Civil War, not a single state had a medical licensure act in effect."[3] Moreover, as the number of medical schools grew, their diplomas came to be viewed as licenses to practice.

In 1821, Georgia became the first state to restrict medical licenses to graduates of medical schools.[4] Opposition was strong, especially from the apprentice-trained physicians; however, as physicians from medical schools began to outnumber those from the apprentice system, the MD degree became the standard of competence. The endorsement of formal medical education over apprenticeship training encouraged an increase in the number of medical schools.

Many of the new medical schools had weak programs and no hospital affiliations. In 1892, Harvard became the first medical school to require 4 years of training. In 1893, Johns Hopkins initiated a 4-year curriculum as part of a pioneering effort to improve medical education. The Johns Hopkins model became the standard for subsequent reform of all medical education.[5]

Many medical schools during this period operated without strict admission requirements, a well-trained faculty, or a place for clinical observation and practice. As a consequence, the quality of the medical degree varied greatly from school to school. Medical societies were organized largely to improve the quality of education and practice. The first such society was the Medical Society of Boston, organized in 1736.[3]

By the turn of the 19th century, most states had medical societies. In 1847, most of those state societies affiliated with the newly formed American Medical Association (AMA). "Though the goal of the AMA at the time was to improve medical education, its early attempts to reform or close some of the weaker medical schools were ineffective."[5] Many of the AMA members opposed closing the weaker schools because they were associated with them and had a vested interest in keeping them open. As a result, attempts to establish a national standard for medical teaching floundered for a few decades.

The Association of American Medical Colleges (AAMC), founded in 1876 by 22 medical schools, also addressed the issue of national standards. The AAMC supported a 4-year curriculum such as the one introduced by the medical schools of Harvard and Johns Hopkins, but it lacked the influence to accomplish the desired reforms.

The Flexner Report and Medical School Reforms

At the beginning of the 20th century, the AMA restructured and became capable of exerting significant pressure for the reform of medical education. In 1904, the organization created a new Council on Medical Education and, at the same time, began the *Journal of the American Medical Association*. The AMA used the journal to publish medical school failure statistics on state board licensing examinations and to group schools by their failure rates.

Strong leadership in the AMA and the AAMC demanded that poor schools improve or leave the association. The most important educational reform accomplishment of the AMA, however, began in 1905, when it obtained the help of the Carnegie Foundation for the Advancement of Teaching to investigate and rate medical schools. Abraham Flexner of the Carnegie Foundation headed a study of the medical schools in the United

States and Canada. Flexner proposed to examine the entrance require-ments at each institution, the size and training of the faculty, endowment fees, the quality of laboratories, and the relationship between the medical schools and hospitals.

In 1909, Flexner started his educational survey of all 155 medical schools in the United States and Canada. He visited each school, inter-viewing the dean and a few faculty members and inspecting laboratories and equipment. After each visit, he summarized the facts observed during his visit and mailed the summary to the dean for verification. The deans and faculty of each school cooperated happily with Flexner in the mis-taken belief that Carnegie was contemplating a contribution to their school.

Flexner's full report, *Medical Education in the United States and Canada,* was published by the Carnegie Foundation in 1910. The report was an accurate and searing description of abuses in the medical schools. Schools were referred to as a "disgrace" and a "plague spot." The assets and liabilities of each school were described in detail, and corrective measures were offered. In the aftermath of this criticism, some schools closed and others consolidated. Flexner had recommended that the number of schools be reduced from 155 to 31, but a decade later, the number was down to only 85.[6]

Not all observations in Flexner's report were negative. Dartmouth, Yale, and Columbia were able to make alterations that improved the quality of their programs. Schools that received praise for excellent performance included Harvard, Western Reserve, McGill, Toronto, and especially Johns Hopkins, which was described as a "model for medical education."[6]

Coming from an independent body, the Flexner report gave increased leverage to medical reformers. Licensing legislation was pursued more vig-orously, and new requirements for the length of medical training and for the quality of laboratories and other facilities were established. The AMA and the AAMC accelerated efforts at reform and, in 1942, established the Liaison Committee on Medical Education to serve as the official accredit-ing body of medical schools.

One of the most important outcomes of Flexner's report was that it stimulated support for medical education from foundations and wealthy individuals. Flexner subsequently joined one of the Rockefeller charities, the General Education Board, which then donated enormous sums to medical education. Schools that received the most favorable ratings from

Flexner shared most of the money. Because most were associated with universities, the university-affiliated medical schools gained significant influence over the direction of medical education.[7]

Academic Medical Centers

Federal research grants of the 1950s and 1960s encouraged the research-oriented medical schools and their teaching hospitals to become the country's centers of scientific and technologic advances in health care. Most of the large tertiary-care hospitals affiliated with the approximately 80 medical schools were attracting patients with complicated medical conditions and getting better results than their smaller unaffiliated counterparts.

Because university medical complexes were increasingly recognized as leading the way toward a more sophisticated and effective health care system, the federal government assisted in extending that expertise through the regional medical program legislation of 1965. One of many federal grant programs of that decade, it funded the development of regional medical programs across the United States to upgrade medical knowledge about the leading causes of death: heart disease, cancer, and stroke. The regional medical programs supported research, continuing professional education, service innovation, regional networking among hospitals and other health care facilities, and dissemination of medical center knowledge and skills among networks of other health care professionals and facilities within designated geographic regions.

University medical complexes, which were the centers of research, teaching, and service innovations, gained the most from the legislation. By 1974, however, the university-based regional medical programs had lost their political support and soon disappeared.

By then, however, the university medical centers were well established as the proponents of cutting-edge advances in research and clinical medicine. Each center was regarded as a regional hub in the overall infrastructure of the health care system. By the early 1980s, federal support had increased the number of medical schools to 127.

Academic medical centers broadened into academic health centers by adding to their complexes such professional schools as nursing, pharmacy, dentistry, and allied health. Together with their large teaching hospitals and other clinical facilities, these academic medical centers became a powerful force in the health care arena.

Academic health centers have become the principal places of education and training for physicians and other health care personnel, the sites for most basic research in medicine, and the clinical settings in which many of the advances in diagnosis and treatment are tested and perfected. The teaching hospitals of academic health centers are also the major providers of the more sophisticated patient care required by trauma centers, burn centers, neonatal intensive care centers, and the technologically advanced treatment of cancer, heart disease, and neurological and other conditions. In addition to their complex tertiary-care services, teaching hospitals in most cities provide much of the primary care for economically disadvantaged populations.

The highly specialized, high-technology nature of academic health centers makes them the most expensive type of health care facility in America's health care system. In addition, care at teaching hospitals is, of necessity, less efficient. Because student physicians order more diagnostic tests and procedures and often have to consult with senior doctors regarding diagnoses and treatment procedures, lengths of stay are longer and, therefore, more costly. Available data suggest that hospitals affiliated with academic health centers are 20% to 30% more expensive than other hospitals;[8] however, because health care has shifted from an era of abundant resources to one of stringent economic constraints, academic medical centers are under increasing pressure to cut back on high-cost activities or face ballooning deficits and questionable survival.[9]

Medical schools have depended on a variety of sources for revenue. A major source for most schools has been the clinical practice of faculty. In the mid-1990s, about one third of the total income of most medical schools came from their faculty practice plans. Research grants and contracts contributed about 18%. Medical schools receive relatively small proportions of their total revenue from state and local government appropriations and from tuition and fees. Endowment revenue varies widely from school to school.[10]

The diverse funding of medical schools means that there is no single source on which they can depend to maintain their fiscal viability. Unlike graduate medical education (GME), which is funded through direct and indirect education payments from Medicare, medical schools rely on their ability to compile successfully the necessary revenues from multiple sources.

The federal government has subsidized GME—the training of resident physicians—through the Medicare program. Serious decreases in Medicare's subsidies to teaching hospitals have significant implications for GME. Because over half of the total patient revenues of academic health center hospitals came from Medicare and Medicaid, reductions in the support from those programs affect academic health centers in two ways.[11] By scaling back subsidies for GME and by encouraging beneficiaries to enroll in managed care plans, these programs reduced both annual revenues and the number of patients receiving care at academic health centers. The result has been severe decreases in the revenue of academic medical centers and significant decreases in the number of patients available for clinical training and research.[9]

Graduate Medical Education Consortia

There are two types of physicians: the MD (Doctor of Medicine) and the DO (Doctor of Osteopathic Medicine). MDs are also known as allopathic physicians. Although both MDs and DOs may use all accepted methods of treatment, including drugs and surgery, DOs place special emphasis on the body's musculoskeletal system. In 2006, there were 125 schools of medicine[12] and 22 accredited colleges and three branch campuses for degrees in osteopathy.[13]

No national agency grants licenses to practice medicine. Instead, after completing a residency, a physician must obtain a license from the medical board of the state where he or she plans to practice. Each state is independent in determining who may practice within the state and may have special requirements or restrictions for licensure.

To provide direct patient care, physicians are required to complete a 3- to 7-year graduate medical program accredited by the Accreditation Council for Graduate Medical Education in one of the recognized medical specialties.[14]

Among approximately 1,500 health care organizations, there are nearly 7,000 residency programs that are loosely held together by accreditation and certification processes, medical schools, program directors, and hospital executives. Given the large number of programs and their loose-knit organization, questions about the quality of the programs and their pertinence to issues of personnel supply and specialty distribution inevitably have been raised. U.S. residency programs were described at the 1992 Macy Foundation conference, "Taking Charge of Graduate Medical Education: To Meet the Nation's Needs in the 21st Century," as "responsive principally to the service needs of hospitals, the interests of the medical specialty societies, the objectives of the residency program directors, and the career preferences of the medical students."[15]

The situation has been addressed with varying success by a number of GME consortia. These consortia are formal associations of medical schools, teaching hospitals, and other organizations involved in the training of residents. The consortia have central coordination and direction that encourages the members to function collectively. The major aims of GME consortia are to improve the structure and governance of residency programs, to increase the ambulatory care training experiences, to address imbalances in physician specialty and location, and to use their collective resources and influence to accomplish those aims.[16]

Whether these consortia succeed in improving the organizational structure and governance of GME and addressing the imbalances in medical specialty production to make the medical workforce more accountable to society's needs or whether medicine's historical reluctance to take decisive actions that alter the status quo will bring government intervention is an open question. As in so many other aspects of health care, it is likely that market forces, rather than policy decisions, will determine the outcomes.

Delineation and Growth of Medical Specialties

As far back as 1866, the issue of medical specialization was debated within the AMA. The questions raised were similar to the concerns expressed today. There was general resistance to the development of medical specialties, prompted both by concern for the quality of patient care and by costs. Questions were raised about whether specialists would fragment care by not treating the whole patient and whether surgeons, trained to operate, would disregard noninvasive alternative medical treatments.

The AMA's slow response to specialty interests prompted specialists to form their own societies and associations. In the last half of the 19th century, organizations arose for physicians interested in ophthalmology, otology, gynecology, obstetrics, and pediatrics. After World War I, with specialization increasing among physicians, specialty hospitals were founded in some cities, and general practitioners found themselves eased out of hospitals by specialists. In response, the American Academy of General Practice was formed in 1947 to advocate for general practice departments in hospitals. It was not until 1969, however, that general practice, now called family medicine, became a recognized specialty.

Despite the growth in the number of specialists, at the time of the Flexner Report, there was no standard for adequate specialty training. The length of specialty training required by various medical schools and hospitals ranged from just a few weeks to 3 years, and the quality of graduating specialists varied from excellent to incompetent. A physician with almost any amount of training could practice as a specialist.

In 1917, the United States Army, in need of physicians, examined the qualifications of those physicians who wished to be classified as specialists. Even though many had practiced for years as specialists, the results were shocking. Very high percentages of physician specialists were rejected by the service as unfit to practice as specialists, and some were deemed unfit to practice in any branch of medicine at all.

The army's finding of highly variable competence among specialists did not surprise leaders in medical education. As improved technology and the development of safer and more effective anesthesia and antiseptic techniques made surgery a more acceptable medical option, the demand grew, and the numbers of surgeons and hospitals increased in response. The American College of Surgeons, established in 1912, set up standards and a board in 1917 for certifying specialists. At the same time, the AMA started inspecting internship sites and produced a listing of approved internship hospitals.

Although both the AMA and the American College of Surgeons began to rate the quality of postgraduate training, they quickly realized that they could not make their findings public. "Conditions were so bad the results were suppressed."[17] In 1924, the Council on Medicine Education began to approve hospitals for residency specialty training programs. For the next 40 years, residency programs were initiated in all kinds of hospitals with little regard for the quality of the training experience. Often poorly planned and supervised, residents' educational experiences were secondary to their obligations as house staff to serve whatever patient load they were assigned. Additionally, because residencies were the responsibility of single-specialty departments, the opportunities for developing expert clinical knowledge and skills depended on how much interest a few attending physicians had in teaching and the type of patient admitted to that specialty service.

Problems in the quality of training resulting from the lack of standards abounded. Reform was needed, and a half century after the Flexner Report, the AMA again requested an outside examination of the medical education process. The AMA commissioned a Citizens Committee on Graduate Medical Education, chaired by John S. Mills, who issued his report in 1966. Key recommendations of the report included the elimination of independent internships and giving the accreditation of residency training programs to institutions rather than to individual medical departments. In 1970, the AMA endorsed the inclusion of the first year of graduate medical education in a program approved by an appropriate residency review committee (RRC). The term "internship" was dropped, and by 1980, the AMA had issued recommendations for broad training in the first postdoctoral year.

The current curriculum requirements for becoming a specialist are well defined and standardized. The physician must graduate from medical school, serve in a residency program in an approved setting, and pass a qualifying examination. The appropriate specialty board then certifies the physician. The boards are sponsored by the major specialty society in the area of study and the appropriate specialty section of the AMA.

Specialty Boards and Residency Performance

Boards were formed for each specialty to ensure a proper instructional program and training period followed by an examination and certification to practice. The American Board of Ophthalmology, established in 1933, was the first specialty board. In the same year, an advisory board for medical specialties was organized. Shortly thereafter, the American Board of Medical Specialties achieved official recognition of specialty boards in medicine. By 1991, there were 24 member boards.

Within the 24 medical specialties, there are now over 100 subspecialties, and the number is increasing as different kinds of specialists train in similar subspecialties. For instance, the specialties of family medicine, internal medicine, and pediatrics all have subspecialties in sports medicine. In addition, advancing technology is creating new subspecialties each year. The specialty areas and a partial list of the growing subspecialties of medicine are presented in Table 5-1.[18]

The usual procedure for subspecialization is for specialists to complete their residency training and become board certified. Then they take another period of training, called a fellowship, which prepares them to subspecialize or conduct research in a specific area.

Each specialty board has a residency review committe (RRC) charged with the responsibility of preserving the quality of GME. In 1928, the AMA published the guidelines for approved residencies and fellowships that set educational standards for residencies. The Accreditation Council for Graduate Medical Education (ACGME), formed in 1972 by the American Board of Medical Specialties, the American Hospital Association, the AMA, AAMC, and the Council of Medical Specialty Societies, extends authority to RRCs to determine the standards for its residencies.

The ACGME supervises and receives reports from each RRC. Thus, "the RRC and all specialties establish guidelines for acceptable standards for graduate medical education. . . . The RRC also controls the number of residents allowed in each program and in general oversees the conduct of the residencies."[19]

In addition to the controls of ACGME and its five parent organizations, numerous influences affect different aspects of residency content and training. These include 24 specialty boards and RRCs, hospital directors, medical school deans, program directors, training directors, faculty, house staff, and specialty societies. The problems inherent in this disjointed system of control will intensify as health care reforms force consideration of changes to accommodate specialty imbalance, physician supply, reductions in funding, managed care, shifts from inpatient to ambulatory care, and the general reconfiguration taking place in the health care industry.

The fastest growing field of medical practice has been developing outside of the aforementioned systems of control over specialty training. Hospitalists are physicians whose sole responsibility is the care of hospitalized patients, and their number is growing. There are now more than 12,000 hospitalists in the United States, and the number is expected to triple before the end of the decade. Hospitalists spend all of their time in hospitals taking care of patients from admission to discharge. They are

Table 5-1 Approved ABMS Member Board General and Subspecialty Certificates

American Specialty Board	Subspecialty Certifications
Allergy and Immunology	Diagnostic Laboratory Immunology
Anesthesiology	Critical Care Medicine
	Pain Medicine
Colon and Rectal Surgery	
Dermatology	Dermatopathology
	Clinical & Laboratory Dermatological Immunology
	Pediatric Dermatology
Emergency Medicine	Medical Toxicology
	Pediatric Emergency Medicine
	Sports Medicine
	Undersea & Hyperbaric Medicine
Family Practice	Adolescent Medicine
	Geriatric Medicine
	Sports Medicine
Internal Medicine	Allergy and Immunology
	Adolescent Medicine
	Cardiovascular Disease
	Critical Care Medicine
	Critical Cardiac Electrophysiology
	Clinical & Laboratory Immunology
	Endocrinology, Diabetes, and Metabolism
	Gastroenterology
	Geriatric Medicine
	Hematology
	Infectious Disease
	Interventional Cardiology
	Medical Oncology
	Nephrology
	Pulmonary Disease
	Rheumatology
	Sports Medicine
Medical Genetics	Molecular Genetic Pathology
Neurological Surgery	
Nuclear Medicine	Cooperates with American Board of Pathology and American Board of Radiology in Radioisotopic Pathology and Nuclear Radiology
Obstetrics and Gynecology	Critical Care Medicine
	Gynecologic Oncology
	Maternal and Fetal Medicine
	Reproductive Endocrinology
Ophthalmology	
Orthopaedic Surgery	Hand Surgery
Otolaryngology	Otology Neurology
	Pediatric Otolaryngology
	Plastic Surgery Within the Head and Neck
Pathology	Blood Banking/Transfusion Medicine
	Chemical Pathology
	Cytopathology
	Dermatopathology
	Forensic Pathology
	Hematology

continues

Table 5-1 *continued*

American Specialty Board	Subspecialty Certifications
	Immunopathology
	Medical Microbiology
	Molecular Genetic Pathology
	Neuropathology
	Pediatric Pathology
Pediatrics	Allergy & Immunology
	Adolescent Medicine
	Critical Laboratory Immunology
	Developmental Behavioral Pediatrics
	Medical Toxicology
	Neonatal-Perinatal Medicine
	Neurodevelopmental Disabilities
	Pediatric Cardiology
	Pediatric Critical Care Medicine
	Pediatric Emergency Medicine
	Pediatric Endocrinology
	Pediatric Gastroendocrinology
	Pediatric Hematology-Oncology
	Pediatric Infectious Diseases
	Pediatric Nephrology
	Pediatric Pulmonology
	Pediatric Rheumatology
	Sports Medicine
Physical Medicine and Rehabilitation	Spinal Cord Injury Medicine
	Pain Medicine
	Pediatric Rehabilitation Medicine
Plastic Surgery	Hand Surgery
	Plastic Surgery Within the Head and Neck
Preventive Medicine	Aerospace Medicine
	Occupational Medicine
	Medical Toxicology
	Public Health & General Preventive Medicine
	Undersea & Hyperbaric Medicine
Psychiatry and Neurology	Addiction Psychiatry
	Child & Adolescent Psychiatry
	Clinical Neurophysiology
	Forensic Psychiatry
	Geriatric Psychiatry
	Neurodevelopmental Disabilities
	Pain Medicine
Radiology	Neuroradiology
	Nuclear Radiology
	Pediatric Radiology
	Vascular and Interventional Radiology
Surgery	Vascular Surgery
	Pediatric Surgery
	Surgery of the Hand
	Surgical Critical Care
Thoracic Surgery	
Urology	

Source: Reprinted with permission from the American Board of Medical Specialties. Approved ABMS Specialty Boards and Certificate Categories may be found on the ABMS website, http://www.abms.org/Who_We_Help/Physicians/specialties.aspx.

present to monitor patients several times a day, order tests, involve consultants as necessary, and in general, coordinate all care during hospital stays. They are expected to care for hospitalized patients in consultation with each patient's primary care physician.

Because there are no specific training requirements for hospitalists, most are trained in internal medicine or, in the case of children's services, pediatrics. For personal reasons, they have chosen to give up private practice and become employees of one or more hospitals or of companies that contract to provide hospitalist services to several hospitals.[20]

The Physician Workforce and U.S. Medical Schools

In the mid-1960s, the federal government expected a national shortage of physicians in the United States. New policies and programs were established to increase the number of physicians. In the 20 years between 1980 and 2000, the total number of physicians in the United States increased from 467,679 to 813,770—an increase of 74%. The physician-to-population ratio increased from 207 to 296 per 100,000 people. More recently, that number has grown to about 900,000 physicians in the United States.

At the same time, there are continuing debates between those who predict physician shortages and those who warn of a physician oversupply. Whether there is a shortage or not, it is the wide geographic variation in physician location rather than the number of physicians that remains a problem. Physicians per 10,000 population actually providing patient care vary from over 35 in Massachusetts to under 16 in Iowa.[21] Regardless of the number of physicians per overall population, the low supply in the less attractive rural and inner-city areas will continue to deny adequate medical care to those populations.

As far back as 1981, the Graduate Medical Education National Advisory Committee predicted an oversupply of physicians. Medical schools, however, did not respond to the warning. Not only did they not reduce their physician output, but they also increased the number of their graduates. Between 1990 and 1997, the number of MD graduates increased by 3.6%, and the much smaller number of DO graduates increased by 32%.

During the same period, the total number of medical residents in accredited residency programs increased even more. The number of residents rose from 82,902 in the 1990–1991 year to 98,143 in the 1997–1998 year.[22] Much of that increase was due to the influx of international medical graduates. Nearly one quarter of the physicians practicing in the United States graduated from medical schools in other countries. Most of those graduates gained entry to the U.S. health care system by completing an accredited medical residency. For more than a decade, the total number of residency positions has continued to increase, with graduates of foreign medical schools making up a larger percentage of the total number.[23]

Between 1990 and 2000, more than 45,000 international medical school graduates (IMGs) entered practice in the United States after serving residencies in U.S. hospitals.[24] In fact, most of the hospitals in the United States depend on IMGs to fill their residency positions. About one fourth of all hospital residencies are filled by IMGs, and consequently, they represent approximately one fourth of the physician workforce in the United States.[24]

In 1998, in response to complaints about the lack of basic clinical and communication skills among some IMGs, a requirement was initiated that they must pass a clinical skill assessment before entering a residency. Although there was a surge of IMG entrants immediately before the requirement went into effect, there has been a significant drop in IMG entrants since the requirement was initiated. As a result, the quality of the applicants has improved while still providing enough IMGs to fill the residency positions not taken by U.S. medical graduates.[25]

Ratios of Generalist to Specialist Physicians and the Changing Demand

Primary care or generalist physicians are widely defined as those who practice family medicine, general internal medicine, and general pediatrics. Physicians practicing obstetrics and gynecology are also sometimes included as primary care practitioners. For years, the numbers of generalist physicians have been considered too low to meet the basic health care needs of large segments of the general population. Additionally, the emphasis on medical diagnosis and treatment by combinations of specialist and subspecialist physicians has been criticized as contributing significantly to the complexity and rising costs of medical care.[26]

In the early 1990s, the growth of managed care raised concerns that the longstanding 60:40 ratio of medical specialists to primary care physicians would leave the United States with an inadequate number of primary care physicians and an oversupply of specialists. Those forecasts led to a number of federal and state policies that encouraged the training of more primary care practitioners. There followed a significant increase in the number of physicians practicing in the primary care fields of family medicine and pediatrics.

In contrast to the early predictions, however, the marketplace demand for medical specialists did not decrease, and the increased supply of primary care physicians appears adequate to meet population needs. In fact, rather than the predicted national oversupply of specialist physicians, many areas of the country are experiencing an inadequate supply of specialists to meet community needs.[27]

The preponderance of medical specialists among all practicing physicians in the United States was not brought about by design. There never has been a master plan to crease a more ideal, or even specific, distribution of specialties within the physician workforce. The number, types, and preparation of physicians have been left to the often independent actions of medical schools, their teaching hospitals, the American Board of Medical Specialties, and the ACGME.

The current ratio of specialists to generalist physicians, about 65:35,[28] is the result of individual career choices made by medical students before graduation. Thus, one of the most important influences of academic health centers is the socialization process that shapes the skills, values, and attitudes of generation after generation of physicians and other health care professionals. It is the educational and training exposures to the different specialty practices and to the practitioners of those specialties that influence a student's personal career objectives and subsequent practice pattern. It is significant in considering the origins of the specialist/generalist imbalance that, until very recently, almost every aspect of most medical school and teaching hospital experiences favored the practice of specialty medicine. Many medical students who had every intention of becoming generalist physicians were induced by exposure to the medical education environment to change their minds.

There are several reasons for the dominant choice of residencies. The hierarchy of respect in the cultures of most academic medical centers tends to denigrate primary care as less intellectually demanding, less prestigious, and requiring less skill than the subspecialties. Although untrue, specialists in medical schools convey the message indirectly—and sometimes directly—to patients, medical students, and other physicians that generalists are not competent to handle the wide range of problems they face. Although generalists cannot have the same expertise in every field that a specialist has in one field, generalists develop a very high level of knowledge in all aspects of primary care and are capable of making appropriate and judicious use of the expertise of specialists when the need arises.

The primary care experience in most medical schools also is skewed when medical students and residents see most patients in tertiary-care hospitals, and work in clinics that are considered of low priority and managed inefficiently, and rarely find a pre-eminent primary care faculty person to serve as a role model. In addition, the differences in working hours, being on-call, income, and public recognition that favor specialists cause many medical students and residents to rethink initial interests in primary care medicine.[29]

Nevertheless, most medical schools encourage medical graduates to accept residencies in one of the primary care fields. Admission committees give preference to candidates for admission that evidence interest in primary care medicine. Family practice departments cultivate promising students, and most medical schools have moved some of their clinical training sites from tertiary-care hospitals to ambulatory service settings and private group practice offices to give students more primary care experience.

Among the most persuasive influences on the practice specialty decisions of graduating medical students are the market conditions that determine the need for and success of potential various medical specialists. Medical students are very much aware of the demand and supply for specialists and subspecialists in urban communities and the opportunities for generalists in managed care environments. They also know that they will have the option to seek further training in a subspecialty at a later date if they aspire to more specialized practice.

Primary Care Physicians

In the early days of managed care, primary care physicians were assigned a new role as gatekeepers of the health care system. Gatekeepers had the responsibility to provide primary care to patients enrolled in managed care plans, to refer them to specialists when the need arises, and to coordinate all of the health services needed by their patients. The term "gatekeeper" was applied because the managed care plans required the primary care physician's approval before they would pay for a visit to a specialist or emergency room.

The gatekeeper role was controversial, however, because the gatekeeper's own reimbursement was often linked to the number of referrals made to specialists. It was common among managed care plans to reduce the income of gatekeepers who cost the plan more for medical specialty care than the plan expected. By pressuring the primary care gatekeepers to limit the number of referrals to more expensive specialist physicians, managed care plans put gatekeepers in uncomfortable, if not unethical, dilemmas.

Primary care gatekeepers had to choose to delay or deny patients the benefit of specialist consultation or treatment or to provide services themselves that are more appropriately delivered by specialists. Either choice may not have been in the best interests of patients. Widespread criticism and a number of lawsuits claiming injury from delay or denial of care prompted managed care organizations to relax or discard the gatekeeper functions of primary care physicians.

Preventive Medicine

The Pew Charitable Trusts created the Pew Health Professions Commission with the "goal of helping health professional schools respond to the changes in the health care system and in the health care needs of Americans."[30] The group published a report in 1991 that outlined what will drive future health care. They concluded that a health-oriented approach that stresses disease prevention will characterize future health care systems. Concerns will be addressed at a community level. This increased emphasis on community health will necessitate changes in medical schools and teaching hospitals and require that learning in a community environment be part of physician training. Physicians will need to be well versed in social and environmental health determinants. Focusing on preventive care and treatment techniques that use technology to the patient's advantage is the challenge facing the new physician.

Medicine and medical education, however, have a history of being incredibly inept in establishing health promotion and disease prevention as a high priority in the U.S. health care system. "Although practicing preventive medicine is a cost saving mechanism, nationwide we spend most health care dollars treating preventable disease."[31] Parameters for prevention are clearly established in many areas, but past studies have shown that only a small percentage of physicians actually adheres to the guidelines.[32]

More recently, however, rising public awareness, media pressure, and enlightened leadership have produced some innovative and productive collaborations between clinical and preventive medicine. In addition to their long history of participating in the public health measures to prevent vaccine-preventable childhood diseases, sexually transmitted diseases, and HIV infection that depend on physician case reporting, immunization, and education, practicing physicians have collaborated in community campaigns for problems such as childhood obesity, diabetes, smoking cessation, cholesterol education, and early cancer detection. For these alliances to expand and grow, however, there will have to be significant changes in all areas of medical education, practice incentives, accountability measures, and financing.[33]

Changing Physician/ Hospital Relationships

Until recently, physicians and hospitals maintained unique, commensal relationships that brought both of them profits from a single source—patient admissions. The independence and autonomy of physicians were respected, and their relationship to the hospital in the care of patients was disregarded by paying the physician separately on a fee-for-service basis and the hospital on the basis of costs incurred. Because hospitals were dependent on physicians to admit patients and make use of the hospitals' resources, hospitals courted physicians by providing them with time, equipment, staff, and other perquisites with little regard for the effects on hospital costs. Additionally, hospitals were challenged to keep their physical facilities attractive, their hotel services efficient, their support services responsive, and their medical staffs as reputable as possible to attract patients and encourage physicians to select their facilities.

In turn, physicians had responsibilities to the institution itself and to the patients they admitted to the hospital. As a component of a hospital's tripartite governance structure, the medical staff organization was responsible to the board of trustees and the administration for a host of organizational activities that require medical expertise. Through the medical staff organization and its committees, physicians have been obligated to provide the knowledge and authority to establish clinical policies and procedures, perform utilization review, ensure quality, and determine the credentialing standards for admission to the hospital's medical staff.[34]

The roles and responsibilities of physicians, however, are changing from when they were the sole determinants of hospital admissions, diagnostic tests and therapeutic procedures, the length of hospital stays, the use of hospital-owned services and other resources, and referrals. Although physicians still admit patients to hospitals, they do so under a broad range of constraints that have markedly affected their independence and autonomy. The spiraling costs of unchecked and mutually beneficial financial and practice relationships of physicians and hospitals have incurred demands from government, employer groups, third-party payers, and managed care plans that have radically altered the business of hospitals and their physician connections. In an environment of constrained resources and competing demands, the relationships between physicians and hospitals are now different and often far more stressful.

Under the prospective payment system, hospitals are at financial risk if the lengths of patient stays or the costs of resource use exceed that allowed for specific patient diagnoses. As a result, hospitals are constantly monitoring and sometimes questioning physician decisions in providing patient care. Albeit indirectly, the administration of the hospital now has a role in clinical decision making, and it is an interaction in which neither party engages enthusiastically.

There are other reasons why physicians can no longer ignore the financial consequences of their clinical decisions. Managed care plans that contract with hospitals to provide services to their members select those hospitals that demonstrate operating efficiency and cost-effectiveness.

Physicians who are not sensitive to the impact of their practice patterns on the financial burden of their hospitals and do not cooperate in keeping them competitive will find themselves increasingly unwelcome on the hospitals' medical staffs.

In addition to these stresses on the internal relationships of hospitals and physicians, there are external conflicts. The new economic environment is causing hospitals and physicians to strain their traditional, long, and fruitful relationship by going into competition with each other. Group practice growth and new technologies that permit many procedures that formerly required inpatient hospitalization to be performed in ambulatory settings have given physicians the financial resources and patient volume to acquire and use these technologies. These entrepreneurial activities have placed physicians in direct competition with hospitals.

In an analogous move, as their inpatient admissions decreased, hospitals have shifted a great many of their activities to community-based ambulatory settings that competed, in some instances, with their own medical staff. Clearly, the competition for patients in the reformed environment has changed traditional hospital–physician relationships.[34]

As was mentioned earlier, one significant change has been the introduction of new hospital-based subspecialty physicians called "hospitalists." In the United States, the hospitalist movement and the term hospitalist were introduced in the mid-1990s. In Europe and Canada, the role of a hospital-based specialist who managed only inpatients has been well established for years.

Unlike hospital-based emergency or critical care specialists, hospitalists may manage patients in any of the inpatient units. Primary care physicians "hand off" their hospitalized patients to hospitalists who serve as physicians of record while those patients are in the hospital. Hospitalists then return the patients to their primary care physician at the time of hospital discharge.

There are several benefits attributed to the use of hospitalists. Hospitalists spend a great deal of time in the hospital, and thus, they are familiar with the hospital systems and can expedite care. They can provide more continuous observation of patients and respond more rapidly to crises and changes in patient condition. Hospitalists also become more expert in recognizing and caring for common inpatient disorders.

The burgeoning hospitalist movement reflects efforts by hospitals to reduce both costs and medical errors, as well as improve the general quality of care. Studies confirm that hospitalists reduce costs by shortening hospital stays, preventing complications, and reducing readmissions. In addition, patients seem more satisfied with hospitalist care than with primary physicians who are able to spend only a few minutes a day with each patient as they fit hospital visits into their busy office schedules.[35]

As with any major changes in clinical practice, the hospitalist concept is not without controversy. Some primary care physicians fear the loss of authority and income and worry that they could ultimately lose hospital privileges. Nevertheless, the hospitalist movement is growing, and hospitalists can choose from a wide selection of employment opportunities.[36]

Cost Containment and the Restructuring of Medical Practice

Historically, physicians were self-employed, engaged in solo practice or with a small number of associates, and received payment on a fee-for-service basis. With the exception of litigated circumstances of alleged malpractice, there was little or no outside accountability for the medical decisions and procedures that occurred during the diagnosis and treatment of patients. It was not until acute concern over the rising cost of health care resulted in cost-containment initiatives that the method of reimbursement for medical services was significantly altered and physicians were subjected to practice parameters and evaluations. Insurance companies, which for decades had simply increased premiums to compensate for escalating charges, began to employ various strategies to hold down costs and stabilize premiums by monitoring physician services rendered.

The introduction of combined, capitated, or other risk-sharing financing and delivery had a dramatic impact on the health care system. Under capitation, health maintenance organizations (HMOs) reimbursed health care providers a set amount per patient. In return, providers were required to provide a comprehensive set of health care services. The old fee-for-service system gave way to capitation payments that provided a base income and could include bonuses or other financial incentives.

In addition to affecting income and methods of payment, managed care, whether or not an HMO, has subjected physicians to utilization reviews. Testing, treatment, and surgery decisions are monitored and evaluated. Physicians have rallied against the loss of authority and income, and some have countered by forming their own preferred provider organizations and independent practitioner organizations. The vast majority of physicians, however, rail against the changes, but continue to subject themselves to the drastically discounted fee-for-service payments and other restrictions of managed care insurers.

Physicians have good reasons to complain. From 1995 to 2003, the average net income of physicians declined 7% after adjusting for inflation, while the incomes of their counterparts in other professions rose by 7%. Primary care physicians, already the lowest paid, saw a 10% decline in their earnings—another reason why medical graduates shun primary care.[37]

Faced with the need to provide quality and price incentives, many managed care organizations are conducting bonus plans that reward both primary care and specialist physicians who follow "best practices" in medical care. Although many physicians welcome the opportunity to augment their income, others consider pay-for-performance as insurer "interference." Clearly, it is in the insurers' best interest to reduce preventable medical complications and other expensive consequences if physicians can be motivated to follow proven treatment protocols. By sharing the ratings of their physicians with patients, managed care organizations can use those ratings to steer patients to the organizations' "preferred" physicians.[38]

Physician practice evaluations based on resource use and patient outcomes will become more widespread as a way of adapting to limited resources. The move to link physician income to practice performance prompted physicians to exert pressure on the AMA to deal with the possibility of loss of income and autonomy. The AMA, however, sidestepped the issue, leaving the methods by which physicians will deal with these changes an open question.

Hold Harmless Clauses

Managed care organizations have affected both the liability risks of their network physicians and their reimbursements through "hold harmless" clauses in their contracts. A common type of hold harmless clause limits physician reimbursement to the fee paid by the managed care organization for covered services. Physicians are prevented from balance billing patients for charges that exceed the insurer's fee scale. "In Tennessee only those HMOs who require physicians to accept this hold harmless clause may obtain a license."[39] Even in the case of an HMO bankruptcy, a physician may be prohibited from balance billing a patient. Other types of hold harmless clauses attempt to shift liability for damages arising from adverse outcomes of medical decisions from the insurer to the physicians. Physicians assume full responsibility, even if the plan was partly at fault because of an error in utilization review.

There is also a hold harmless clause that gives the managed care organization the right to do a background check on the physician. The information obtained from this check may be released without liability to the plans owned, managed, or administered by the managed care organization.

As might be expected, the number and extent of these hold harmless clauses in managed care organization contracts have presented numerous legal problems for participating physicians.

Clinical Practice Guidelines

Just as managed care has impinged on physician practice autonomy, so has the development of practice guidelines. Their growing acceptance as the means to more cost-effective and efficient health care has raised concerns about further intrusions by outside forces into the process of clinical decision making. Practice guidelines are defined as "systematically developed statements to assist practitioner and patient decisions about appropriate health care for specific clinical circumstances."[40]

Clinical practice guidelines evolved in the late 1970s and early 1980s after publication of data showing wide variations in the applications of medical procedures in regions in the United States and increased use of questionable, inappropriate, and unnecessary services that added significantly to the spiraling costs of health care. These studies are discussed in detail in Chapter 11, but it is important to note here that the variations in the level of health care interventions were so great as to suggest that physicians were unaware of the relative effectiveness of various procedures and that patients were not benefiting from much of the care they received.

Health care researchers conjectured that assessments of the outcomes or relative effectiveness of various medical procedures would lead to practice guidelines and eliminate ineffective, unnecessary, or inappropriate procedures and their related costs. To this end, Congress created the Agency for Health Care Policy and Research in 1989. The agency was directed to fund outcomes research and start developing practice guidelines. After a slow start, the agency started releasing practice guidelines for specific conditions. Although fewer than 2 dozen guidelines had been released by 1995, the agency's efforts sparked a great deal of guideline development by other institutions and agencies.[41] The RAND Corporation, medical specialty societies, HMOs, insurers, and others have now produced over 1,600 practice parameters.[42]

Although a number of specialty societies have developed and promoted practice guidelines as a service to their members, many physicians feel that practice guidelines threaten their autonomy. After years of making clinical decisions without outside scrutiny or interference, practice guidelines appear to be yet another means for third-party payers and policy makers to make physicians document their performance and demonstrate their cost-effectiveness.

Acceptance of practice guidelines seems to be dependent on who developed them and how they are presented. The guidelines that are trusted the most have been developed by the physicians' own organizations, such as the AMA or a specialty society. Guidelines developed by insurers or pharmaceutical firms are trusted the least.

The type of practice in which physicians are engaged is also a factor in guideline acceptance. Physicians most deeply involved in managed care, such as those in staff or group model HMOs, are most likely to believe that guidelines will improve the quality of patient care.[43]

The widespread application of clinical practice guidelines is expected to have a significant effect on medical practice. The nature of that effect is difficult to predict, however. Guidelines are considered by some to be the means to prevent unnecessary and negligent events and to clarify when negligence has occurred. Others think that employers, insurers, providers, and others who base treatment and payment decisions on practice guidelines are likely to face complicated legal questions if harm results. In any case, with government agencies, health systems, third-party payers, specialty societies, and managed care organizations promoting the use of guidelines, it is certain that they will become an integral part of medical practice.

Physician Report Cards

As recently as the mid-1970s, the code of ethics of the AMA explicitly prohibited "information that would point out differences between doctors." Thirty-two states had passed laws supporting the AMA's position. The laws were intended to prevent misleading or competitive advertising of office hours, charges, or services. The position of organized medicine, however, reflected a long history of protecting physician performance from public scrutiny.[44]

Subsequently, the state laws supporting the AMA's position were determined to be violations of the First Amendment. Passage of freedom of information acts that prohibited governments from hiding information from the public removed the barriers that prevented the public from comparing the performance of physicians. In 1986, when the Health Care Financing Administration released hospital-specific mortality rates for Medicare patients, the dam was broken. In December 1991, *Newsday* published the first information regarding physician performance ever made public. Never again would the public be denied access to government data about the quality of medical care. The *Newsday* publication was based on New York State's pioneering effort to compare and publish hospital-specific, severity-adjusted heart surgery mortality rates. Although New York State had intended to publish the names of only the hospitals involved, a *Newsday* freedom of information request, supported by the State Supreme Court, forced release of the rankings of the heart surgeons involved.[45]

Within less than a decade, the contentious matter of exposing the comparative performance of physicians on a wide spectrum of variables has been resolved in favor of the consumers of medical care. Although physicians have protested and lobbied against each additional revelation as inaccurate, unfair, and misleading, consumer groups are winning out. A dozen states have passed legislation that gives the public access to physician information, including disciplinary records, malpractice actions, and whether a physician has lost privileges at a hospital. Florida has gone so far as to release the exact amount of every malpractice payment going back to the 1980s and allows the public to request a summary of each case that includes the patient's allegations.[46]

Medical societies in general support physician-profiling programs that report a physician's education, training, licensure, and membership in professional societies, state disciplinary actions, and serious misdemeanor convictions. They object strongly to medical malpractice and hospital disciplinary information as not true indicators of the quality of care.

Information technology has made it possible to assemble and adjust performance data so that service entities, be they physicians, hospitals, or managed care plans, can be compared on a wide variety of parameters of importance to consumers. Concise and relevant information on the quality of services provided can be invaluable to patients reviewing their options. Report cards allow the public to see information regarding the comparative performance of physicians and hospitals. It is also important to recognize that report cards have introduced incentives that encourage providers to improve their performance. Physicians want good report cards, and their behavior changes rapidly when they realize that their colleagues are doing better than they are.

Internet sites have greatly facilitated access to report card information. Health Grades, Inc. provides a consumer website, www.healthgrades.com, that provides quality ratings and profiles for over 5,000 hospitals, 620,000 physicians, and 16,000 nursing homes. In addition, information is available on other health care providers such as home health agencies, chiropractors, fertility clinics, and assisted living residences.[47]

The Escalating Costs of Malpractice Insurance

The steeply rising costs of medical liability insurance are a growing concern for practicing physicians, medical schools, and teaching hospitals. In the last decade, schools of medicine and hospitals have seen their liability premium costs increase from 6 to 10 times—from thousands to millions. In some states, physicians, especially specialists, have seen their premiums triple or quadruple in just a few years.

Rising liability insurance costs reflect steep increases in the amount of malpractice jury awards. Also, during an economic downturn, insurance companies that depended on investment income are forced to raise premiums to keep their businesses viable.

In any case, the effect has been demoralizing to many physicians. Physicians are leaving high-premium states, choosing to retire early, or reducing high-risk aspects of their practice to lower their insurance costs. Many communities are deprived of certain medical services, such as obstetrics, as a result. It appears that legislative limits placed on jury awards will be required to resolve the problem.

Growing Concern About Ethical Issues

Two developments have focused attention on a number of issues of medical ethics. Rather than concerns about unethical or unprofessional conduct, these ethical issues reflect the practice dilemmas faced by physicians working in the rapidly changing health care environment. The first set of ethical concerns relates to the various policies promoted by managed care organizations. Efforts of such organizations to manage the financing, costs, accessibility, or quality of the care delivered cause them to subject physicians to a range of guidelines, treatment parameters, peer reviews, and financial incentives and penalties. Cost-avoidance policies that require preauthorization for the more expensive procedures, substitution of less expensive tests, and restraint of hospitalization in favor of alternative ambulatory services raise questions about increased risks to patients.

Interestingly, an opposite set of ethical concerns could be raised about the risk to patients subjected to the practices of fee-for-service traditional medicine, which the managed care policies try to avoid—unnecessary hospitalizations, needless or inappropriate tests and procedures, ineffective treatments, and uncoordinated care by multiple providers. There is no question, however, that particular control strategies of managed care present related ethical issues. Increasingly, physicians admit that they exaggerate the severity of an illness to help patients get necessary care. Systems that encourage deceitful practices, be they fee-for-service or managed care, diminish the professional standards of medicine.

The second development that is creating vexing ethical issues is the remarkable advance in technologic capability that has occurred in the last few years. Medicine's ability to save more severely brain-injured patients, increasingly premature infants, terminally ill or brain-dead patients, and others with no promise of functional survival has increased the need for ethical guidelines. At present, individual physicians can decide how they will advise families of such patients. If the family and the physician cannot agree about treatment, there is no set procedure for deciding what to do. These and other ethical dilemmas brought about by the technologic advances in medicine present formidable challenges to the ethics committees of hospitals and professional organizations.

Among the most critical of future ethical issues are those related to advances in the field of molecular biology and gene manipulation and therapy. International research efforts, such as the Human Genome Project and the discovery and characterization of molecular correlates of human health and disease, with all of their potential use and abuse ramifications, present a mind-boggling ethical challenge. The future use of individual genetic blueprints for diagnosis and treatment as well as for predicting future medical events has scientists, policy makers, and ethicists concerned about potential runaway applications of the technology. Amidst all the potential benefits of this amazing scientific advance are fears of the unethical application of the technology.

Physicians and the Internet

Patients are not the only ones using the Internet to obtain online health information. Recent studies found that after a slow start, 70% of U.S. physicians are now using the Internet to access the sites of peer-reviewed research, medical publishers, medical societies, and health care provider organizations.[48] The number of new medical websites has been growing at the rate of 10% per month, listing information about everything from medical meetings around the world to the disease-specific displays of pharmaceutical companies to quality information provided by national medical organizations. In addition, physicians themselves have developed personal websites to establish their credentials, explain their practice specialties, and attract patients and referrals.

In addition to information on professional meetings and seminars and the latest developments in clinical practice, physicians can obtain the latest data from more than 4,000 clinical trials. The U.S. National Institutes of Health website, www.ClinicalTrials.gov, allows physicians as well as the public to learn about federal, university, and private medical studies at more than 47,000 locations nationwide. Information is provided about the research locations, designs, purpose, criteria for participation, and diseases or treatments under study.

The Internet release of that information long before it can be evaluated as suitable for publication through established methods and published in one of the traditional peer-reviewed medical journals has set off a heated debate between the leading figures in academic medicine and advocates of open access.

The Future of Medical Practice

Medicine has made astounding progress in the last half century. An increasing number of highly specialized physicians and support personnel, working in concert, achieve marvels of technical accomplishment. Yet the overall success of American medicine as measured by overall health system performance place the United States 37th in the world according to the World Health Organization.[49] These rankings are usually explained away by pointing to the heterogeneity of the United States population as compared with those of other developed countries. Nevertheless, underlying the impressive motivation and clinical competence of American physicians and the outstanding technology available to them is a system that was organized for a much earlier period in medical history. For instance, the incredibly complex character of current American medicine, with a few notable exceptions, still relies on the slow hand-offs of personal and clinical information from one physician to another or between and among other care providers. Sometimes the information does not move at all or gets misplaced. It is an incongruity of a highly sophisticated diagnostic and treatment structure that many physicians and hospitals still rely on barely legible handwritten notes to record patient assessments, treatment modalities, and patient responses.

Communication among providers and between providers and patients remains problematic as medical technology progresses and time pressures on physicians increase. The National Board of Medical Examiners has addressed one aspect of the patient communication problem. Starting with the 2005 class of graduating medical students, a requirement of graduation is the passing a "clinical-skills assessment" test. The day-long test, with actors playing the part of patients with common illnesses, will test a graduate's ability to communicate with patients, gather information, perform physical examinations, and diagnose illnesses.[49]

It is ironic that just at the time when scientific and technologic advances have prepared the U.S. health care system to make its greatest contributions to the prevention and treatment of disease, the financing and delivery problems of the system are in frustrating disorder. Unfortunately, until those problems are solved, health care never will be able to achieve the full potential of its scientific and technical capacity. In the midst of all of the changes that are taking place, one circumstance seems abundantly clear: Physicians and their professional organizations are incapable of resolving the problems they now face.

Physicians can work closely with the hospitals to serve their mutual needs. They can contract with managed care organizations to continue to serve the enrollees who were previously their fee-for-service patients. They can join the various provider networks to retain some negotiating power among the shifting market forces, but they cannot solve the problems that affect them the most because those are the problems of the larger society. Even if all of the participants in the system—the providers, consumers, payers, insurers, and managed care organizations—try to solve the health system problems, they cannot do it. This situation is occurring at a crucial time in the evolution of medical care: the components of the system are struggling for long-term viability, if not survival, in an environment that is changing rapidly.

The imbalance among the access, cost, and quality of health care that provoked the market-driven reforms evolved from an entrepreneurial system that tried constantly to improve an already superb ability to diagnose and treat the ills of individual patients while failing dismally to address the needs of the larger society. The more sophisticated the medical care technology became, the more indifferent providers seemed to become toward meeting the health needs of populations rather than individuals.

Now, the health care system's problems of cost, access, and quality have demonstrated, at great expense, that it is not enough for physicians and other health professionals to serve the individuals they choose, one patient at a time. The education and socialization of health professionals has failed when many, if not most, feel no obligation to address the health needs of groups of people in ways that benefit public health and decrease the need for costly medical interventions.

Most physicians and other health care professionals in clinical practice have not been adequately prepared to exercise their potential to prevent disease, address the problems of unequal access to competent care, and assume accountability for the effectiveness of their therapies. The high level of autonomy physicians enjoyed for decades is rapidly disappearing because they failed to bring their salient knowledge and skills to bear on relevant societal problems. The power to direct the course of health care in the United States has rapidly shifted from the providers to the insurers and purchasers.

Instead of fighting to retain the status quo in battles already lost, physicians and other health care professionals should be making it clear to the larger society that the dynamics driving the health care revolution cannot be dealt with separately by vested interests. Medicine is not solely responsible for inventing more health care than people want to pay for. Medicine responded to the public desire to have the best and the most of medical services, but medicine now has a responsibility to make the public understand that the problem is beyond those within the system. As politically onerous as it might be, U.S. citizens and their representatives have to assume the responsibility for carefully and deliberately creating a new form of health care organization that will ensure a coherent, efficient, and effective health care delivery system. Until that happens, physicians will continue to lose the authority, autonomy, and status that formerly characterized the practice of medicine.

References

1. Raffel MW, Raffel NK. *The U.S. Health System: Origins and Functions.* 4th ed. Albany, NY: Delmar Publishers; 1994.
2. Jones RS. Organized medicine in the United States. *Ann Surg.* 1993;217:423.
3. Jones RS. Organized medicine in the United States. *Ann Surg.* 1993;217:424.
4. Raffel MW, Raffel NK. *The U.S. Health System: Origins and Functions.* 4th ed. Albany, NY: Delmar Publishers; 1994:5.
5. Raffel MW, Raffel NK. *The U.S. Health System: Origins and Functions.* 4th ed. Albany, NY: Delmar Publishers; 1994:6.
6. Raffel MW, Raffel NK. *The U.S. Health System: Origins and Functions.* 4th ed. Albany, NY: Delmar Publishers; 1994:11.
7. Raffel MW, Raffel NK. *The U.S. Health System: Origins and Functions.* 4th ed. Albany, NY: Delmar Publishers; 1994:12.
8. Anderson GF, Greenberg G, Lisk, CK, et al. Academic health centers: exploring a financial paradox. *Health Affairs.* 1999;18:163.
9. Their S, Keohane N. How can we assure the survival of academic health center? *Chronicle of Higher Education.* 1998:A640.
10. AMA-CME Report. 10-A-98. Available from http://www.ama-assn.org/meetings/public/annual_98/reports/cme.rpt10.htm. Accessed August 14, 2000.
11. Academic Health Centers Summary. Task Force on Academic Health Centers. Available from http://www.cmwt.org/progsumm/ahcs_summ.asp. Accessed August 14, 2000.
12. Association of American Medical Colleges, AAMC Accredited Medical Schools. Available from http://www.aamc.org/medicalschools.htm. Accessed November 25, 2006.

13. American Association of Colleges of Osteopathic Medicine, AACOM Accredited Colleges of Osteopathic Medicine. Available from http://www.aacom.org/colleges/. Accessed November 25, 2006.

14. National Resident Matching Program. About Residency. Available from http://www.eraspo5.aamc.org/nmrp.index.htm. Accessed August 7, 2000.

15. Morris TQ, Sirica CM. *Taking Charge of Graduate Medical Education: To Meet the Nation's Needs in the 21st Century.* Proceedings of a conference sponsored by the Josiah Macy, Jr. Foundation. New York, June 1992.

16. Kelly JV, Larned, FS, Smits, HL, et al. Graduate medical education consortia: expectations and experiences. *Acad Med.* 1994;12:931–943.

17. Raffel MW, Raffel NK. *The U.S. Health System: Origins and Functions.* 4th ed. Albany, NY: Delmar Publishers; 1994:16.

18. American Board of Medical Specialties. *Annual Report and Reference Handbook—2002.* Evanston, IL: American Board of Medical Specialties; 2002:111–114.

19. Jones RS. Organized medicine in the United States. *Ann Surg.* 1993;217:427.

20. The New England Journal of Medicine. *Here Come the Hospitalists.* Available from http://www.nejmjobs.org/career-resources/here-come-the-hospitalists, aspx. Accessed November 27, 2006

21. National Center for Health Statistics. *United States 2004 with Chartbook on Trends in Health of Americans.* Hyattsville, MD: Centers for Disease Control and Prevention; 2004.

22. Daugherty RM, Jr. Adjusting the Size of the Education Pipeline. American Medical Association—Medical Schools Section: Council of Medical Education CME Report 6 1-98. Available from http://www.ama-assn.org/annual 99/reports/cmerpts/rtf/cmerep10.rtf. Accessed August 6, 2000.

23. National Center for Health Statistics, Bureau of Health Professions. Table 107, First-Year Enrollment and Graduates of Health Professions Schools and Number of Schools According to Profession: United States, Selected Years 1980-98. Available from http://www.cdc.gov/nchs/products/pubs/pubd/hus/tables/99hus107.pdf. Accessed August 14, 2000.

24. Whelan GP, Gary NE, Kostis J, et al. The changing pool of international medical graduates seeking certification training in US graduate medical education programs. *JAMA.* 2002;288:1079–1084.

25. U.S. Department of Labor, Bureau of Labor Statistics. Occupation outlook handbook, 2004–2005 ed. Available from http://www.bls.gov/oco/ocos074, htm. Accessed December 27, 2004.

26. Cooper RA. Seeking a balanced physician work force for the 21st century. *JAMA.* 1994;272:680–687.

27. Salsberg ES, Forte GJ. Trends in the physicians workforce, 1980–2000. *Health Affairs.* September/October 2002;21:165–173.

28. U.S. Department of Labor, Bureau of Labor Statistics. Occupational outlook handbook 2001–2002 ed. Available from http://www.bls.gov/oco/ocos074. htm. Accessed July 22, 2000.

29. Steiner E, Stoken JM. Overcoming barriers to generalism in medicine: the residents' perspective. *Acad Med.* 1995;70:589–594.

30. O'Neil EH. Education as part of the health care solution. *JAMA*. 1992;268: 1146.
31. Inwald SA, Winters FD. Emphasizing a preventive medicine orientation during primary care/family practice residency training. *J Am Osteopath Assoc*. 1995;95:267.
32. Inwald SA, Winters, FD. Emphasizing a preventive medicine orientation during primary care/family practice residency training. *J Am Osteopath Assoc*. 1995;95:268.
33. McGinnis JM. Can public health and medicine partner in the public interest? *Health Affairs*. 2006;25:1044, 1052.
34. Kovner AR. *Health Care Delivery in the United States*. 5th ed. New York: Springer Publishing Co; 1995:429–430.
35. Gregory D, Baigelman, W, Wilson, IB, et al. Hospital economics of the hospitalist. *Health Serv Res*. 2003;38:905–918.
36. Coile RC, Jr. Hospitalists redefine the future of inpatient medicine. *CQOnline*. Available from http://www.cost-quality.com/restpast/vbi4a2html. Accessed August 28, 2002.
37. Abelson R. Report of the center for health system change. *New York Times*. June 22, 2006, C3.
38. Lanaro L. Pay-for-performance reaches out to specialists. *The Wall Street Journal*. December 15, 2003, D-3.
39. Overlook ME. Managed care and the infamous hold harmless clause. *J Tennessee Med Assoc*. 1993;86:454.
40. Institute of Medicine. United States Committee on Clinical Practice Guidelines. In: Field MJ, Lohr KN, eds. *Guidelines for Clinical Practice: From Development to Use*. Washington, DC: National Academy Press, 1992:63.
41. Agency for Health Care Policy and Research. AHCPR clinical practice guideline topics. *Agency for Health Care Policy and Research News Report*. (March 1994).
42. Toepp MC, Kuznets, N. *Directory of Practice Parameters: Titles, Sources, and Updates*. 1994 ed. Chicago, IL: American Medical Association Office of Quality Assurance and Medical Review; 1994:vi.
43. Sisk JE. How are health care organizations using clinical guidelines? *Health Affairs*. 1998;17:91–109.
44. Millenson ML. *Demanding Medical Excellence*. Chicago, IL: University of Chicago Press; 1997:173.
45. Millenson ML. *Demanding Medical Excellence*. Chicago, IL: University of Chicago Press; 1997:193.
46. Special report, docs fight to hide lawsuits. *New York Daily News, Sports Final*. April 17, 2000, 12.
47. The Healthcare Report Cards, Inc. Web site grades 5,000 U.S. hospitals in critical medical specialties. *Health Industry Today*. 1999;62:10.
48. Physician use of internet explodes. *Health Manage Technol*. 1999;20:8–9.
49. Efrati E. New requirement for medical students: dealing with patients. *The Wall Street Journal*. June 10, 2004, B1.

CHAPTER 6

Health Care Personnel

This chapter defines the major health care professions, with particular emphasis on their educational preparation, credentials, numbers, and roles in the health service system. The factors that influence demand for the various health care providers and the workforce issues that divide them are also reviewed. The chapter concludes with a discussion of the development of health workforce policy and some expectations for the future.

As one of the nation's largest and most important industries, health care is also one of the largest employment sectors. The Department of Labor estimates that 13.8 million people, or approximately 10% of the U.S. workforce, are employed in the health care industry (Table 6-1). In the next decade, more new jobs, about 3.6 million, will be created in health care than in any other industry.[1]

Although hospitals are still a major employer, recent employment growth has been among health maintenance organizations, ambulatory clinics and services, home health providers, and offices of health practitioners.

Health Professions

There are more than 200 occupations and professions among the over 13 million workers in the health care field. As the system continues to change, making use of new technology, expanding in some sectors and contracting in others, additional vocations will appear. The personnel of those new vocations will be required to possess more specialized knowledge and more sophisticated skills.

Table 6-1 Percent Distribution of Health Care Employment by Setting

Offices and clinics of:	Percent Distribution
Physicians	12.3
Dentists	5.7
Other Practitioners	3.5
Outpatient care centers	6.4
Home health care services	5.4
Other health care services*	6.9
Hospitals	41.5
Nursing care facilities	13.8
Residential care without nursing	4.4
All health service sites	100.0

*Includes ambulance services, blood banks, diagnostic centers, and others.

Source: Reprinted from U.S. Department of Labor, Bureau of Labor Statistics.

Specialization to attain higher levels of technical competence also reduces the flexibility of providers to develop more efficient staffing patterns. Specialization among the workforce increases personnel costs as additional employees are required to perform specific tasks. Smaller service facilities, especially in rural areas, are burdened most by the need for infrequently used specialists.

As a result, there is growing acceptance of multiskilled health practitioners. Hospitals, in particular, are employing individuals trained in more than one skill. A large number of combinations are feasible: occupational therapy assistants are also serving as physical therapy assistants; radiologic technologists are performing ultrasound; and a variety of nonclinical personnel are performing phlebotomy.

The expansion of home health care services is also contributing to job growth. Technological advances now permit sophisticated medical procedures to be performed in home settings. Cost constraints force people to forego or shorten hospital stays, and the larger number and increased longevity of aging Americans will increase the need for the home care services of nurses, therapists, and aides.

Credentialing and Regulating Health Professionals

Government regulation of the health professions is considered necessary to protect the public from incompetent and unethical practitioners.

Because each state assumes and exercises most of that responsibility for itself, how health care occupations are regulated and the manner in which regulation is carried out vary from state to state. About 50 health occupations are regulated throughout the United States.

Regulatory restrictions limit health care service agencies in how they may use personnel and limit their ability to explore innovative ways to provide patient care. Similarly, regulatory restrictions influence educational programs to focus curricula on what has been prescribed by regulatory boards and their related accrediting bodies, even when those practice patterns have been replaced by more advanced procedures. Many states have taken steps to revise their credentialing systems to provide greater flexibility and responsiveness to fast-changing health care technology.[2]

The health care occupations have been regulated by one of three procedures: state licensure, state or national certification, or state or national registration. In licensure, the state law defines the scope of practice to be regulated and the educational and testing requirements that must be met to engage in that practice. Licensure, the most restrictive of the three types of regulation, is intended to restrict entry or practice in certain occupations and to prevent the use of professional titles by those without predetermined qualifications. For example, it is illegal for individuals to perform procedures defined in the statutes as medicine or dentistry or to call themselves physicians or dentists without the appropriate license.

Most licensure boards are composed primarily of practitioners whose concern is for setting standards and assessing competence for initial entrance into the field. Except by requiring attendance at continuing education courses, licensure boards have done very little about ensuring continuing competence, dealing with impaired practitioners, or disciplining wayward members of their professions; however, they do have the power to censure, warn members, or even revoke licenses.

Certification is the regulating process under which a state or voluntary professional organization, such as a national board, attests to the educational achievements and performance abilities of persons in a health care field of practice. It is a much less restrictive regulation than licensing and means that the individual has obtained advanced or specialized training in that area of practice. When applied to such fields as psychology and social work, certification does not make it illegal for unqualified individuals to engage in activities within the scope of practice in those fields as long as they do not claim or use the titles of certified psychologist or social worker. Certification allows the public, employers, and third-party payers to determine which practitioners are appropriately qualified in their specialty or occupation.

Certification generally has no provision for regulating impaired or misbehaving practitioners other than putting them on probation or dropping them from certification. Unlike licensure, certification has no legal basis for preventing an impaired or professionally delinquent individual from practicing. It is a weakness of certification that it is left to third-party payers or employers to insist on only certified practitioners.

Registration began as a mechanism to facilitate contacts and relationships among members of a profession and potential employers or the public. It is the least rigorous of regulatory processes, ranging from simple listings or registries of persons offering a service, such as private duty nurses, to national registration programs of professional or occupational groups that require educational and testing qualifications. Because most registration programs are voluntary, they have little to do with continuing competence or disciplinary actions.[3]

Health Care Occupations

Although space does not allow for the description of all or even most of the occupations in health care, several major health care vocations are outlined here. Because Chapter 5 is devoted to medical education and practice, the information regarding physicians in this chapter is purposely limited.

Physicians

There are 125 accredited medical schools in the United States that award the Doctor of Medicine (MD) degree. Their enrollment has increased slightly over the last several years. In 2006, they graduated 17,370 students. The number of women enrolled in U.S. medical schools has more than doubled in the last 20 years. In 2006, the graduating class was 49% female. The number of minority students enrolled in medical schools nearly tripled during the same period. In 2006, 6.8% of the medical school graduates were black, 7.1% Hispanic, 18.8% Asian, 3.3% either foreign, American Indian, or of mixed or unknown race, and the remaining 65% white.[4]

There are 22 accredited colleges and three branch campuses that confer the Doctor of Osteopathy degree (DO). In the last 2 decades, their enrollment has nearly doubled, and they now graduate about 2,400 students per year. Doctors of medicine and doctors of osteopathy share the same privileges in most U.S. hospitals. The 47,000 doctors of osteopathy practicing in the United States make up about 5% of all the physicians in the country.[5]

Although medical education in the United States begins in undergraduate medical school, it continues intensively for as many as 8 years of graduate medical training. Most states require 1 year of graduate medical education before a physician can be licensed. That year, which used to be called an internship, is now considered the first of 3 years of residency training regarded by the medical profession as the minimum needed to practice medicine.

Residency training prepares a physician to practice a medical specialty. In a period of 3 to 8 years, depending on the specialty, residency qualifies a physician for certification in 1 of 24 medical specialty boards. Further residency training, often called a fellowship, can lead to a certificate in 1 of over 100 subspecialties. A listing of these medical specialties and subspecialties is in Chapter 5.

Because U.S. medical schools consistently graduate about 5,000 fewer new physicians per year than are employed as first-year residents, the gap is filled by physicians trained in medical schools outside of the United States. The annual number of foreign nationals who graduate from medical school outside the United States and then enter this country to practice each year increased rapidly until a hands-on clinical skills assessment was required in 1998. The responsibility for evaluating the credentials of International Medical Graduates (IMGs) entering the United States to enter residency programs lies with the Educational Commission for Foreign Medical Graduates, a private nonprofit organization sponsored by major U.S. medical organizations, including the American Association of Medical Colleges.

Although the more stringent certification process and the heightened security concerns after the tragic events of September 11th may have deterred some IMGs from pursuing the opportunity to train in the United States, the number entering this country annually, about 6,000, is more than adequate to meet the annual shortfall of U.S. medical school graduates.[6]

The impetus for this influx is the demand for resident house officers in both teaching and nonteaching hospitals. All but the most prestigious hospitals, particularly those in rural or inner-city areas, depend heavily on foreign medical graduates to staff their clinical services. Future planning for the physician workforce in the context of the projected shortage of physicians will have to be sensitive to the future role of foreign medical graduates, particularly in underserved areas.[7]

After finishing their residency training, most of these IMGs remain in the United States to practice. As a result, IMGs now constitute about one-quarter of the active U.S. physician workforce. There is also a relatively stable group of about 1,350 U.S. citizens who attend medical schools outside the country and return to practice each year.

About one third of the over 700,000 practicing physicians in the United States are in primary care, general pediatrics, general or family practice, or general internal medicine practice. Two-thirds of this country's physicians limit their practice to one of the many medical specialties.[8]

The number and size of managed care organizations that depended on primary care physicians to minimize patient referrals to specialists and subspecialists temporarily altered the usual ratio of specialist to generalist physicians. Because managed care organizations relaxed those restrictions in response to intense public and physician disapproval, however, medical specialists are again in demand. In fact, there are serious shortages in certain medical specialties that affect the efficiency and quality of medical care in various geographic areas. Depending on the region of the country, radiologists, obstetricians, anesthesiologists, gastroenterologists, gerontologists, cardiologists, urologists, pulmonologists, orthopedic and general surgeons, hematologists, oncologists, and a variety of intensive care physicians may be in short supply.[9]

Nursing

Nursing was a common employment position for women during the 19th century through association with a religious or benevolent group. A physician, Ann Preston, organized the first training program for nurses in the United States in 1861 at Philadelphia's Woman's Hospital. Training was open to all women "who wished greater proficiency in their domestic responsibilities."[10]

At the turn of the century, hundreds of new hospitals were built under the aegis of religious orders, ethnic groups, industrialists, and elite groups of civic-minded individuals. Because student nurses were a constantly renewable source of low-cost workers to staff the wards, even some of the smallest hospitals maintained nursing schools.[11] Hospital nursing school programs, therefore, were primarily sequences of on-the-job training rather than academic courses. As the programs evolved, stronger academic components were introduced, eventually leading to baccalaureate degrees instead of hospital diplomas.

World War I had a profound effect on the nursing profession. Before the war, nursing was divided into three domains—public health, private duty, and hospital. Public health nursing was the elite pursuit and was recognized as instrumental in the campaign against tuberculosis and promoting infant welfare. Only a few nurses worked for hospitals. In 1920, over 70% of nurses worked in private duty, about half in patients' homes and half for private patients in hospitals.

The war emphasized the drama and effectiveness of hospitals, and it soon became the center of nursing education in the increasingly specialized acute-care medical environment. The social medicine and public health aspects of nursing were subjugated to the image of nursing as a symbol of patriotism, national sacrifice, and efficiency. The war experience established nurses as dedicated associates in hospital science. Nursing leaders promoted the idea of upgrading nursing through high-quality hospital nursing schools, preferably associated with universities. The choice to idealize the role of the nurse as dedicated and deferential to the physician specialist in the hospital marginalized the independent role of the nurse in social medicine and public health.[12]

World War II brought increased funding for the educational preparation of nurses. Later, the Nurse Training Act of 1964, the Health Manpower Act of 1968, and the Nurse Training Act of 1971 added substantially to the federal support of nursing education.[13] Nevertheless, state funding provides the largest support for nursing schools, some 80% of which are in colleges and universities.

Different levels of nursing education were developed at a variety of educational institutions. A registered nurse (RN) could be trained in a 2-year associate degree program at a community college or a junior college, a 2- to 3-year diploma program offered through a hospital, or a 4- to 5-year bachelor of science degree program at a university or college.

The increasing complexity in health care forced specialization in nursing as it did in medicine. Nurses with a bachelor's degree may undertake advanced studies in several clinical areas to develop the needed competence for teaching, supervision, or advanced practice. Clinical nurse specialists in hospitals play important liaison roles between the medical practitioners in narrow and highly technical subspecialties, the patients, and supportive nursing services. By the 1960s, master's degree and doctoral programs were developed for nurses who wished to specialize.

The number of RNs in the United States increased by over 1 million between 1980 and 2000. The increase slowed considerably during the last 4 years of that period as nurse dissatisfaction with working conditions became widely known. The latest survey of the RN population conducted in 2004 and reported in 2006 indicated that there was a new high of 2.9 million RNs in the United States and that 83% of those nurses were actively employed. The average age had climbed to 46.8 years, the highest average age since records have been kept in 1960. Only 8% were less than 30 year old compared with 25% in 1980.[14]

It has been estimated that about one third of the increase in the number of nurses in the U.S. since the 1990s was due to the influx of nurses born outside of the United States.[15] Nurses are encouraged to leave their home countries and work in the United States for the opportunity to earn more money, enjoy a higher standard of living, and advance their education.

Over 60% of employed nurses have been working in hospitals. The following table illustrates the distribution of nurses in the United States by field of employment. The data were obtained during the national sample survey of RNs conducted in 2000 (Table 6-2).[16]

One of the major changes occurring in nursing is in the type of program that nurses enter to obtain their basic education. Almost 90% of nurses now receive their basic education in an institution of higher education compared with 20% in 1960. RNs with master's or doctorate degrees rose to 376,901, an increase of 37% since 1980.[14]

Nurses began to specialize during the 1950s. After World War II, nurses were in short supply, and hospitals began to group the least physiologically stable patients in one nursing unit for intensive care. The more competent nurses cared for the sickest patients, but instead of lowering the need for nurses, the critical care nurse specialty began, and the need for staff nurses continued to grow.

There are now more than 50 U.S. schools that have at least one of the three types of doctoral programs in nursing. The doctor of nursing (ND) is the first professional doctoral degree building on liberal arts or scientific education and preparing the student to take the state licensing exam to

Table 6-2 Percent Distribution of Employed Registered Nurses by Setting in 2000

Setting	Percent Distribution
Hospital	62.1
Nursing home	8.4
Ambulatory care setting	8.1
Home health	6.5
Community/Public Health	4.8
Student health service	2.9
Nursing education	2.3
Occupational health	1.0
Other	3.9
Total	100.0

Source: Data from U.S. Department of Health and Human Services, Health Resources and Service Administration, Bureau of Health Professions, National Center for Health Workforce Analysis, 2000 National Sample Survey of Registered Nurses.

practice as an RN. The doctor of nursing science (DNS and DNSc) degrees are professional doctorates that prepare the nurse for advanced clinical practice. The nursing PhD is an academic degree with requirements similar to the PhD in other fields—extensive preparation in a narrow field and a dissertation.[17]

During the 1980s, the importance of nursing research was recognized by the addition of the National Center for Nursing Research within the National Institutes of Health.

Men comprise a small percentage of the nurse population, although their numbers are increasing. In 2000, only about 5.4% of RNs were men. By 2004, the number of men in nursing reached 9.5% of all nurses. Rapid increases are also occurring in the numbers of RNs identifying themselves as members of a minority group. By 2002, one of every five nurses was of a minority group.[18]

Hospital consolidations in response to market pressures and the widespread acceptance of managed care are affecting nursing employment in several ways. Hospital workforces have been reorganized to adjust to fiscal restraints, reductions in the number of admissions, and shortened lengths of stay. At the same time, increases in the intensity of nursing care required by the more complicated illnesses of the patients who are admitted to hospitals suggest the need for higher nurse–patient ratios. Thus, although many hospitals employ fewer nurses for inpatient care, those retained are expected to maintain clinically sophisticated nursing skills, monitor lesser trained persons employed to provide direct patient care, and manage nursing units filled with seriously ill patients.

Fewer nurses taking care of more severely ill patients during even shorter hospital stays, combined with the need to supervise nonprofessional and unlicensed personnel performing nursing tasks, has increased nursing workloads, lowered morale, and raised serious concerns about the declining quality of care.

Not surprisingly, concerns for the quality of care, frustration with unresponsive hospital managers, and burnout from working in understaffed facilities have made hospital nursing a less attractive career. As a result, many competent nurses have retired or sought employment in noninpatient settings. Nurses formerly employed in serving hospitals have been absorbed in ambulatory service facilities such as surgery centers and group practices. Others have chosen to reorient themselves to the quite different job requirements of nurses in home care organizations and long-term care facilities.

Although there remain important concerns about the continued aging of the currently employed RN population and the difficulty schools of nursing are experiencing in expanding nursing enrollment, there are promising developments. There has been a recent increase in the number of nursing graduates taking the national licensure exam, and hospitals are developing innovative ways to increase enrollment in schools of nursing. For instance, North Carolina Baptist Hospital in Winston-Salem has created a steady supply of nurses by paying all educational expenses for 45 nursing students each year in return for a 3-year commitment to the hospital. Other facilities are offering attractive sign-on bonuses to recruit new graduates. In addition, many schools of nursing are adding accelerated programs as a way to bring nurses to the workforce more quickly.[19]

The Robert Wood Johnson Foundation, which has a long history of supporting nurses, is addressing one of the roots of the problem. Its projects are directed at changing the frustrating nursing work environment through alterations of both physical facilities and hospital cultures. The changes are intended to decrease the amount of time nurses spend on nonnursing tasks to permit them to focus on the more satisfying responsibilities of maintaining the quality of patient care.[20]

If, however, these and other strategies fail to relieve the shortage of nurses, the demand for nurses will exceed the supply. The current shortage of nurses, which is estimated to be about 6% of jobs unfilled, is projected to grow to 15% in 2015 and 29% in 2020 (Figure 6-1).

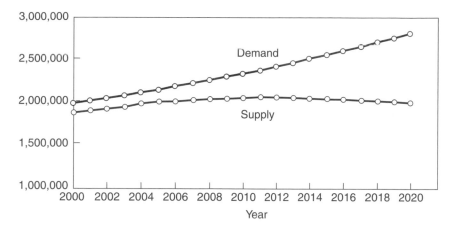

FIGURE 6-1 National Supply and Demand Projections of FTE Registered Nurses, 2000 to 2020.
Source: U.S. Department of Health and Human Services, Health Resources and Service Administration, Bureau of Health Professions, RN Supply and Demand Projections.

Licensed Practical Nurses

A licensed practical nurse (LPN) works under the direct supervision of an RN or physician. One-year LPN training is offered at about 1,100 state-approved technical or vocational schools or community or junior colleges. Programs include both classroom study and supervised clinical practice. Like RNs, LPNs must pass a national licensing examination.

Since 2002, when 28% of the over 700,000 LPNs worked in hospitals, employment in hospitals is decreasing. The reduction in inpatient days and the substitution of unlicensed personnel have decreased the number of LPNs in hospitals by almost 10,000 per year. The demand for LPNs in the other work settings, however, is increasing. Nursing homes employ 26% of the LPNs, and another 12% are employed in physician offices and clinics. The remainder works in home health care, residential care facilities, schools, and government agencies.[21]

Nurse Practitioners

Nurse practitioners are RNs with advanced education and clinical experience. Most nurse practitioners specialize. Neonatal nurse practitioners work with newborns. Pediatric nurse practitioners treat children from infancy through adolescence. School nurse practitioners serve students in elementary and secondary schools, colleges, and universities. Adult and family nurse practitioners are generalists who serve adults and families. Occupational health nurse practitioners work in industry providing on-the-job care. Psychiatric nurse practitioners serve people with mental or emotional problems. Geriatric nurse practitioners care for older adults.[22]

The earliest nurse practitioners were nurse midwives and nurse anesthetists. Nurse midwives examine women throughout pregnancy, educate them about labor and birth, assist them in managing labor and birth, deliver the infant, and care for the newborn and mother. A nurse midwife usually is an RN who completes a 1- or 2-year master's degree program in nurse midwifery. They are licensed by the state and may also be required to be certified by the American College of Nurse Midwives. Currently, almost all of the midwife-assisted births take place in a hospital or birthing clinic.

The roots for the nurse anesthetist specialty go back over a century, when nurses administered anesthesia in Catholic hospitals. Early training was provided in hospitals, but in 1945, the American Association of Nurse Anesthetists established a certification program. Nurse anesthetists are now required to have a master's degree from an accredited school and must pass the national certification examination. Most nurse anesthetists work with physician anesthesiologists in hospitals, ambulatory surgery centers, and urgent care centers providing comprehensive care to patients who need anesthesia. Approximately 20% of anesthesia being administered to patients is by nurse anesthetists working alone.[23]

The current nurse practitioner movement began in the 1960s because of the shortage of physicians. The goal was to have specially prepared nurses augment the supply of physicians by working as primary care providers in pediatrics, adult health, geriatrics, and obstetrics. Nurse practitioners had to overcome some resistance from organized medicine and legal difficulties caused by restrictions in most state nurse practice acts, which included a prohibition against nurses diagnosing and treating patients. Nurse practitioners sought state-by-state changes in nurse practice acts, and by 1975, most states had started certifying or accepting the national certification of nurse practitioners, nurse midwives, and nurse anesthetists.[24]

Two-thirds of the first 131 nurse practitioner programs, were certificate programs, and one-third were master's programs. The certificate programs ranged from 3 to 24 months, with an average of about 8 months. The master's programs, which ranged from 10 to 21 months, averaged 15 months. The programs specialized primarily in training for practice in pediatrics, midwifery, maternity, family medicine, adult health, or psychiatry. As in most ventures into uncharted territory, several approaches to nurse practitioner preparation were tested. Eventually, it was accepted that a nurse practitioner should be an RN with a master's degree. National certification and recertification are necessary.[25]

Efforts at health care cost containment have increased the demand for cost-effective nurse practitioners. Managed care organizations have been particularly successful in using nurse practitioners and physician assistants to bolster their complement of staff physicians. Rural hospitals, with limited reserves of physicians, make substantial use of nurse practitioners and physician assistants. Rural hospital executives consider the use of nurse practitioners and physician assistants to be a cost-effective means to provide an expanded scope of services and to improve access to primary care.[26]

Nurse practitioners and physician assistants also are heavily involved in emergency department care. They manage a wide range of conditions in about 4% of all emergency department visits in the United States.[27]

The high regard for nurse practitioners among both other medical personnel and the public is evidenced by the fact that there are now over 300 master's and post-master's programs in the United States for the preparation of nurse practitioners.[28]

Clinical Nurse Specialist

A different, but related, type of advanced nursing practice is the clinical nurse specialist. Just as the role of nurse practitioners evolved over several decades to meet demands for increased access to primary health care, so too did the role of the clinical nurse specialist, which was developed in response to the specialized nursing care needs of increasingly complex patients.[29] Like specialist physicians, clinical nurse specialists are advanced practice specialists with in-depth knowledge and skills that make them valuable adjunct practitioners in specialized clinical settings.

As a result, there are now 218 master's programs for the advanced preparation of clinical nurse specialists.[30]

Dentistry

Dentistry in early America was primitive. Tooth extraction was performed by either an itinerant tooth drawer, the neighborhood doctor or barber, or in many cases, the local blacksmith. Because there were no regulations, anyone could practice dentistry, and skilled craftsmen and artisans turned their talents to dental practice.

During the 19th century, most people turned to their local physicians, some of whom practiced dentistry as their principal occupation, for dental care. Until about 1850, almost all prominent dentists were medical doctors who had chosen dentistry rather than general medicine as their vocation.[31] It was also in the 19th century that dentistry began its emergence from a trade to a profession. Dental schools were established to replace preceptorships, and dental practitioners participated in developing laws to regulate the profession.[32]

In 1840, the State of Maryland chartered the first dental school, the Baltimore College of Dental Surgery. The course of study lasted 2 years, the same as that required for a medical degree. By 1884, 28 dental colleges existed. Although a few were affiliated with universities, most were privately owned. New York took the lead in regulating the profession by licensure. The state's dental society was empowered in 1868 to establish a board of censors to examine candidates. In time, it became the State Board of Dental Examiners. By the end of the century, most other states also had passed licensure laws.

The mix of university-affiliated and independent dental schools resulted in significant variations in the quality of dental education. In 1922, 12 years after the Carnegie Foundation for the Advancement of Teaching had issued the Flexner report evaluating U.S. medical education, the foundation created a commission to examine dental education. The commission's report appeared in 1926 and resulted in a complete reorganization of dental education in the United States.[33]

World War II brought about profound changes in Americans' attitudes toward dentistry. Citizens were shocked to learn that the dental health of the nation's young men was deplorable. Among the first 2 million draftees summoned by the Selective Service System, one of five lacked even the minimum standard of 12 functioning teeth. The Selective Service had to eliminate all dental standards to avoid mass disqualification of selectees. As a consequence, after the war, the United States made a vigorous effort to improve the dental health of the country's population.

Before World War II, dentists were not involved in public health, and few dental schools taught anything on the subject. A decade after the first graduate course of study in dental public health was established in the 1940s by the University of Michigan, the new field of public health dentistry emerged in the United States. Today, a number of schools have established courses leading to advanced degrees in the field, and there is an American Board of Dental Public Health to certify them as specialists.

The U.S. Public Health Service established the National Institute of Dental Research (NIDR) in 1948. Ultimately incorporated into the National Institutes of Health, the National Institute of Dental Research played a major role in furthering basic and applied dental research.

Also beneficial to dentistry during the postwar years was the increase in insurance group plans that provide payment for routine dental care and, in certain instances, more extensive dentistry at an additional premium. By 1980, almost 100 million Americans were covered, to some degree, by a dental insurance plan, and today, it is a common employee benefit.

The overall number of dentists per U.S. citizen reached its highest point in 1987 but will continue to decrease in the coming decades. There have been major decreases in the annual number of dental graduates, while the general population continues to increase.

Nine practice specialties have developed in dentistry:

1. Dental public health
2. Endodontics
3. Oral and maxillofacial pathology
4. Oral and maxillofacial radiology
5. Oral and maxillofacial surgery
6. Orthodontics and dentofacial orthopedics
7. Pediatric dentistry
8. Periodontics
9. Prosthodontics

Unlike in medicine, more than 85% of the 150,000 practicing dentists in the United States are general practitioners.[34] There are 56 U.S. dental schools in the United States, a decrease of 5 since 1980. These dental schools graduate about 4,300 dentists per year, a drop of over 1,200 per year in the last 2 decades. Graduates receive a Doctor of Dental Surgery (DDS) degree or its equivalent, a Doctor of Dental Medicine (DMD).

The demographic composition of America's dental profession is also changing. From a low of 13% in 1980, minorities now constitute one third of the annual enrollment in dental schools. Women are also more prominent in dental school enrollment. Female dental students, once a rarity in dental schools, now comprise about one half of first-year enrollments.[35]

Overall, dentists are working fewer hours for increased earnings. Dentistry has successfully resisted managed care and capitated payments and remains a "cottage industry." With most dentists in solo practice choosing to serve only those with dental insurance or the fiscal means to pay prevailing fees, many of the population groups with the greatest need for dental services will continue to be underserved. Neither dental education nor the current practice model places high priority on the creation of a dental safety net for underserved populations.[36]

Pharmacy

Pharmaceutical practice dates back to ancient Egypt, Rome, and Greece. The first apothecaries appeared in Europe during the 12th century, and by 1546, the Senate of the city of Nuremberg, Germany, recognized the value of standardizing drugs to ensure uniformity in filling prescriptions.[37]

Hospital pharmacists were apprentice physicians in early America. In 1765, John Morgan proposed that medicine and pharmacy be separate, and by 1811, the New York Hospital had a full-time pharmaceutical practitioner.[38] The American Pharmaceutical Association was organized on October 7, 1852. Professional training programs were developed for pharmacists, and by 1864, there were eight colleges of pharmacy in the United States.[37]

Eighty-nine colleges of pharmacy are now accredited to confer degrees by the American Council on Pharmaceutical Education. Pharmacy programs grant a Doctor of Pharmacy (PharmD) degree after at least 6 years of postsecondary study. The PharmD degree has replaced the Bachelor of Pharmacy degree, which is no longer awarded. Sixty-seven colleges of pharmacy also offer a master's or PhD degree after completion of a PharmD program for pharmacists who want more laboratory or research experience to do research for a drug company or teach at a university. After graduation, each pharmacist is licensed by passing a state examination and completing an internship with a licensed pharmacist. Schools of pharmacy graduate about 8,000 students annually. The number of active pharmacists in the United States is now well over 200,000, an increase of over 50,000 since 1980.[39]

In 1976, the American Pharmaceutical Association created the Board of Pharmaceutical Specialties. It has approved nuclear pharmacy, clinical pharmacy, nutritional support pharmacy, and pharmacotherapy as specialties in which pharmacists may be certified.[40]

Sixty percent of pharmacists work in community pharmacies, many of which are owned by large commercial chains. There, they may supervise other employees, manage overall business needs, computerize patients' records, and advise physicians and patients about drug dosage, side effects, and interaction with other medications. Twenty-five percent of pharmacists work in hospitals, and the balance are employed by clinics, nursing homes, health maintenance organizations, and the federal government.

Employment of pharmacists is expected to grow faster than the average for all occupations because of the increased pharmaceutical needs of an aging population and the increased use of medications. The need for pharmacists is increasing as they become more involved in drug therapy decision making and patient counseling. Although enrollment in pharmacy programs is growing as students are attracted by high salaries and good job prospects, employment opportunities are expected to exceed applicants through the year 2012.[39]

Podiatric Medicine

Podiatric medicine is specifically concerned with the diagnosis and treatment of diseases and injuries of the lower leg and foot. Podiatrists can prescribe drugs; order radiographs, laboratory tests, and physical therapy; set fractures; and perform surgery. They also fit corrective inserts called orthotics, design plaster casts and strappings to correct deformities, and design custom-made shoes.

There are seven accredited schools in the United States where students can apply after graduating from college. Graduates of these professional schools obtain a Doctor of Podiatric Medicine (DPM) degree. The 4 years of professional training is similar to that for physicians. A residency is not required, but most podiatrists spend 2 or more years completing a residency in a hospital after they graduate. Podiatrists may also take postgraduate training and become board-certified in the specialties of orthopedics, primary medicine, or surgery. All doctors of podiatric medicine must be licensed by the state in which they practice. It is probably in the care of older adults, enabling people to live at home and function independently as long as possible, that podiatric medicine makes its greatest public health contribution.

Podiatric care is more dependent on disposable income than other medical services. Medicare and most private health insurance programs cover acute medical and surgical foot services, as well as diagnostic radiographs and leg braces; however, routine foot care ordinarily is not covered.[41]

Chiropractors

Chiropractors treat the whole body without the use of drugs or surgery. Special care is given to the spine, as chiropractors believe that misalignment or irritations of spinal nerves interfere with normal body functions. Daniel David Palmer of Iowa was a "magnetic healer" in the late 19th century who believed that disease and maladies are the result of nerve interference caused by misaligned vertebrae. He and his son, B. J. Palmer, created the first chiropractic school to teach their philosophies of health. Today there are 15 chiropractic programs and 2 chiropractic institutions. Students need at least an associate degree before applying to one of the accredited chiropractic programs or colleges. After completion of the Doctor of Chiropractic (DC) degree, all states require chiropractors to be licensed to practice. About 2,500 graduates of chiropractic programs enter the growing profession each year, bringing the number of active chiropractors to approximately 70,000.[42]

Chiropractors follow a holistic approach that recognizes exercise, diet, rest, environment, and heredity as factors affecting each patient. Chiropractors use radiographs to examine a patient's spine and compare it with "ideal" posture. Manipulations, typically with hand thrusts or with a chiropractic tool called an activator, are given to patients. Some recent studies have shown that, although chiropractic treatment generally costs more than medical treatment by a primary care physician, patients still see the chiropractor more often and for a longer period of time.[43]

Physicians have long questioned chiropractic practice because of the lack of scientific data that suggest the efficacy of chiropractic treatments.

Nevertheless, patients are generally satisfied with chiropractic care, and for specific conditions causing back pain, chiropractors achieve outcomes comparable to those of physicians.

Chiropractic practice has strong public support, and chiropractors have used that patronage to make significant gains in legal and legislative areas. Regardless of medicine's questions about chiropractic's lack of scientifically proven effectiveness, chiropractors achieved Medicare coverage and participate in most managed care, and many other insurance policies contain some form of chiropractic coverage.

Optometry

A Doctor of Optometry (OD) examines patients' eyes to diagnose vision problems and eye disease, prescribes drugs for treatment, and prescribes and fits eyeglasses and contact lenses. An optometrist should not be confused with an ophthalmologist or an optician. An ophthalmologist is a physician who specializes in the treatment of eye diseases and injuries and uses drugs, surgery, or the prescription of corrective lenses to correct vision deficiencies. An optician is a licensed health professional who fits eyeglasses or contact lenses to individual patients as prescribed by ophthalmologists.

Optometrists must graduate from 1 of the 17 accredited 4-year colleges of optometry and pass both written and clinical state board examinations to obtain a license to practice.[44] More than 1,300 students graduate each year to swell the current number of active optometrists to over 34,000.

One-year residency programs are available for optometrists who wish to specialize in family practice optometry, pediatric optometry, geriatric optometry, occupational vision care, low-vision rehabilitation, vision therapy, contact lenses, hospital-based optometry, or sports vision.

Optometrists usually work in private practice, but many are now forming small group practices. Optometrists can hire opticians and optometric assistants to help them increase their productivity and thus care for more patients. "Persons over 45 visit optometrists and ophthalmologists more frequently because of the onset of vision problems in middle age and the increased likelihood of cataracts, glaucoma, diabetes and hypertension in old age." Because more than half of the people in the United States wear glasses or contact lenses and there is a constant need for eye care by the majority of the aging population, growth in the field of optometry is expected to remain consistent.[45]

Health Care Administrators

Like any other business, health care needs good management to keep it running smoothly. Health care administrators are managers who plan, organize, direct, control, or coordinate medicine and health services in hospitals, clinics, nursing care facilities, and physicians' offices. The majority of health care administrators are employed in hospital settings, but others work for insurers, clinics, or medical group practices. Employment opportunities are numerous because there are over a quarter of a million jobs for health care administrators.

Bachelor's, master's, and doctoral degree programs in health care administration are offered by a wide variety of colleges and universities. At least 70 schools have accredited programs leading to a master's degree in health services administration. There also are short certificate or diploma programs, usually lasting less than 1 year, in health services administration or in medical office management.[46]

Allied Health Personnel

Unlike professionals in medicine, dentistry, nursing, and pharmacy, allied health personnel represent a varied and complex array of health care disciplines. Their roles in providing health care are not generally recognized or well understood by the public. Allied health personnel support, complement, or supplement the professional functions of physicians, dentists, or other health professionals in delivering health care to patients, and they assist in environmental health control, health promotion, and disease prevention. A number of more recent categories of health care specialists were created to implement the new procedures, equipment, and diagnostic, surgical, and therapeutic techniques that proliferated during the last 3 decades. There are now over 200 allied health occupations and specialties.[47]

The range of allied health professions may be understood best by classifying them according to the functions they serve. They may be grouped into the following four categories:

1. Laboratory technologists and technicians
2. Therapeutic science practitioners
3. Behavioral scientists
4. Support services

It should be recognized, however, that some allied health disciplines should be included in more than one of these functional classifications.

Technicians and Technologists

There are a rapidly growing number of technicians and technologists, including such major categories as cardiovascular technicians and technologists, clinical laboratory technicians, emergency medical technicians, health information technicians, nuclear medicine technologists, cytotechnologists, histologic technicians and technologists, surgical technologists, occupational safety and health technicians, pharmacy technicians, and many more. Because space does not allow for a discussion of all or even most of these important health vocations, the following descriptions include only several representative disciplines in this allied health category.

Laboratory Technologists and Technicians

Clinical laboratory technologists and technicians have a critically important role in the diagnosis of disease, monitoring of physiologic function and the effectiveness of intervention, and application of highly technical procedures. Technologists, also known as clinical laboratory scientists or medical technologists, usually have a bachelor's degree in one of the life sciences. Clinical laboratory technicians, also known as medical technicians or medical laboratory technicians, generally need an associate's degree or a certificate.

Among their roles, clinical laboratory personnel analyze body fluids, tissues, and cells checking for bacteria and other microorganisms; analyze chemical content; test drug levels in blood to monitor the effectiveness of treatment; and match blood for transfusion.

The National Accrediting Agency for Clinical Laboratory Sciences accredits 467 programs for clinical laboratory technologists and technicians. Employed graduates of those programs number over 300,000. More than 50% of those employed work in hospitals. Most of the others work in physician offices or diagnostic laboratories. Faster than average employment growth is expected because of population growth and development of new laboratory tests.[48]

Radiologic Technology. A radiologic technologist works under the supervision of a radiologist, a physician who specializes in the use and interpretation of radiographs. The radiologic technologist will use radiographs, fluoroscopic equipment, and high-tech imaging machines such as ultrasonography, computed tomography, magnetic resonance imaging, and positron emission tomography units to produce films that allow physicians to study the internal organs and bones of their patients. Formal training programs in radiography range in length from 1 to 4 years and lead to a certificate, associate's degree, or bachelor's degree. Two-year associate's degrees are most prevalent. The Joint Review Committee on Education in Radiology has accredited over 600 formal programs in 2003.[49]

Technological advances and the growth and aging of the nation's population continue to increase the demand for diagnostic imaging. As a result, the vacancy rate for radiologic technologists is the highest in any field of health care. The U.S. Department of Labor predicts that employment opportunities for radiologic technologists will grow faster than the average for all health care occupations through 2014.[50]

Nuclear Medicine Technology. Nuclear medicine technologists use diagnostic imaging techniques to detect and map radioactive drugs in the human body. They administer radioactive pharmaceuticals to patients and then monitor the characteristics and functions of tissues or organs in which they localize. Abnormal areas show higher or lower concentrations of radioactivity than normal ones do.

Nuclear medicine technologists are prepared in 1-year certificate programs offered by hospitals to those who are already radiologic technologists, medical technologists, or RNs or who are in 2- to 4-year programs offered in university schools of allied health. Nuclear medicine technologists must meet the minimum federal standards on the administration of radioactive drugs and the operation of radiation detection equipment. In addition, about half of all states require technologists to be licensed. Technologists also may obtain voluntary professional certification or registration.[51]

Therapeutic Science Practitioners

Practitioners of the therapeutic sciences are essential to the treatment and rehabilitation of patients with diseases and injuries of all kinds. Physical therapists, occupational therapists, speech pathology and audiology therapists, radiation therapists, and respiratory therapists are only some of the allied health disciplines in this category.

Physical Therapy. Physical therapists provide services that help restore function, improve mobility, relieve pain, and prevent or limit physical disabilities of patients suffering from injuries or disease. They restore, maintain, and promote overall fitness and health. They review patients' medical histories and measure patients' strength, range of motion, balance, coordination, muscle performance, and motor function. They then develop and implement treatment plans that include exercises to develop flexibility, strength, and endurance. They also may give patients exercises to do at home.

Physical therapists may also use electrical stimulation, hot or cold compresses, and ultrasound to relieve pain and reduce swelling. They also teach patients to use assistive and adaptive devices, such as crutches, prostheses, and wheelchairs. Physical therapists supervise physical therapy assistants to aid them in meeting the needs of an increasing number of patients. Physical therapy assistants earn associate's degrees and take a national certifying examination.

Physical therapists often consult and practice with physicians, dentists, nurses, educators, social workers, and occupational or speech therapists. They may practice as generalists or specialize in areas such as pediatrics, geriatrics, orthopedics, sports medicine, neurology, or cardiopulmonary physical therapy.

There were 205 accredited physical therapy programs in 2006. Of those, 115 offered master's degrees and 90 offered doctoral degrees. The Commission on Accreditation in Physical Therapy Education no longer accredits physical therapy programs that do not provide at least master's-level degrees.

Employment opportunities have grown rapidly in the physical therapy field, and the demand now exceeds the supply. Physical therapists have demonstrated their value in the rehabilitation of injured, diseased, or otherwise debilitated patients and are in increasing demand as the population ages.[52]

Occupational Therapy. Occupational therapists (OTs) assist patients in recovering from accidents, injuries, or diseases to improve their ability to perform tasks in their daily living and working environments. A wide range of patients work with occupational therapists, from those with irreversible physical disabilities to those with mental disabilities or disorders. Occupational therapists assist patients in caring for their daily needs such as dressing, cooking, and eating. They also use physical exercises and other activities to increase strength and dexterity, visual acuity, and hand–eye coordination. Occupational therapists instruct in the use of adaptive equipment such as wheelchairs, splints, and aids for eating and dressing. They may also design or make special equipment needed at home or at work. Therapists may collaborate with clients and employers to modify work environments so that clients can maintain employment.

A bachelor's degree in occupational therapy was the minimum requirement for entry into this field, but beginning in 2007, a master's degree or higher is now required.

Most occupational therapists are employed by hospitals, but many also work in offices, nursing homes, community mental health centers, adult day care programs, rehabilitation centers, and residential care facilities. Private practice is currently the fastest growing sector of this profession. As the population ages and patients with critical problems survive more frequently, the demand for occupational therapists will continue to increase.[53]

Speech-Language Pathology. Speech-language pathologists, sometimes called speech therapists, treat patients with speech problems, swallowing, and other disorders in hospitals, schools, clinics, and private practice. About one half of all speech pathologists are employed in the education system—from preschools to universities.

About 233 colleges and universities offer graduate programs in speech-language pathology. A master's degree is the standard practice requirement. Speech-language pathologists use written and oral tests and special instruments to diagnose the nature of the impairment and develop an individualized plan of care. They may teach the use of alternative communication methods, including automated devices and sign language.

The number of speech-language pathologists, now numbering about 130,000, is expected to grow rapidly as the population ages. Older age groups are prone to medical conditions that result in speech, language, and swallowing problems.[54]

Physician Assistant. The emergence of physician assistants (PAs) closely parallels the creation of nurse practitioners. In the 1960s, there was a shortage of health care providers. Duke University initiated the first PA program in 1961. It was a new provider model designed to benefit from the experience and expertise of the many hospital corpsmen and medics that were discharged from the armed forces. As the flow of returning corpsmen and medics tapered off, individuals without prior health care training were accepted into PA programs. The Medex program, which began at the University of Washington and was later adopted at a number of other universities, is well known. It was designed to train general assistants to family medicine physicians and internists.

Today there are at least 135 education programs for physician assistants. Sixty-eight offer a master's degree and the rest offer a bachelor or associate's degree. Most PAs have at least a bachelor's degree. PAs provide health care services under the supervision of a physician. Unlike medical assistants who perform routine clinical and clerical tasks, PAs are formally trained to provide diagnostic, preventive, and therapeutic health care services as delegated by the physician. PAs take medical histories, order and interpret laboratory tests and X-rays, make diagnoses, and prescribe medications as allowed in 47 states and the District of Columbia.

Many PAs are employed in specialties such as internal medicine, pediatrics, family medicine, orthopedics, and emergency medicine. Others specialize in surgery and may provide preoperative and postoperative care and act as first or second assistants during major surgery.

The U.S. Department of Labor projects a significant increase in the employment of PAs because of an expected expansion of the health care industry and an emphasis on cost containment.[55]

Behavioral Scientists

Behavioral scientists are crucial in the social, psychological, and community and patient educational activities related to health maintenance, prevention of disease, and accommodation of patients to disability. They include professionals in social work, health education, community mental health, alcoholism and drug abuse services, and other health and human service areas.[56]

Social Work. Social workers counsel patients and families and assist them in addressing the personal, economic, and social problems associated with illness and disability. They arrange for community-based services as necessary to meet patient needs after discharge from a health facility. A bachelor's degree is required from an accredited college program; however, a master's degree from an accredited graduate school of social work is often the standard requirement for employment.

Social workers provide social services in hospitals and other health-related settings that interact with managed care organizations that strive to contain costs. Medical and public health social workers provide patients and families with psychosocial support in cases of acute, chronic, or terminal illnesses. Mental health and substance abuse social workers assess and treat persons with mental illness or those who abuse alcohol, tobacco, or other drugs.

The most recent tally by the Council on Social Work Education listed 435 bachelor's programs, 149 master's in social work degree programs, and 78 doctoral programs. Employment of social workers is expected to grow faster than the average of other occupations, especially for those with backgrounds in gerontology and substance abuse treatment.[57]

Rehabilitation Counselor. A rehabilitation counselor gives personalized counseling, emotional support, and rehabilitation therapy to patients limited by physical or emotional disabilities. Patients may be recovering from illness or injury, have psychiatric problems, or have intellectual deficits. After an injury or illness is stabilized, the rehabilitation counselor will test the patient's motor ability, skill level, interests, and psychologic makeup and develop an appropriate training or retraining plan. The goal is to maximize the patient's ability to function in society.

A master's degree is often required to be licensed or certified as a rehabilitation counselor. The Commission on Rehabilitation Counselor Certification offers voluntary certification. The need for rehabilitation counselors is expected to grow as the population ages and medical technology saves more lives. In addition, legislation requiring equal employment rights for persons with disabilities will increase the demand for counselors to prepare such people for employment.[58]

Support Services

Support services are necessary for the highly complex and sophisticated system of health care to function. Specialists who provide services frequently work behind the scenes, performing administrative and management duties and often working closely with the actual providers of health care services. Health information administrators, dental laboratory technologists, electroencephalographic technologists, food service administrators, surgical technologists, and environmental health technologists are some of the allied health professionals in this category, and they serve to illustrate the diverse nature of the required support disciplines in allied health.

Health Information Administrators

Health information administrators are responsible for the activities and functions of the medical records departments of hospitals, skilled nursing facilities, managed care organizations, rehabilitation centers, ambulatory care facilities, and a number of other health care operations. They are accountable for planning and maintaining an information system that permits patient data to be received, recorded, stored, and retrieved easily to assist in diagnosis and treatment. These data may also be used to track disease patterns, provide information for medical research, assist staff in evaluating the quality of patient care, and verify insurance claims. Health information administrators supervise the staff in the medical records department and are responsible for the confidentiality of all the information within their departments.

A bachelor's degree in health information administration is the entry-level credential. The Council of Certification of the American Health Information Management Association gives a national accreditation examination for Registered Health Information Administrator. Currently, there are over 50 programs preparing health information administrators and over 150 programs training medical records and health information technologists/technicians. The U.S. Department of Labor estimates a 49% increase in the employment of these health information personnel by 2010.[59]

Career Advancement in Allied Health

The entry-level degree for practice in the allied health fields ranges from the certificate or associate's degree in some disciplines to the bachelor's degree in others and the master's or doctoral degree in still others. Two-year programs that offer associate's degrees or certificates produce allied health personnel who, for the most part, perform under the supervision of those with more advanced training. Because the allied health fields offer so diverse an array of programs, the opportunity for career advancement through educational "laddering" is probably without equal.

It is commonplace for graduates of allied health programs to practice for a period of time and then advance their careers by entering higher level programs and achieving more advanced degrees. For example, it is not unusual for occupational therapists or physical therapists with bachelor's degrees to pursue master's degrees and doctorates in related fields and then become researchers, university faculty, and more advanced clinical practitioners. Allied health practitioners are uniquely positioned to achieve career goals at the highest level of their competence.[60]

Alternative Therapists

Rather than diminishing the public's interest in alternative forms of health care, the increasing sophistication of scientific medicine seems to have fostered a more receptive climate for implausible and inexplicable forms of therapy. Across the country, and notably on the West Coast and in the Midwest, there is widespread interest in complementary and alternative medicine (CAM). CAM is defined as "a group of diverse medical and health care systems, practices, and products that are not presently considered to be part of conventional medicine." Complementary medicine and alternative medicine differ from each other. Complementary medicine is used together with conventional medicine. Alternative medicine is used in place of conventional medicine.[61]

In 1992, with one-third of Americans resorting to alternative medical therapies at the time, the National Institutes of Health created an Office of Alternative Medicine to examine whether alternative therapies work. The more perplexing question of how they work was to be investigated later. In 1998, when more than 40% of Americans reported the use of alternative or complementary therapies, the Office of Alternative Medicine was elevated to the National Center for Complementary and Alternative Medicine and its mandate expanded.

A 2004 press release of the National Center provided the findings of a 2002 national health interview survey that queried respondents about 27 types of complementary and alternative treatments—10 requiring the services of a provider, such as an acupuncturist or chiropractor, and 17 non-provider types, such as herbs, megavitamins, and special diets. The survey found that the U.S. public spent $36 billion to $47 billion that year on CAM therapies. Of that amount, $12 to $20 billion was spent "out of pocket" to professional CAM providers; $5 billion was spent on herbal products alone.[62]

The center is also engaged in the first international study of traditional medicines, including ancient Chinese and American Indian methods.

The plan proposes the first National Institutes of Health study of botanicals that will sort through 1,500 medicinal herbs for evaluation. Unusual therapies, such as telepathic healing, that are on the far fringes of medical practice will also be investigated.[63]

Because estimates of alternative treatment use by cancer patients range from a low of 9% to as high as 50%, the American Cancer Society has a Committee on Unproven Methods of Cancer Treatment that maintains a list of 23 questionable cancer treatment modalities. The use of alternative therapies by cancer patients is usually with family and physician knowledge. About 50% of the patients using unproven therapies continue following conventional treatment as well.[64]

Many alternative therapies involve lifestyle programs, such as macrobiotics, natural food diets, yoga, and other stress-reducing techniques. Others focus on mind–body techniques, including biofeedback, visualization, music therapy, and prayer. Still others are traditional practices of other cultures—acupuncture, homeopathy, and microdose pharmacology.

Along with alternative techniques comes a new class of alternative practitioners. To name a few, there are certified trager practitioners, who rock and cradle the patient's body for relaxation and mental clarity; doctors of naturopathy (NDs), who use natural healing methods that include diet, herbal medicine, and homeopathy; advanced certified rolfers, who use deep massage to restore the body's natural alignment; and registered polarity practitioners, who use touch and advice on diet, self-awareness, and exercise to balance energy flow. In spite of the fact that medical societies strongly oppose naturopathy, considering the practice "unscientific" and "irrational," naturopathic doctors have made great strides in the last few years. Although they do not have medical degrees and are trained in loosely monitored schools, they are able to generate strong public support within state legislatures. Twelve states already license naturopaths and seven more are contemplating licensing legislation. Several of these states allow naturopaths to prescribe conventional drugs, deliver babies, and perform minor surgery.[65]

The gains of naturopaths and other alternative practitioners reflect the public's frustration with much of conventional medicine, high drug prices, and media reports of disproved treatments. The interest of insurance companies in alternative forms of medicine is also important. Insurers say that when traditional medicine is ineffective and an alternative form of therapy, such as acupuncture for a condition such as chronic pain, costs less and satisfies the patient, they will pay for it. As a result, several states now require insurance companies to cover naturopathic procedures and others, such as acupuncture.[66]

Factors That Influence Demand for Health Personnel

Without attempting to include all of the interrelated factors that influence demand for various types of health personnel, it is important to recognize some major determinants of the size and nature of the health care employment sector. Regardless of the potential for legislatively mandated reforms of the health care system, the number and skill requirements of each discipline within the health care workforce will depend on the interdependence of the following factors.

Changing Nature of Disease, Disability, and Treatment

The aging of the population and advances in the treatment of acute and life-threatening conditions will result in an increasing survival of people with chronic illness or disabilities. The growing number of patients with deteriorating mental capacities, cardiac conditions, cancer, stroke, head and spinal cord injuries, neonatal deficits, and congenital disorders will significantly increase the demand for workers who provide and support prolonged medical treatment, rehabilitation, and nursing home or custodial care.

Physician Supply

Although many categories of health personnel perform independently of physicians, most of the decisions regarding the use of health care resources, acceptance of other therapeutic modalities, and treatment provided by nonphysicians are made by physicians. It is important to recognize, therefore, that the anticipated changes in the numbers and types of physicians will have a direct impact on the demand for many other types of health care personnel.

Technology

Medical and nonmedical technology used in the provision of health care has important implications for the number and skill requirements of the health care workforce. Advances in computerization, information systems, miniaturization, radiologic imaging, and laser technology have the potential to both increase and decrease the demand for various kinds of personnel. Some technologies, such as transluminal coronary angioplasty, have led to the elimination of more laborious medical interventions. Others, such as sophisticated patient monitoring systems, have facilitated the shifts to new service settings, such as ambulatory surgical centers. Also, automation of clinical laboratory testing has reduced the need for laboratory personnel. Thus, the mix of skills and the numbers of personnel ebb and flow with the discovery and application of new service modalities.

Expansion of Home Care

Health care reforms are likely to continue the shift in health service delivery sites from acute-care hospitals to ambulatory, home care, and long-term care settings. With the emphasis on cost-containment and an array of high-technology devices that contribute to more efficient techniques for providing nursing care and occupational, physical, and respiratory therapy in the home, the home care component of the health care industry is expected to expand significantly in the next decade. In addition, there is a growing body of evidence that therapy provided in the home helps patients recover faster and reduces hospital readmissions. It is anticipated that the growing number of managed care organizations that emphasize offering the most appropriate services in the most appropriate settings will encourage an expansion of home-delivered services to take advantage of the economies and benefits of that service option.

The expansion of home care, however, will be accompanied by new professional challenges. As hospitals discharge patients earlier in their recovery and as physicians grow more comfortable in depending on home care for patients they might otherwise have hospitalized, more specialized knowledge and skills will be required of home care service providers, and the quality, as well as the economy of care will become of increasing concern.

Corporatization of Health Care

It appears that the solo practice of medicine, dentistry, podiatry, and other health professions is fast becoming a practice pattern of the past. The increase in group practices; the development of several forms of provider organizations; the evolution of hospital networks; the assembly of vertically integrated systems that link hospitals, nursing homes, home care, and other services; and the diversification of health providers into various health-related corporate ventures all reflect the corporatization of health care.

The effect already has been pronounced. In the last 2 decades, employment in physicians' offices far outpaced the growth of the health care industry as a whole. In addition, the introduction of the corporate approach to health care is likely to increase the need for business managers, fiscal staff, planners, data analysts, and other types of personnel more commonly found in large business organizations than in health care facilities.[67]

Health Care Workforce Issues

Policy makers at every level of government, insurers, educators, providers, and consumers have a vested interest in the issues that pertain to the health care workforce. Those issues have been clearly defined in a publication of the Association of Academic Health Centers as follows:[68]

- The adequacy of supply of various health professionals, such as nurses, allied health professionals, primary care physicians, and geriatricians
- The geographic distribution of health professionals, especially their shortage in rural and underserved urban areas
- The underrepresentation of minorities in all health professions, in both primary and specialty care, as well as in the health profession's educational programs
- The potential supply and poor distribution of specialty physicians
- The questions about the appropriate scope of practice for various health professionals and concern about legal restrictions on scope of practice for nonphysician practitioners
- The concern about the quality and relevance of the health profession's educational programs; whether educational institutions are producing the health professionals needed for an effective and productive workforce in the 21st century

- The costs associated with educating health professionals and the impact that changes in the health care delivery system may have on the financing of health profession's education
- The competency testing of health care professionals
- The redefinition of health professions as technology and the delivery system change, and various professions reconsider the credentials needed to practice within the profession
- The concern about the supply of faculty to train health professionals

The Health Workforce in a Chaotic System

During the 21st century, the aging of the population, the shifting nature of diseases, health care reforms, new technology, managed care, and economic factors will significantly change the demand for services provided by different types of practitioners. The market for services will expand in some disciplines and contract in others. It will be necessary to modify the roles and scope of practice of many of the health care professions to adapt to changing service patterns. Yet the lack of any single body in the United States being responsible for making data-based demand/supply projections and policy decisions leaves these important issues to be addressed piecemeal by a number of interested bodies.

Federal and state governments, educational institutions, professional organizations, insurers, and provider institutions have separate and often conflicting interests in health workforce education and training, regulation, financing, entry-level preparation, and scope of practice. The various levels at which policy decisions are made and the disparate interests that influence those decisions present major obstacles to ensuring a coherent, efficient, and rational health workforce in the United States. Nevertheless, those policies supported the production of an enormous number of health professionals to serve the health care system of the late 20th century.

Until the 1990s, the assumptions that guided health workforce policy—like those of foreign and defense policy—seemed self-evident to the people who made policy for spending and taxation. Debates about public financing for health profession education were almost always about when, rather than whether, it is desirable to increase public spending. Educators of health professionals and their allies had considerably warmer relationships with budget officials and senior legislators than, for example, enthusiasts for public health, services for the mentally ill, or more spending for the poor.[69]

With health workforce policies influenced independently by federal and state governments, educational institutions, insurers, the professions, and the competitive health care marketplace, the next few years are certain to be increasingly chaotic. Driven by an ever more cost-conscious health care market, rapid changes will continue in the organization and financing of health care. As occurred in the case of hospital nursing, those unpredictable changes may force health services personnel to make unwelcome adaptations to different work settings and service responsibilities.

Nevertheless, an aging population and technologic advances will have a significant effect on the health care industry over the next decade. Already one of the largest industries in the United States, employment in health care will continue to enjoy significant growth.[70]

References

1. U.S. Department of Labor, Bureau of Labor Statistics. http://www.bls.gov. Accessed July 5, 2007.
2. Collier SN. Report of the State Issues Task Force. *Pew Health Professions Commission State Issues Task Force.* 1991:1–9.
3. Collier SN. Report of the State Issues Task Force. *Pew Health Professions Commission State Issues Task Force.* 1991:7.
4. American Association of Medical Colleges. FACTS-applications, matriculation and graduates. Available from http://www.aamc.org/data/facts/2006/2003to2006detmat.htm. Accessed January 3, 2007.
5. American Association of Colleges of Osteopathic Medicine. Available from http://www.aacom.org. Accessed January 3, 2007.
6. Bouldet JR, Morcini JJ, Whelan GP, et al. The international medical graduate pipeline: recent trends in certification and residency training. *Health Affairs.* 2006;25:469–477.
7. Salsberg ES, Forte GJ. Trends in the physicians workforce, 1980–2000. *Health Affairs.* 2002;21:165–173.
8. National Center for Health Statistics, Health, United States. Chartbook on trends in the health of Americans. Hyattville, MD: Author; 2006:357.
9. O'Brien P. All a women's life can bring: the domestic roots of nursing in Philadelphia, 1830–1885. *Nursing Res.* 1987;36:12–17.

10. Stevens R. *In Sickness and in Wealth: American Hospitals in the Twentieth Century.* New York, NY: Basic Books; 1989:17.

11. Stevens R. *In Sickness and in Wealth: American Hospitals in the Twentieth Century.* New York, NY: Basic Books; 1989:96–98.

12. Kovner C. Nursing. In Kovner AR, ed. *Health Care Delivery in the United States.* New York, NY: Springer Publishing; 1995:101–121.

13. Lamm RD. The coming dislocation in the health professions. *Healthcare Forum.* 1996;39:558–562.

14. U.S. Department of Health and Human Services, Health Resources and Services Administration. Available from http://bhpr.hrsa.gov./nursing/. Accessed July 5, 2007.

15. Buerhaus PI, Staiger DO, Auerbach DI, et al. Is the current shortage of hospital nurses ending? *Health Affairs* 2003;22:191–198.

16. U.S. Department of Health and Human Services, Health Resources and Services Administration, Bureau of Health Professions. *United States Health Workforce Personnel Factbook.* Washington, DC: U.S. Government Printing Office; 1999:73, 74.

17. *Health, United States, 2004 with Chartbook on Trends in the Health of Americans.* Washington, DC: U.S. Government Printing Office; 2004:316.

18. Accelerated Nursing Programs. *Trustee.* Center for Healthcare Governance. Chicago, IL: American Hospital Association; 2007:3.

19. Hassmiller SB, Cozine M. Addressing the nurse shortage to improve the quality of care. *Health Affairs.* 2006;1:268–274.

20. Robert Wood Johnson Foundation. A new era of nursing: transforming care at the bedside. Available from http://www.rwf.org/pr/product. Accessed June 3, 2007.

21. Bureau of Labor Statistics, U.S. Department of Labor. Occupational outlook handbook, 2004–2005 edition, licensed practical and licensed vocational nurses. Available from http://www.bls.gov/oco/ocos102.htm. Accessed January 18, 2005.

22. 2000 National Occupation and Employment and Wage Estimates, Bureau of Labor Statistics. Available from http://www.bls.gov/oco/ocos102.htm. Accessed October 7, 2002.

23. Bullough B, Bullough VI. *Nursing Issues for the Nineties and Beyond.* New York, NY: Springer Publishing Co; 1944:15.

24. Sultz HA, Henry OM, Sullivan JA, et al. *Nurse Practitioners, USA.* Lexington, MA: Lexington Books; 1979:215–229.

25. Krein SL. The employment and use of nurse practitioners and physician assistants by rural hospitals. *Rural Health.* 1997;13:45–58.

26. Hooker RS, McKaig L. Emergency department uses of physician assistants and nurse practitioners: a national survey. *Am J Emerg Med.* 1996;14: 245–249.

27. U.S. Department of Labor, Bureau of Labor Statistics, Occupational outlook handbook. Available from http://.bls.gov/oco/ocos083.htm. Accessed January 5, 2007.

28. Dunn I. A literature review of advanced clinical nursing in the United States of America. *J Adv Nursing.* 1997;25:814–819.

29. Snow C. Home-care firms fill chronic-care niche. *Mod Healthcare.* 1996; 26:50.

30. Indiana School of Nursing. Available from http://nursing.iupui.edu/Academic Programs/default.asp?/Academic Programs. Accessed, July 5, 2007.

31. Ring M. *Dentistry: An Illustrated History.* New York, NY: Harry N. Abrams; 1985:203.

32. Loevy HT, Kowitz AA. Dental development in the midwest of America. *Int Dental J.* 1992;12:157–164.

33. Ring M. *Dentistry: An Illustrated History.* New York, NY: Harry N. Abrams; 1985:283–284.

34. Bureau of Labor Statistics. U.S. Department of Labor, occupational outlook handbook, 2006–2007 edition, dentists. Available from http://www.bls.gov/oco/ocos072.htm. Accessed January 6, 2007.

35. U.S. Department of Health & Human Services, Health Resources and Services Administration, Bureau of Health Professions. *United States Health Workforce Personnel Factbook.* Washington, DC: U.S. Government Printing Office; 1999:63.

36. Mertz E, O'Nell E. The growing challenge of providing oral health care services to all Americans. *Health Affairs.* 2002;21:65–77.

37. Gable FB. *Opportunities in Pharmacy Careers.* Lincolnwood, IL: NTC Publishing Group; 1993:10–14.

38. Higby GJ. American hospital pharmacy from the Colonial Period to the 1930s. *Am J Hosp Pharm.* 1994;51:2817–2823.

39. U.S. Department of Labor, Bureau of Labor Statistics. Occupational outlook handbook. 2006–2007 edition, pharmacists. Available from http://www.bls.gov/oco/ocos079.htm. Accessed January 6, 2007.

40. Maddox RR. Specialization and pharmacy's future. *Ann Pharmacother.* 1990; 24:637–639.

41. U.S. Department of Labor, Bureau of Labor Statistics. Occupational outlook handbook. 2006–2007 edition, podiatrists. Available from http://www.bls.gov/oco/ocos079.htm. Accessed January 6, 2007.

42. U.S. Department of Labor, Bureau of Labor Statistics. Occupational outlook handbook. 2006–2007 edition, chiropractors. Available from http://www.bls.gov/oco/ocos079.htm. Accessed January 8, 2007.

43. Shekelle MM, Rachel L. An epidemiologic study of episodes of back pain care. *Spine.* 1995;20:168.

44. U.S. Department of Labor, Bureau of Labor Statistics. Occupational outlook handbook. 2006–2007 edition, optometrists. Available from http://www.bls.gov/oco/ocos079.htm. Accessed January 8, 2007.

45. U.S. Department of Labor, Bureau of Labor Statistics. Occupational outlook handbook. 2006–2007 edition, health care administrators. Available from http://www.bls.gov/oco/ocos079.htm. Accessed January 8, 2007.

46. New York State Department of Health. *Final Report of the New York State Labor: Health Industry Task Force on Health Personnel.* Albany, NY: New York State Department of Health; 1989:1–71.

47. Sultz HA. *Allied Health Personnel. Consultant Report to the Labor-Health Industry Task Force on Health Personnel.* Albany, NY: New York State Department of Health; 1987.

48. U.S. Department of Labor, Bureau of Labor Statistics. Occupational outlook handbook. 2006–2007 edition, clinical laboratory technologists and technicians. Available from http://www.bls.gov/oco/ocos079.htm. Accessed January 9, 2007.

49. U.S. Department of Labor, Bureau of Labor Statistics. Occupational outlook handbook. 2006–2007 edition, radiologic technologists. Available from http://www.bls.gov/oco/ocos079.htm. Accessed January 9, 2007.

50. U.S. Department of Labor, Bureau of Labor Statistics. Occupational outlook handbook. 2006–2007 edition, radiological technologists and technicians. Available from http://www.bls.gov/oco/ocos/05.htm. Accessed December 6, 2007.

51. U.S. Department of Labor, Bureau of Labor Statistics. Occupational outlook handbook. 2006–2007 edition, nuclear medicine technologists. Available from http://www.bls.gov/oco/ocos079.htm. Accessed January 10, 2007.

52. U.S. Department of Labor, Bureau of Labor Statistics. Occupational outlook handbook. 2006–2007 edition, physical therapists. Available from http://www.bls.gov/oco/ocos079.htm. Accessed January 11, 2007.

53. U.S. Department of Labor, Bureau of Labor Statistics. Occupational outlook handbook. 2006–2007 edition, occupational therapists. Available from http://www.bls.gov/oco/ocos079.htm. Accessed January 11, 2007.

54. U.S. Department of Labor, Bureau of Labor Statistics. Occupational outlook handbook. 2006–2007 edition, speech-language pathologists. Available from http://www.bls.gov/oco/ocos079.htm. Accessed January 11, 2007.

55. U.S. Department of Labor, Bureau of Labor Statistics. Occupational outlook handbook. 2006–2007 edition, physicians assistants. Available from http://www.bls.gov/oco/ocos079.htm. Accessed January 9, 2007.

56. Sultz HA. *Allied Health Personnel. Consultant Report to the Labor-Health Industry Task Force on Health Personnel.* Albany, NY: New York State Department of Health; 1987.

57. U.S. Department of Labor, Bureau of Labor Statistics. Occupational outlook handbook. 2006–2007 edition, social workers. Available from http://www.bls.gov/oco/ocos079.htm. Accessed January 9, 2007.

58. U.S. Department of Labor, Bureau of Labor Statistics. Occupational outlook handbook. 2006–2007 edition, counselors. Available from http://www.bls.gov/oco/ocos079.htm. Accessed January 12, 2007.

59. U.S. Department of Labor, Bureau of Labor Statistics. Occupational outlook handbook. 2006–2007 edition, health information administrators. Available from http://www.bls.gov/oco/ocos079.htm. Accessed January 12, 2007.

60. Sultz HA. *Allied Health Personnel. Consultant Report to the Labor-Health Industry Task Force on Health Personnel.* Albany, NY: New York State Department of Health; 1987.

61. National Center for Complementary and Alternative Medicine. National Institutes of Health. Available from http://nccam.nih.gov/health/whatiscam/#sup1. Accessed April 13, 2004.

62. National Center for Complementary and Alternative Medicine. National Institutes of Health. Press Release 2004. More Than One-Third of U.S. Adults Use Complementary and Alternative Medicine. Available from http://nccam.nih.gov. Accessed May 27, 2004.

63. U.S. National Institutes of Health, National Center for Complementary and Alternative Medicine, Annual Report. Available from http://nccam.nih.gov. Accessed April 21, 2000.

64. McGinnis LS. Alternative therapies, 1990: An overview. *Cancer.* 1991; 67:1788–1792.

65. Petersen A. States grant herb doctors new powers. *Wall Street Journal.* August 22, 2002, D1.

66. Rubenstein S. Alternative health plans widen. *Wall Street Journal.* August 22, 2004, D7.

67. United States Department of Labor. *The American Workforce: 1992–2005.* Washington, DC: Bureau of Labor Statistics; 1994:96–119.

68. McLaughlin CJ. Health work force issues and policy-making roles. In Larson PF, Osterweis M, and Rubin ER, eds. *Health Work Force Issues for the 21st Century.* Washington, DC: Association of Academic Health Centers; 1994:1–3.

69. Fox DM. The Political History of Health Workforce Policy. In: Osterweis M, McLaughlin CJ, Manasse HR, et al., eds. *The U.S. Health Workforce: Power, Politics, and Policy.* Washington, DC: Association of Academic Health Centers; 1996:31–46.

70. Career Guide to Industries 2002–2003. Health Services, Bureau of Labor Statistics, U.S. Department of Labor. Available from http://stats.bls.gov.oco/cg/cgs035.htm. Accessed October 8, 2002.

Financing Health Care

This chapter reviews the most currently available data on national health care expenditures and sources of payment and provides a historical overview of the developments that played major roles in creating the national health care reimbursement infrastructure. Major factors that affect health care costs are identified and discussed. Significant trends in health care spending are reviewed, along with underlying reasons for evolving changes. The roles of government as a payer and provider of services are presented with an overview of continuing efforts to link costs with quality.

The financing of the U.S. health care system has evolved from a variety of influences, including provider, employer, purchaser, consumer, and political factors. These influences continue to produce major tensions in ongoing debates about the role and responsibility of the government as payer, the financial responsibilities of consumers, the relationships of costs to quality, the impact of payment systems on quality, and the overall effects managed care has on health care delivery. Controlling the rising costs of health care and dealing with the estimated 47 million Americans who are uninsured or underinsured are two of the most challenging issues. Managed care is central to a discussion of health care financing. Linking the delivery of and payment for services, it is now the predominant form of health insurance. Managed care has reshaped how health care services are delivered and paid for in the United States.

Health Care Expenditures in Perspective

National health care expenditures in 2005 totaled $1.99 trillion, 16% of the gross domestic product and approximately $6,700 per person (Figure 7-1). The rate of growth between 2004 and 2005 was 6.9%, the slowest growth rate since 1999.[1] In contrast, between 1980 and 1990, average annual growth rates exceeded 10%.[2]

Managed care's focus on controlling utilization was a major factor in slowing spending growth. Throughout the decade of the 1990s, market factors that enabled large purchasers of health insurance to negotiate arrangements aggressively with providers contributed significantly to the impact of expenditure-cutting managed care initiatives. Beginning in the 1980s and continuing through the 1990s, restrictions imposed on hospital and physician practices through prospective payment and restrictive fee schedules also contributed to the decline in health care expenditure growth. Since 2000, enactment of the Balanced Budget Refinement Act, the Medicare, Medicaid and SCHIP Benefits Improvement and Protection Act, and the Medicare Prescription Drug, Improvement, and Modernization Act (MMA) have contributed to increased government spending relative to the private sector. In 2005, government's share of total national health care expenditures was 45.4%, $902.7 billion.[1]

Major factors that result in increased health care expenditures include the following:

- More advanced and more types of technology
- Growth in the population of older adults
- Emphasis on specialty medicine
- The uninsured and underinsured
- Labor intensity
- Reimbursement system incentives

An overview of each factor follows.

New Diagnostic and Treatment Technology

The array of medical interventions and diagnostic modalities has increased exponentially in the past 30 years, including a vast expansion of pharmaceuticals to treat acute and chronic conditions. The availability of new treatments and diagnostic techniques contributed to increased costs.

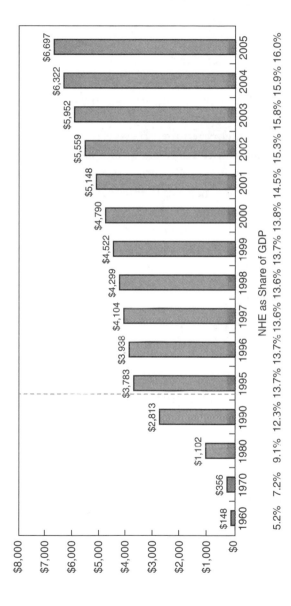

FIGURE 7-1 National Health Expenditures per Capita and Their Share of the Gross Domestic Product, 1960–2005.
Source: Centers for Medicare and Medicaid Services, Office of the Actuary, National Health Statistics Group.

The development of angioplasty as a routine treatment for blocked coronary blood vessels is one example. The capacity of diagnostic modalities such as magnetic resonance imaging is being continuously upgraded and enhanced through new, computerized technology that is significantly expanding its applications. Many other diagnostic, therapeutic, and surgical techniques are undergoing revolutionary changes resulting from the availability of new equipment and computer-aided technologies. Advances of these types come at a significant price, however. Information technology and computer-aided innovations require expensive software and hardware, new patient care equipment, and highly trained personnel. The large capital investments required drive economic and professional imperatives for their use. Historically, the health care reimbursement system required neither documentation of the necessity for the use of technologic interventions nor estimates of their benefit. The tendency to favor broad, rather than discretionary use, grew with the number of interventions available. Managed care organizations (MCOs), which require preapprovals, procedure authorizations, and physician economic incentives, continue the effort to dampen the overuse of technology and avoid unnecessary interventions.

The addition of new pharmacologic agents, increased access to drug coverage through Medicare and managed care, and "direct to consumer" marketing of prescription drugs via television, radio, and print media combined to make the rise in prescription drug spending a focal point of national attention;[3] however, in 2005, the prescription drug expenditure growth rate declined to 5.8% from the 2004 rate of 8.6% due to increased use of generics, changes in therapy, and a major decline in Medicaid prescription drug spending.[1]

Aging Population

Growth in the number of older adults is another major factor in rising health care expenditures. The U.S. Administration on Aging reports that since 1900, the percentage of Americans 65 years old or older has tripled with a 12-fold increase in numbers, reaching 36.3 million in 2005.[4] The age group of 85 years old or older is expected to reach 8.9 million by 2030.[4]

Persons over the age of 65 years are the major consumers of inpatient hospital care. These individuals account for more than one third of all hospital stays and one half of all days of care in hospitals.[5,6] In addition, the aging of the baby-boomers born between 1946 and 1964 is expected to have a profound effect on health care services consumption beginning with the second decade of the 21st century.[7] These demographic developments have major implications for future health care spending.

The Growth of Specialized Medicine

Growth in specialized medicine occurred as medical science and technology advanced. Americans' preference for specialty care resulted in high utilization and rapidly rising costs. Unlike other developed nations, where physician specialists represent half or fewer of physicians in general practice, approximately 60% of practicing physicians in the United States are specialists.[8] The high value that Americans place on advanced technology made specialty care synonymous with high-quality care. This perception may be accurate when the most appropriate treatment choice for an illness requires a specialist's services, but because specialists' services are generally more costly, their inappropriate use generates unnecessary expense. The use of more costly specialists for primary care needs also tends to cause higher use both of diagnostic and therapeutic services than may be necessary for appropriate treatment. Historically, the health insurance models prevalent in the United States carried no prohibitions against self-referrals to specialty care. Patients freely referred themselves to specialists based on their own interpretations of symptoms.

The Uninsured and Underinsured

Among all developed countries of the world, the United States has the highest proportion of population with no health insurance coverage. In 2007, the U.S. Bureau of the Census estimated that 47 million Americans had no health insurance, an increase of approximately 2.2 million uninsured persons over the prior year.[9] Nearly all uninsured adults are employed. Less than one-fifth of all uninsured individuals have no connection to the workforce[10] (Figure 7-2).

The lack of health insurance or insufficient coverage carries major consequences by affecting the ability of individuals to receive timely and

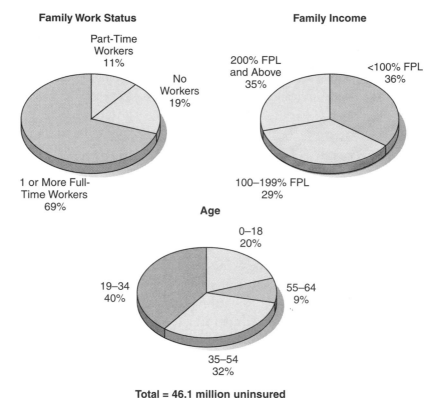

Total = 46.1 million uninsured

The federal poverty level was $19,971 for a family of four in 2005.
Data may not total 100% due to rounding.

FIGURE 7-2 Characteristics of the Uninsured.
Source: The Uninsured: A Primer (#7451-02). The Henry J. Kaiser Family
Foundation, October 2006. *This information was reprinted with permission
from the Henry J. Kaiser Family Foundation. The Kaiser Family Foundation,
based in Menlo Park, California, is a nonprofit, private operating foundation
focusing on the major health care issues facing the nation and is not
associated with Kaiser Permanente or Kaiser Industries.*

needed care for prevention, as well as for acute and chronic conditions. A
lack of insurance coverage drives individuals to seek care in hospital emergency departments at costs higher than care provided at the physician's
office or other ambulatory settings. Furthermore, uninsured or underinsured individuals tend to be low users of preventive services and are
known to delay seeking care, even for acute conditions. These behaviors

often result in increased illness severity and more complications, adding to diagnostic and treatment costs. Uninsured Americans are much more likely than insured individuals to enter care in the late stages of disease, require avoidable hospitalizations, and lack preventive care.[10] Providers absorb increased costs as free care. Insurers pass costs on to the insured in the form of higher premiums, and citizens pay higher taxes to support public hospitals or public insurance programs.[11]

A Labor-Intensive Industry

Health care is a labor-intensive industry. It is one of the largest industries in the United States, employing approximately 13.5 million workers, many of whom represent some of the most highly educated, trained, and compensated individuals in the workforce. The U.S. Department of Labor reports that approximately 27% of all wage and salary jobs created by 2014 will be in health services.[12]

Among the most important factors that continue to produce high employment demands are technologic advances and continued growth in the aging population with more intense and diverse health care needs.

Economic Incentives That Fuel Rising Costs

Both private and government health care financing mechanisms are recognized as major contributors to rising costs. Until the widespread introduction of prospective payment and managed care in the 1980s, government and private third-party payers paid largely on a piecework, fee-for-service, retrospective basis. This system created economic incentives favoring high utilization among both physicians and hospitals. In combination with other factors fueling increased consumption of health care resources, these economic incentives created by the health care financing system played major roles in the rapid rate of expenditure growth. Later sections of this chapter review the history of failed attempts to change the health care financing system, providing a foundation for managed care's emergence as the predominant form of health care financing in the United States.

Components of Health Care Expenditures

Figure 7-3 depicts the major expenditure components of the national health care dollar.[13] Of the total $1.99 trillion in 2005 health care expenditures, the largest portion, $611.6 billion, or 30%, was spent on hospital care. The next largest component of expenditures was physician services, totaling $421.2 billion, or 21% of the health care dollar. Prescription drugs consumed a total of $200.7 billion or 10%. Administration and net costs of private health insurance were $143.0 billion, or 7%. Nursing home care provided in free-standing, non–hospital-based facilities, at $121.9 billion, represented 6% of expenditures.[14]

Sources of Health Care Payment

Figure 7-4 depicts the major payment sources for national health care expenditures.[15] Private health insurance funds 35% of expenditures, totaling $694.4 billion in 2005. Contributing $342.0 billion, Medicare

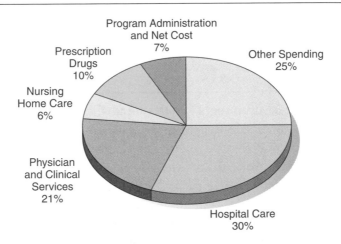

Note: Other spending includes dentist services, other professional services, home health, durable medical products, over-the-counter medicines and sundries, public health, other personal health care, research and structures, and equipment.

FIGURE 7-3 The Nation's Health Care Dollar 2005: Where it Went. *Source:* Centers for Medicare and Medicaid Services, Office of the Actuary, National Health Statistics Group.

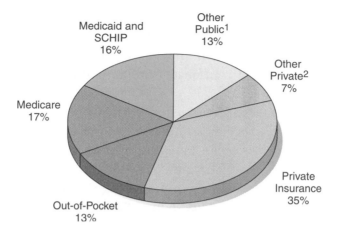

¹Other Public includes program such as workers' compensation, public health activity, Department of Defense, Department of Veterans Affairs, Indian Health Service, State and local hospital subsidies, and school health.
²Other Private includes industrial in-plant, privately funded construction, and non-patient revenues, including philanthropy.
Note: Numbers shown may not add to 100.0 because of rounding.

FIGURE 7-4 The Nation's Health Care Dollar 2005: Where it Came From.
Source: Centers for Medicare and Medicaid Services, Office of the Actuary, National Health Statistics Group.

funds 17% of total expenditures and at $313.1 billion, Medicaid, including the State Children's Health Insurance Program, funds 16%. Other public funds, including federal, state, and local sources, contribute $247.5 billion or 13%. Private, out-of-pocket payments of $249.4 billion constitute 13% of expenditures, whereas other private funds contribute $141.2 billion, or 7%.[1] Public funds contributed a total of 46%, or $914.3 billion, to total national health care expenditures in 2005.

Evolution of Health Insurance and Managed Care

Health insurance is the primary source of payment for health care costs in the United States. As a mechanism that helps protect individuals from financial devastation when expensive care is required, insurance helps decrease risks of costly delays in seeking treatment for conditions that might otherwise become more serious and more costly. National debates about health care reform and the need for universal coverage continuously highlight the impact of inadequate or no insurance for over 47 million Americans.

The U.S. system of health insurance currently includes numerous private entities that provide either indemnity coverage (reimbursement to those insured) or coverage on a prepaid, managed care basis. The federal Medicare program, serving Americans aged 65 years old or older, and the joint federal–state Medicaid program for low-income individuals are the primary government-funded health insurance programs.

The historic definition of insurance, by which it is still commonly understood, is a mechanism through which individuals pay an advance sum to a pool in which payments from numerous individuals offset the cost of a possible future costly event. Central to this definition is that events insured against are rare or unlikely to occur for a particular individual but may be predicted for a group with a fair level of accuracy. This latter understanding is the basis for payment or premium setting that helps to keep the costs of coverage reasonable for individual participants by pooling risks.

As early as the mid-1800s, a movement began to insure workers against lost wages resulting from injuries. Later, insurance to cover lost wages resulting from catastrophic illness was added to accident policies. It was not until the 1930s that health insurance began paying part or all of the costs of medical treatment to providers. Throughout the 1930s and early 1940s, the voluntary hospital sector and employers, in part responding to hospitals' difficulty in collecting payment from individuals who lacked financial resources, organized group hospital prepayment plans. This response reflected hospitals' dependence on private, out-of-pocket payments. In 1935, private payments from individuals accounted for over 70% of hospital income.[16] Today, personal, out-of-pocket payments represent only approximately 3% of expenditures for hospital care.[17]

The Development of Blue Cross and Blue Shield

In 1930, a group of Baylor University teachers contracted with Baylor Hospital in Dallas, Texas to provide coverage for hospital expenses.[18] This arrangement created a model for the development of what was to become Blue Cross, a private, not-for-profit insurance empire that grew over the succeeding 4 decades into the dominant form of health insurance in the United States. The Blue Shield plans providing physician payments began shortly after Blue Cross, and by the early 1940s, numerous Blue Shield plans were operating across the country. In 1946, the American Medical Association (AMA) financed the Association Medical Care Plans, which later became the National Association of Blue Shield Plans.

These developments, through which health insurance was transformed from a mechanism to reimburse individuals for lost wages resulting from injury or illness to one that reimbursed providers for the costs of medical care, carried major implications. The basic concept of health insurance is antithetical to the central premise of insurance. Whereas insurance originally guarded against the low risk of a rare occurrence, such as premature death, and unpredictable events such as accidents, the new medical care insurance model provided coverage for predictable, routine uses of the health care system as well as unforeseen and unpredictable illnesses or injuries. Coverage for routine use of health care services added a new dimension to the concept of insurance. Perhaps the term "assurance" more appropriately describes the health care payment system that evolved. In the United Kingdom, "assurance" is used to denote coverage for contingencies that must eventually happen (e.g., life assurance), whereas "insurance" is reserved for coverage of those contingencies (e.g., fire and theft) that may never occur.[19]

The establishment and subsequent proliferation of the "Blues" signaled a new era in U.S. health care delivery and financing. They played a significant role in establishing hospitals as the centers of medical care proliferation and technology, and by reimbursing for expensive services, they put hospital care easily within the reach of middle-class working Americans for the first time. The insulation from costs of care provided by the Blues had a major impact on utilization. By the late 1930s, annual hospital admission rates for Blue Cross enrollees were 50% higher on average than for the nation as a whole.[20] In addition to contributing to increased utilization of hospital services by removing financial barriers, the Blue Cross movement had other lasting impacts on national policy making. Rosemary Stevens noted, "In the United States, the brave new world of medicine was specialized, interventionist, mechanistic and expensive—at least as interpreted, through prepayment, for workers in major organizations."[21] By 1940, the Blue Cross movement represented a major financing alternative, countering forces that had long lobbied politically for a form of national health insurance, a concept opposed vehemently by private medicine. The plans also stimulated the American Hospital Association and local hospitals to consider providing similar forms of reimbursement for low-income populations, modeled after the Blue Cross benefits recognizing private, semiprivate, and ward care. This latter movement, which continued for the next 20 years, focused attention on government as a potential source of insurance that was designed for low-income populations, the unemployed, or sporadic seasonal workers and that was modeled along Blue Cross lines.[22]

Uniform features of all Blue Cross plans included not-for-profit status, supervision by state insurance departments, direct payments through contract arrangements with providers, and the use of community rating, in which all individuals in a defined group pay single premiums without regard to age, gender, occupation, and health status. Community rating helped ensure nondiscrimination against groups with varying risk characteristics in order to provide coverage at reasonable rates for the community as a whole; however, as commercial insurers entered the health care insurance marketplace, using "experience rating," basing premiums on historically documented patterns of utilization, Blue Cross plans, to remain competitive, began offering a variety of benefit packages. Ultimately, the Blue Cross plans were compelled to switch to experience-rating schemes to avoid attracting a disproportionate share of high-risk individuals for whom commercial insurance was prohibitively expensive.[23]

The Costs of Expanding Technology

Beginning in the 1950s, health care technology expanded rapidly. Hospitals became high-technology centers, consuming increasing resources in care delivery and capital to expand capacity and add technology. Physician expenditures also spiraled upward, and costly specialty care burgeoned. By 1970, the U.S. health care delivery system had emerged as the world's undisputed leader in high-technology and sophisticated medicine, but not without high costs. In 1960, national hospital care expenditures totaled $9.2 billion; by 1970, they had increased threefold, totaling $27.6 billion.[17] Physician service expenditures saw parallel growth. In 1960, they totaled $5.4 billion, and by 1970, they reached $14 billion.[17] National economic factors could not explain these increases as the rates of hospital and physician expenditure growth vastly outstripped inflation and growth in the gross domestic product. Since the 1940s, when employers offset post-World War II wage controls with fully paid health insurance benefits, working Americans had been insulated from health care costs. They grew to expect and demand what they perceived as the "best" care. For most, affordability or costs did not enter into the decision-making equation. Physicians' treatment recommendations were uninhibited by economic considerations among their well-insured patients. The length of hospital stay and the use of consultant specialists and tests were at the physicians' sole discretion, with few, if any, financial implications for the patient.

Health Maintenance Organizations and Managed Care

Since 1900, the U.S. government had participated in relatively minor ways in providing and insuring medical care (e.g., workers' compensation benefits, welfare programs of the Social Security Administration). In 1965, however, the federal government committed to becoming a major payer with the passage of Medicare and Medicaid amendments to the Social Security Act. In the years after Medicare and Medicaid enactment, Congress and state governments tried with marginal success to slow the growth of health care expenditures; however, the delivery system identified new ways to optimize reimbursement, including cost shifting, increases in utilization, and justifications for added technology and personnel. In addition, emerging environmental factors such as increasing poverty, the HIV/AIDS epidemic, inflation, and increasing substance abuse and violence added to health care costs.

By the 1960s, rapid increases in health care expenditure growth accompanied by quality concerns captured the attention of health and government policy makers and of industry as the major purchasers of health care benefits. President Nixon and the U.S. Congress enacted the Health Maintenance Organization Act (HMO) Act of 1973. Although many employer groups had used principles of managed care for decades through contracts with health care providers to serve employees on a prepaid basis, provisions of the HMO Act opened participation to the employer-based market allowing the rapid proliferation of managed care plans.

The HMO Act of 1973 provided loans and grants for the planning, development, and implementation of combined insurance and health care delivery organizations and required that a comprehensive array of preventive and primary care services be included in the HMO arrangement.

The legislation also mandated that employers with 25 or more employees offer an HMO option if one was available in their area and required employers to contribute to employees' HMO premiums in an amount equal to what they contributed to indemnity plan premiums. Initially, this employer mandate helped stimulate the growth of HMO membership in regions where federally funded and qualified plans were first established.

As authorized by the 1973 legislation, HMOs were organizations that combined providers and insurers into one organizational entity. As originally established, members of HMOs usually were required to obtain all of their medical care within the organization.

Initially, there were two major types of HMOs. The first was a staff model and was the type most commonly established from the initial HMO legislation. It employed groups of physicians to provide the majority of ambulatory care needs of its members. HMOs often provided some specialty services within the organization or contracted for services with community specialists. In the staff model, the HMO also operated the facilities in which its physicians practiced, providing on-site ancillary support services, such as radiology, laboratory, and pharmacy services. The HMO usually purchased hospital care and other services for its members through fee-for-service or prepaid contracted arrangements. Staff model HMOs were referred to as "closed panel" because they employed the physicians who provided the majority of their members' care, and those physicians did not provide services outside the HMO membership. Similarly, community-based physicians could not participate in HMO member care without authorization by the HMO.

The second type of HMO stimulated by the 1973 legislation was the individual practice association (IPA). IPAs are physician organizations comprised of community-based independent physicians in solo or group practices that provide services to HMO members. An IPA HMO, therefore, did not operate facilities in which members received care, but rather provided its members services through private physician office practices. Like the staff model HMO, the IPA HMO purchased hospital care and specialty services not available through IPA-participating physicians from other area providers on a prepaid or fee-for-service basis. Some IPA HMOs allowed physicians to have a nonexclusive relationship that permitted treatment of nonmembers as well as members; however, HMO relationships with an IPA also could be established on an exclusive basis. In this scenario, an HMO took the initiative in recruiting and organizing community physicians into an IPA to serve its members. Because the HMO was the organizing force in such an arrangement, it was common for the HMO to require exclusivity by the IPA, limiting its services only to that HMO's membership.[24]

The staff model and IPA-type organizations illustrate two major types of HMOs, but each type spawned several hybrids since the 1973 HMO Act. Other forms of MCOs emerged throughout the 1980s in response to national cost and quality concerns. Peter Kongstvedt identifies three additional HMO models as the most common: group practice, network, and direct contract.[25] In a group practice model, an HMO contracts with a multispecialty group practice to provide all the physician services required by HMO enrollees. The physicians remain independent—employed by their group rather than the HMO. Such an arrangement may or may not be exclusive.

In the network model, the HMO contracts with more than one group practice and may maintain contracts with several physician groups representing both primary care and specialty practices. The direct contract model HMOs maintain contractual relationships with individual physicians, in contrast to the physician groups as in the IPA and network models. The direct contract approach gave the HMO the advantages of maintaining a higher level of control over fee arrangements by reducing physicians' negotiating power to an individual basis and avoiding the risk of lost services to its members by contractual termination of a large group of providers.

All forms of managed care entail interdependence between the provision of and payment for health care. Managed care is population, rather than individual, oriented. It is a system through which care providing groups or networks take responsibility and share financial risk with an insurer for a specified population's medical care and health maintenance. The population basis enables the insurer to determine actuarially, projected use of services related to age, gender, and other factors. Service utilization estimates provide a basis for expected costs over a defined period.

Estimates enable the insurer to establish premiums for benefit coverage. Miller and Luft described the other characteristic of managed care plans—the provider network—as "the single most important feature distinguishing a managed care from an indemnity (fee-for-service) plan."[26] This feature is key to insurers' ability to exert influence over the delivery, use, and costs of services.

By linking the insurance of and delivery of services, managed care reverses the financial incentives of providers in the fee-for-service model. Fee for service is essentially a piecework, pay-as-you-go system in which the care provider is financially rewarded for high service utilization. Managed care uses the concept of prepayment, in which providers are paid a preset amount in advance for all services their insured population is projected to need in a given period. Capitation, a method that pays providers for services on a per-member-per-month basis, is a common form of prepayment. The provider receives payment whether or not services are used. If a physician exceeds the predetermined payment level, he or she may suffer a financial penalty. Similarly, if the physician uses fewer resources than predicted, he or she may retain the excess as profit.

Fee-for-service payments that withhold a portion of the customary fee are another form of payment that seeks to provide financial incentives for efficient resource management. In the withhold scheme, physicians are provided a target amount of resources, usually on an annual basis, to provide a pre-established array of services to a defined population. If the physician meets the target, the withheld amount is returned to the physician. If the physician exceeds the target, a financial penalty in the form of retention of all or a percentage of the withheld fees is incurred.

There are many other forms of physician payment in managed care systems that address the direction of financial incentives to promote efficient resource use. The key element of all such physician prepayment arrangements is to encourage cost-conscious, efficient, and effective care.

From its earliest roots in the prepaid health plans of more than 70 years ago, the goal of managed care has been to control costs by controlling service utilization. To achieve cost control, managed care plans rely on transferring some measure of financial risk from insurers to care providers and often, beneficiaries. Transfers of financial risk to beneficiaries most commonly take the form of co-payments and deductibles. Co-payments require that beneficiaries pay a set fee each time they receive a covered service, such as a co-payment for each physician office visit. A deductible requires beneficiaries to meet a predetermined, out-of-pocket expenditure level before the MCO assumes payment responsibility for the balance of charges.

Managed care is the predominant form of health insurance in the United States. Employers provide the primary source of health insurance, covering approximately 158 million Americans under the age of 65 years. Nearly all businesses with at least 200 workers offer health insurance to their employees, but less than half of employers with fewer than 10 workers do so.[27] The majority of employees in companies offering health care coverage subscribe to one or more managed care plans with only a small fraction subscribing to conventional plans. As enrollment in managed care accelerated throughout the 1980s and 1990s, concerns emerged about MCO restrictions on consumer choice of providers and services. In response, MCOs spawned point-of-service (POS) plans that allow members to use providers outside the MCOs' approved provider networks. To exercise this choice, POS members are charged co-payments and deductibles higher than those charged for in-network services. In 2005, POS plans represented 15% of covered employee enrollment.[28] Another form of managed care arrangement, preferred provider organizations (PPOs), were formed by physicians and hospitals to serve the needs of private, third-party payers, and self-insured firms. Through these arrangements, PPOs guarantee a certain volume of business to hospitals and physicians in return for a negotiated discount in fees. PPOs offer attractive features to both physicians and hospitals. Physicians are not required to share in financial risk as a condition of participation, and PPOs reimburse physicians on the fee-for-service basis to which they are accustomed. By providing predictable admission volume, PPOs help hospitals to shore up declining occupancy rates and attenuate the competition for admissions with other hospitals. To control costs, PPOs use negotiated discount fees, requirements that members receive care exclusively from contracted providers (or incur financial penalty), requirements for preauthorization of hospital admission, and second opinions for major procedures. PPOs maintain systems of utilization review and review of hospital lengths of stay as both a prospective and retrospective means to control costs and advocate for more efficient service utilization by hospitals and physicians. Currently, PPOs are the most popular managed care plans, encompassing over 60% of employer-covered workers[28] (Figure 7-5).

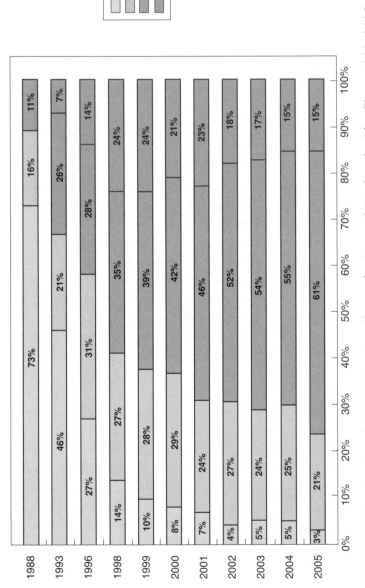

FIGURE 7-5 Distribution of Health Plan Enrollment for Covered Workers by Plan Type, 1988–2005.
Source: Employer Health Benefits Annual Survey (#7315). The Henry J. Kaiser Foundation & Health Research and Educational Trust, September 2005. *This information was reprinted with permission from the Henry J. Kaiser Family Foundation. The Kaiser Family Foundation, based in Menlo Park, California, is a nonprofit, private operating foundation focusing on the major health care issues facing the nation and is not associated with Kaiser Permanente or Kaiser Industries.*

The organizational forms of managed care have continued evolving because of changing marketplace conditions, including purchaser preferences, beneficiary demands, and other factors. The emergence of PPOs as the most popular employee choice and the decline of staff model HMOs are notable developments. PPOs represented a means to involve payers and providers in negotiating fees and monitoring utilization while giving beneficiaries more choice. The decline of the staff model HMO resulted from many factors, including beneficiary demands for more provider choice, large capital outlays associated with facility maintenance and expansion, and increased competition from IPA models. In 1988, staff models constituted about 42% of MCO membership. Currently, they represent less than 1%.[29] MCOs continue offering diversified products and services to maintain the highest appeal to employer purchasers seeking cost savings and quality. Another trend has been MCOs' increased use of clinical practice guidelines that provide uniform protocols for the treatment of specified medical conditions (see Chapter 11). MCOs advocate guidelines as one means to promote consistency in clinical practice and reduce costs. Guidelines are assumed by many to promote the quality of clinical outcomes by helping to decrease variability in provider practices.

Four decades of research suggest that higher health care expenditures do not always contribute to the quality of care and that savings could result from a higher level of scrutiny of the appropriateness of medical interventions. Both directly, by changing reimbursement incentives, and indirectly, by instituting quality control measures to standardize care and decrease variations in the treatment of common illnesses, managed care principles resulted in major shifts in the patient, provider, and payer relationships.

Because physicians are the predominant influence over the use of virtually all patient care resources, managed care emphasizes the primary physician's role as the "gatekeeper" who controls patient entry to all other levels of care. In response to patient demands for easier access to specialty services, some MCOs have relented on specialty referral requirements, but all continue to encourage avoidance of unnecessary use of high-cost services by appropriate and timely treatment at the primary level.

Developments in Managed Care

The surge in managed care enrollment throughout the 1990s and decreases in premiums significantly contributed to a decline in the average annual growth of national health care expenditures;[30] however, after 4 years of decline, health insurance premiums increased 8.2% in 1998, more than double the increase of the 3 prior years.[31] The insurance "underwriting cycle," in which insurers underprice during periods of market development, and then increase premiums later to restore profitability is noted as a major reason for increases. Managed care plans realized high profitability in the early 1990s, when large-scale migration occurred from conventional health insurance.

Between 2006 and 2007, growth in health insurance premiums was 6.1%, the slowest rate since 1999[27]; however, since 2001, premium increases exceeded the 3.7% increase in wages and the overall inflation rate during the same period.[32] (Figure 7-6) Since 2001, family coverage premiums have increased by 78%, whereas wages have increased 19% and inflation 17%.[32] Workers now contribute 10% more toward their employer-sponsored coverage than in 2005, and the annual premium for family coverage exceeds the gross earnings ($10,715) of a full-time minimum wage worker.[33]

The rise in premiums carries significant implications. Higher premiums and requirements for larger employee contributions cause workers to drop coverage. This effect increases in severity as the annual earnings of employees decrease, meaning that lower wage workers who can least afford the risk of high health care costs are the most likely to become uninsured. Employers also seek to control costs through "benefit buy-downs." Methods include reducing the scope of benefits, increasing co-payments and/or co-insurance, and increasing co-pays for prescription drugs.[34] Some experts estimate that every one percent increase in premiums produces a net increase of 164,000 uninsured individuals.[35]

The Managed Care Backlash

In what is termed the managed care "backlash" that began in the late '90s, organized medicine, other health care providers, and consumers railed against MCO policies on choice of providers, referrals, and other practices that were viewed as unduly restrictive. A presidential commission was established to review the need for guidelines in the managed care industry.[36] In 1998, the president imposed patient protection requirements on private insurance companies providing health coverage to

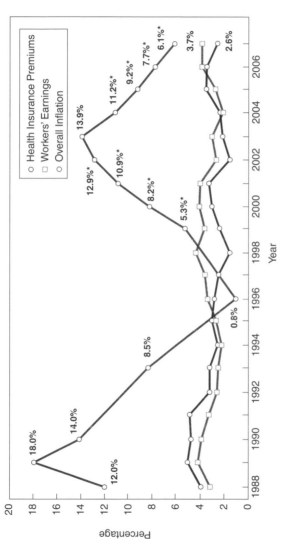

*Estimate is statistically different from estimate for the previous year shown (p < .05). No statistical tests are conducted for year prior to 1999.

Note: Data on premium increases reflect the cost of health insurance premiums for a family of four. The average premium increase is weighted by covered workers.

FIGURE 7-6 Increases in Health Insurance Premiums Compared to Other Indicators, 1988–2007.
Source: Trends in Health Care Costs and Spending (#7692). The Henry J. Kaiser Family Foundation, September 2007. *This information was reprinted with permission from the Henry J. Kaiser Family Foundation. The Kaiser Family Foundation, based in Menlo Park, California, is a nonprofit, private operating foundation focusing on the major health care issues facing the nation and is not associated with Kaiser Permanente or Kaiser Industries.*

federal workers.[37] Public dissatisfaction with constraints over the right to receive care deemed necessary and the freedom of physicians to refer patients to specialists received wide publicity. Public concerns driving sentiments toward more government regulation of the managed care industry included the belief that managed care was hurting the quality of patient care and that the managed care industry was not doing as good a job for patients as other sectors of the health care industry. First introduced in 1998 to the 105th Congress as the Bipartisan Patient Protection Act, the bill under similar title (now in the 110th Congress, The Bipartisan Consensus Managed Care Improvement Act of 2007) has failed to attain passage. The states took the lead in the patients' rights arena. Since 1998, state legislatures have enacted over 900 laws and regulations addressing both consumer and provider protections.[38]

In another response to the managed care "backlash," increasing numbers of employers began allowing employees to make personal decisions about their coverage, dubbed "consumer-driven" health plans (CDHP). The ultimate goal of the CDHP is cost savings, relying on the assumption that if employees take more responsibility for health care decisions, they will exercise more cost consciousness. The typical CDHP consists of either a health reimbursement arrangement (HRA) or a health savings account (HSA).[39] Eligibility for an HSA requires the employee's enrollment in a high-deductible health insurance plan. Because the plan deductible typically exceeds the employer contribution, the employee is at risk for higher out-of-pocket costs. Employers and employees may contribute to the HSA up to a qualified amount. CDHPs provide comparative information to employees in Web-based and traditional formats to increase knowledge about their health care choices and associated costs. In the HSA-high deductible arrangement, the employee draws on the HSA to purchase care until the account is exhausted, when the policy's major medical provision activates. The second type of plan allows employees to design their own provider networks and benefits, based on anticipated needs and costs. The third uses Web-based information to enable employees to choose from established groupings of provider networks and benefits to "customize" coverage. In 2006, approximately 4 million workers, only about 5% of those obtaining health benefits from their employers, participated in CDHPs.[39] Predictions vary widely regarding the future of such arrangements in the health insurance marketplace.

Since the mid-1990s, MCOs have undergone many changes in their operating policies, mergers, and consolidations. The most prominent changes have come as responses to provider and consumer demands reflected by state-enacted patient protection legislation, a loosening of early restrictions on patient choice of provider, provider specialty referrals, and patient access to information about operating policies, especially regarding denials of payment. A 5-year literature analysis of MCO performance indicates that MCOs overall did not accomplish their early promises to change clinical practice and improve quality while lowering costs. Findings suggest that a systematic revamping of information systems, coupled with appropriate incentives and revised clinical processes, will be required to produce the desired changes in cost and quality performance.[40]

Managed Care Organizations and Quality

Nationally, the most influential managed care quality assurance organization is the National Committee on Quality Assurance (NCQA). The NCQA formed in 1979 as two managed care trade organizations, the American Managed Care and Review Association and Group Health Association of America, merged under the title of the American Association of Health Plans. The title was later changed to the NCQA. In 1990, the NCQA became an independent, not-for-profit organization deriving its revenue primarily from fees for accreditation services.[41] The organization also publishes and markets a compendium of quality indicators on 250 health plans serving 50 million Americans.[42]

The NCQA evaluates participating organizations on a voluntary request basis. NCQA programs include accreditation for MCOs, PPOs, managed behavioral health care organizations, new health plans, and disease management programs. The NCQA provides certification for organizations that verify provider credentials, physician organizations, utilization management organizations, and disease management organizations and programs. It also provides physician recognition programs for performance excellence in the areas of diabetes, heart/stroke, and back pain management.[43] Accreditation of MCOs entails rigorous reviews of all aspects of the respective organizations including online surveys and onsite reviews of key clinical and administrative processes. The review focuses on six major areas: management, physician credentials, member rights and responsibilities, preventive health services, utilization, and medical records. Beginning in 1999, the NCQA began including outcomes of care and measures of clinical processes in accreditation reviews, increasing the likelihood that accreditation status will accurately reflect the quality of care delivered.[44]

The Health Plan Employer Data and Information Set (HEDIS) evolved from a partnership among health plans, employers, and the NCQA in 1989.[45] It provides a standardized method for managed care organizations to collect, calculate, and report information about their performance to allow employers, other purchasers, and consumers to compare different plans. HEDIS has evolved through several stages of development and continuously refines its measurements through a rigorous review and independent audits. The data set contains 71 measures of MCO performance, divided among eight domains:[46]

1. Effectiveness of care
2. Accessibility and availability of care
3. Satisfaction with care
4. Health plan stability
5. Use of service
6. Cost of care
7. Informed health choices
8. Health plan descriptive information

The HEDIS also incorporates the Consumer Assessment of Health Plans Survey, which addresses enrollee satisfaction.[47] The HEDIS reports are referred to as MCO "report cards." They are available to the public on the Web.[48]

The Centers for Medicare and Medicaid Services requires that all Medicare Advantage–managed care plans publicly report HEDIS data, and the NCQA requires all accredited plans to allow public reporting of their clinical quality data. A number of states also require plans providing Medicaid–managed care to report HEDIS data.[49]

The NCQA/HEDIS data provide an important means of accountability to the employer purchasers and consumers of health care and feedback to its providers that is critical in efforts to achieve improvement. In 2005, 536 HMOs and POS plans reported data for more than 62 million

Americans. For the first time in 2005, more than 80 PPOs reported data for an additional 14 million enrollees.[50] Benchmarked against the performance of the top 10% of all participating health plans, these data disclose quality disparities and gaps that inform purchasers, plan administrators, and policy makers. Comparisons allow the calculation of numbers of avoidable illnesses and deaths for several of the most common, costly, and deadly health conditions.[51]

MCOs also apply numerous internal techniques to manage quality, many of which directly or indirectly relate to physician performance. They focus much attention on the quality of the institutional providers, especially on the hospitals with which they contract for services. Database systems may track the use of services on both a prospective and retrospective basis to control resource use and monitor quality. Through disease management programs, many MCOs are attempting to control costs and improve care quality for individuals with chronic and costly conditions through methods such as evidence-based clinical guidelines, patient self-management education, disease registries, risk stratification, proactive outreach, and performance feedback to providers. Programs may also include personnel in the form of clinical specialists who provide monitoring and support to patients with disease management issues. Several states and the federal government are also using disease management programs for Medicaid and Medicare recipients.[52]

Self-Funded Insurance Programs

Since the late 1970s, self-funding (full or partial) and self-insurance of employee health benefits became increasingly common among large employers. Through the self-funded mechanism, the employer (or other group, such as a union or trade association) collects premiums and pools these into a fund or account from which it pays claims against medical benefits instead of using a commercial carrier. Self-insured plans often use the services of an actuarial firm to set premium rates and a third-party administrator (TPA) to administer benefits, pay claims, and collect data on utilization. Many TPAs also provide case management services for potentially extraordinarily expensive cases to help coordinate care and control employer risk of catastrophic expenses.

Self-insurance offers significant advantages to employers, such as avoiding additional administrative and other charges made by commercial carriers. By self-funding benefits, employers also can avoid premium taxes and accrue interest on the cash reserves held in the benefit account. A major stimulus to the development of self-insurance programs has been their exemption from the Employee Retirement and Income Security Act of 1974 (ERISA), which mandates minimum benefits under state law. This exemption allowed employers much greater flexibility in designing benefit packages and provided one mechanism to control benefit costs.

Major controversies continue to arise from the ERISA exemption of self-insured employer plans. One controversy is based in states' interpretation of their responsibilities for consumer protection through regulation of the types and scope of required coverage in employer-provided plans. ERISA has historically preempted such regulation. Another major area of dispute centers on the states' losses of premium revenue taxes as they struggle with growing financial burdens of uncompensated care and caring for uninsured populations. An additional area of controversy and legal actions surrounding ERISA is its prohibition against employees suing employer-provided health plans over matters involving coverage decisions. Under ERISA, organizations that administer employer-based health benefit plans maintain a degree of legal immunity from litigation and liability for withholding coverage or failing to provide necessary care. In 2004, the U.S. Supreme Court upheld an Appeals Court decision that beneficiaries of employment-related managed care plans cannot hold the plans accountable for damages when injured as a result of coverage denial decisions.[53]

Government as a Source of Payment: System in Name Only

Federal and state government and to a lesser extent local government finance health care services. Federal funding originally focused on specific population groups, providing health care for those in government service, their dependents, and particular population groups, such as Native Americans. Today, a combination of public programs, chief among them the federal Medicare program and joint federal–state Medicaid program, constitutes almost half of total national care expenditures.[17]

Government payment for health services includes federal support of U.S. Public Health Service hospitals, the Indian Health Service, state and local inpatient psychiatric and other long-term care facilities, services of the Veterans Affairs hospitals and health services, services provided by the Department of Defense to military personnel and their dependents, workers' compensation, public health activities, and other government-sponsored service grants and initiatives.

In the absence of a comprehensive national health and social services policy, government's role in financing health care services can be described as a system only in the loosest interpretation of that term. It may be more accurate to describe government's various roles in health care financing as a mosaic of individual programs of reimbursement, direct payments to vendors, grants, matching funds, and subsidies. Some financing programs are interrelated or interdependent, representing tiers, first-pocket, or second-pocket approaches; others are totally independent of each other. Many are overlapping in their intent; some, like the Medicaid program, are conglomerates of federal and state source funds with policy making subject to federal, state, and local administrative and legislative influences.

As a source of health care service payments, the system of financing operates primarily in a vendor/purchaser relationship, with government contracting with health care services providers rather than providing services directly. A prime example is the Medicare program, in which the federal government purchases hospital, home health, nursing home, physician, and other medical services under contract with suppliers. The Medicaid system operates similarly. This vendor/purchaser arrangement stands in contrast to arrangements such as that in Great Britain, with a comprehensive program of national health insurance in which the government is both the payer and operator of the system. America's history of fierce resistance from the private sector, both organized medicine and, to an extent, the voluntary medicine and hospital system, has resisted enactment of a comprehensive national health care system. Private sector lobby resistance can be traced from the early 20th century's attempts to provide some form of national health insurance through the failure of the Clinton administration's National Health Security Act in 1994.

Medicare and Medicaid, comprising the majority of public spending on health, are discussed below. Chapter 10 discusses other government-financed programs.

Medicare

Were it not for the successful opposition of the private sector led by the AMA, the Social Security Act of 1935, the most significant piece of social legislation ever enacted by the federal government, would have included a form of national health insurance. It was not to be for another 30 years, during which time many presidential and congressional acts for national health insurance had been proposed and defeated, that Congress enacted Medicare, "Health Insurance for the Aged," Title XVIII of the Social Security Act, in 1965. Medicare became only the second mandated health insurance program in the United States, after workers' compensation. Today, the Medicare program covers 44 million Americans, including most 65 years of age and older, younger individuals who receive Social Security Disability Insurance (SSDI) benefits, and individuals with end-stage kidney disease and Lou Gehrig's disease following their eligibility for SSDI. Projected 2006 expenditures total $374 billion, approximately 14% of the federal budget.[54]

The enactment of Medicare legislation was a historical benchmark. By giving every American 65 years of age or older covered by the Social Security system entitlement to a range of medical benefits, it signaled government's entry into the personal care financing arena. On the federal level, the Medicare program was established under the aegis of the Social Security Administration, and hospital payment was contracted to local intermediaries chosen by hospitals. Over 90% of hospitals chose their local Blue Cross association as the intermediary. In response to organized medicine's opposition to government certification, the Social Security Administration agreed to accreditation by the private Joint Commission on Accreditation of Hospitals as meeting the certification requirement for Medicare participation.[55] Describing the enactment of Medicare as a "watershed," Rosemary Stevens wrote the following:[55]

> Thus with the stroke of a pen, the elderly acquired hospital benefits, the hospitals acquired cost reimbursement for these benefits, the Blue Cross Association was precipitated into prominence as a major national organization (since the national contract was to be with the association, with subcontracting to local plans), and the Joint Commission was given formal government recognition.

The Medicare amendment stated that there should be "prohibition against any federal interference with the practice of medicine or the way medical services were provided."[56] Ultimately, however, the government's acceptance of responsibility for payment for the care of older adults generated a flood of regulations to address cost and quality control of the services and products for which it was now a major payer.

As originally implemented, the Medicare program consisted of two parts, which differed in sources of funding and benefits. Part A provided benefits for care provided in the hospital, outpatient diagnostic services, extended care facilities, short-term care at home required by an illness for which the patient was hospitalized, and Supplemental Medical Insurance. This portion of coverage was mandatory and was funded by Social Security payroll taxes. Part B was structured as a voluntary program covering physician services and services ordered by physicians, such as outpatient diagnostic tests, medical equipment and supplies, and home health services. This portion was funded from beneficiary premium payments, matched by general federal revenues.

The Balanced Budget Act of 1997 added Part C, known as Medicare + Choice, allowing MCOs to administer Medicare contracts. In 2003, the Medicare Prescription Drug, Improvement, and Modernization Act changed Part C to "Medicare Advantage," revising the administration of Medicare managed care programs and adding a new Part D for prescription drug coverage.

From the outset, Medicare coverage was not fully comprehensive and that remains true today. Beneficiaries are required to share costs through a system of deductibles and coinsurance. For Part A, the deductible requires beneficiaries to reach a set amount in personal outlays for hospitalization each 12-month period, and coinsurance requires that patients cover 20% of hospitalization costs. The program also limits total compensated days of hospital care on a lifetime pool of days. For Part B coverage, monthly premiums are deducted from Social Security payments. These limitations gave rise to a variety of private supplemental, or "Medi-gap," policies, designed to cover Medicare coinsurance and deductibles.[57]

From its inception, Medicare spending surpassed projections. Although hospital costs for the growing older adult population increased more rapidly than expected, the rise over projected Medicare expenses could not be explained in major part by that phenomenon. A 1976 study by the U.S. Human Resources Administration reviewed the first 10 years of Medicare hospital expenses. The study attributed less than 10% of increases to growing utilization and the growing older adult population. Almost one-fourth of the increase over projected hospital costs was attributed to general inflation and two thirds to huge growth in hospital payroll and nonpayroll expenses, including profits.[56]

Like Blue Cross, Medicare's hospital reimbursement mechanism was cost based and retrospective on a per-day-of-stay basis. While facilitating the rapid incorporation of almost 20 million beneficiaries into the new benefit system, cost-based reimbursement also fueled utilization in an era of rapidly advancing medical technology. Paid on a retrospective basis for costs incurred, hospitals had a strong incentive toward utilization of services with no incentives for efficiency.

In the decade after Medicare and Medicaid enactment, several amendments to the Social Security Act made significant changes to both programs. In general, amendments of the first 5 years increased the types of covered services and expanded the population of eligible persons. During the later period, amendments addressed a rising tide of concerns about the costs and quality of the programs.

Cost Control and Quality Initiatives

Many initiatives attempted to slow spiraling costs and address quality concerns. They were largely unsuccessful. In 1966, Congress enacted the Comprehensive Health Planning Act (CHP) to support states in conducting local health planning to ensure adequate facilities and services and avoid duplications.[58] In 1974, the Health Planning Resources and Development Act replaced the CHP with Health Systems Agencies (HSAs) to develop plans for local health resources based on quantified population needs. The act also required all states to obtain approval from a state planning agency before starting any major capital project and several states adopted certificate-of-need legislation for this purpose. Congress repealed the federal mandate in 1987, but 36 states still maintain some form of certificate-of-need program, strongly focused on development of physician-owned facilities such as ambulatory surgery and diagnostic imaging centers.[59] HSAs were unsuccessful in materially influencing decisions about service or technology expansion, as decisions were dominated by institutional and economic interests. Concurrent with attempts to slow cost increases through a planning approach, a number of other legislative initiatives took shape that were directly related to concerns over Medicare costs and service quality.

Professional standards review organizations (PSROs) established in 1972 signaled the first federal attempt to review care provided under Medicare, Medicaid, and certain other federally-funded health care programs.[60] Each local PSRO was a not-for-profit organization composed of a representative group of local physicians who performed record reviews and made payment recommendations to the local Medicare intermediary. Plagued by questionable effectiveness and high administrative costs, PSROs were replaced by peer review organizations (PROs).[61] In 2001, peer review organizations were renamed quality improvement organizations as part of broad quality improvement initiatives of the Centers for Medicare and Medicaid Services.

In addition to the expansion of services and facilities occurring in the voluntary hospital sector, investor-owned for-profit hospitals saw the opportunity for expansion offered by Medicare's guarantee of full-cost reimbursement. By 1970, there were 29 investor-owned for-profit hospital chains. Both not-for-profit and for-profit hospital enterprises proliferated without the controlling impact of market competition. By 1980, over 90% of hospital expenditures were flowing through organized third parties: government, Blue Cross, or commercial insurers.

The Omnibus Budget Reconciliation Acts of 1980 and 1981 (OBRA) again amended the Medicare legislation with a strong focus on reducing hospitalizations and lengths of hospital stay. Amendments advocated home health services as an alternative to hospitalization by eliminating the limit on the annual number of reimbursable home health care visits, a 3-day hospitalization requirement for home health visit coverage eligibility, and the need for occupational therapy as a requirement for initial entitlement to home health care services. The prior exclusion from Medicare participation of proprietary home health care agencies in states that did not require agency licensure was also lifted.

Diagnosis-Related Groups

In 1983, Congress enacted a case payment system that radically changed hospital reimbursement under Medicare. In the new scheme, reimbursement for hospital operating costs shifted from the retrospective to prospective mode. The diagnosis-related groups (DRGs) were developed for the Health Care Financing Administration as a patient classification scheme that provided a means of relating the type of patients a hospital treated (i.e., its case mix) to the costs. The DRG payment system based hospital payments on established fees for services required to treat specific diagnoses rather than discreet units of services. The DRGs work by grouping the 10,000+ International Classification of Disease codes into approximately 500 patient categories. Patients within each category are similar clinically and in terms of resource use.[62] DRGs form a manageable, clinically coherent set of patient classes that relate a hospital's case mix to the resource demands and associated costs experienced by the hospital. The payment an individual hospital receives under this system is ultimately calculated using input from a host of other data known to impact costs, such as hospital teaching status and wage data for its geographic location.

The DRG system changed hospital incentives from consuming resources toward efficiency and effectiveness. Instead of financially rewarding hospitals for high use of services through retrospective reimbursement, the DRG system provided incentives for the hospital to spend only what was needed to achieve optimal patient outcomes. If outcomes could be achieved at a cost lower than the preset payment, the hospital realized an excess payment for those cases. If the hospital spent more to treat cases than allowed, it absorbed the excess costs. The DRG system also made financial provisions for cases classified as "outliers" due to complications. The DRG system did not build in allowances to the payment rate for direct medical education expenses for teaching hospitals, hospital outpatient expenses, or capital expenditures. These continued to be reimbursed on a cost basis.

The principle of case-based prospective payment soon was adopted in varying forms by numerous states and private third-party payers as a basis for their hospital reimbursement systems.

Implementation of the prospective payment system raised numerous concerns among hospitals, health care providers, and consumers about its possible effects. Concerns included fears about premature hospital discharges, hospitals' questionable ability to streamline services to conform with preset payments, and the home health care industry's capacity to adapt to the anticipated increase in cases.

"Quicker and sicker" was the slogan popularized by the media during the first years of the prospective payment system to characterize the drive for shorter hospital stays. The media also popularized the term "patient dumping," referring to documented cases of hospitals' inappropriately transferring patients at high risk of long, expensive, and potentially unprofitable service needs to other hospitals.

Postimplementation research on the impact of the prospective payment system demonstrated that many early concerns were unfounded and that DRGs did have a measurable impact on the overall growth of Medicare spending. Also, advancements in medical care and technology of the 1980s increased resources available to treat Medicare patients. For example, until 1983, growth rates in Medicare expenditures for inpatient and outpatient services had increased at comparable rates. Beginning in 1983, Medicare outpatient services covered under Part B (hospital outpatient services and physician services not included in the prospective payment system) increased dramatically, in part offsetting impacts of prospective payment on total Medicare spending.[63] Medical advancements and changing physician practice patterns also affected costs in the inpatient setting.[64] The impact of the prospective payment system on patient care quality, as demonstrated by comparisons of selected quality indicators before and after the system's implementation, was the subject of extensive research. The federal Prospective Payment Assessment Commission (ProPAC) was established to monitor the effects of the prospective system, and empirical studies reviewed hospital readmission rates as one quality indicator.

On balance, the studies revealed few effects on Medicare patient readmission rates attributable to the new method of hospital payment.[64] The RAND Corporation also conducted several studies of another indicator of patient care quality, in-hospital mortality rates. The studies reviewed almost 17,000 records of Medicare patients admitted to hospitals for five common diagnoses. Findings included a drop of 24% in the average length of hospital stay for these conditions and an overall improvement in mortality rates among the diagnoses studied.[65]

Concerns about patient dumping were formally addressed in 1985 by the Consolidated Omnibus Budget Reconciliation Act and were refined by the Emergency Medical Treatment and Labor Act of 1986 (EMTALA), which required hospitals to provide care to everyone who presented in their emergency departments, regardless of ability to pay. Stiff financial penalties, as well as risk of the loss of Medicare certification by hospitals inappropriately transferring patients, accompanied the EMTALA provisions.[66]

Evidence indicates that the prospective payment system slowed hospital cost growth during the early years after implementation, largely through reductions in lengths of stay, hospital personnel, and new medical technologies; however, total Medicare cost growth later reaccelerated, in part because of increased volume in outpatient spending and other factors whose impact have not been clearly determined.[65] Concerns about the capacity of the home health care industry to meet anticipated increases in demand dissipated quickly. Both the not-for-profit and proprietary sectors of the industry responded by creating new or expanding existing home health care services as components of vertically integrated systems. In the early years of the prospective payment system, hospitals did not experience the predicted negative financial impact, and they actually posted substantial profits.[65] In fact, the federal government partially justified subsequent reductions in prospective payment on the basis that early payments were too high relative to costs.[66] It has even been suggested that the large surpluses generated by not-for-profit hospitals in the early years of prospective payment fueled hospital costs by making new surpluses available for investment.[67]

From the outset, the prospective payment system's cost-containment effectiveness was limited by its application to only inpatient hospital care for Medicare recipients. Aggressive shifting of Medicare-covered services to the outpatient setting and shifting hospital costs onto private pay patients were two major reactions that dampened the prospective payment system's cost-containment results.

Physician Reimbursement

Medicare physician reimbursement through Medicare Part B was fee-for-service, based on prevailing fees within a specified geographic area. The Medicare physician payment rate of increase averaged 18% annually between 1975 and 1987 and provoked legislative action.[68] Medicare first enacted a temporary price freeze for physician services.[69] Assessments of the price freeze suggested that physicians offset the lower fees by increasing the volume of services.[69] This raised the issue of whether physicians respond to fee pressures by using more services to compensate for lower reimbursement. Concerns over absolute cost increases and overuse of costly specialty care prompted additional congressional cost-containment action.

The OBRA of 1989 established a new method of Medicare physician reimbursement that became effective in 1992.[70] The method used a resource-based relative value scale (RBRVS) to replace the fee-for-service reimbursement system. The RBRVS system was an attempt to contain costs by instituting the same payments for the same services, whether performed by a generalist or specialist physician. The RBRVS system included three components: a measure of total work performed, an allowance for medical practice costs, and an allowance for malpractice insurance expense. The system assigned each service a specified number of relative value units, multiplied by a national conversion factor to arrive at the fee. The relative value units were adjusted for geographic area variations in costs. The hoped-for results were reductions in the numbers of expensive procedures and lowering the incentive for physicians to specialize. The RBRVS continues in use. A committee involving the AMA and national medical specialty societies makes recommendations for annual updates.[70]

The Balanced Budget Act of 1997

Medicare reforms enacted by the prospective payment system and regulatory efforts of the 1980s and influences of managed care, market competition, technology advances, and consumerism produced unprecedented changes in physician practice patterns, hospitals' affinities for technology, and consumer expectations of hospital care. The Medicare prospective payment system even succeeded in demonstrating that "more is not necessarily better," as lengths of stay and service intensity declined to accommodate the DRG framework, with no demonstrable negative impact on the overall quality of patient care. Then, in the early 1990s, the nation witnessed one of the most vigorously debated issues of the century: the Clinton administration's National Health Security Act. Although the act never reached a congressional vote, many months of debate thrust national concerns about increased Medicare spending, lack of access to services, beneficiary costs, and provider choice into the public spotlight. Popular and political sensitivities to these issues continued to rise against the backdrop of an escalating national dialogue about predictions of the potential insolvency of the Hospital Insurance Trust Fund.[71]

Several trends supported the need for major changes in the Medicare system. First, the Congressional Budget Office was projecting that

Medicare costs would grow at approximately 9% per year while the economy would expand at approximately 5%, suggesting that the Medicare program would soon require cuts in other government programs, major increases in taxes, or larger budget deficits.[72]

Second, the structure of the Medicare program was becoming rapidly outmoded. Medicare remained a fee-for-service indemnity program, whereas employer-sponsored plans, Medicaid, and private insurance plans were rapidly embracing managed care principles. Recognition was growing that a program of Medicare's relative size in terms of total national health care expenditures could not resist current trends in health care financing and consumer sensitivity.

Third, Medicare coverage left significant gaps requiring co-pays and co-insurance that many beneficiaries were unable to fill with supplemental "Medi-gap" insurance policies. Although some Medicare beneficiaries were eligible for Medicaid subsidies of these expenses, subsidies created additional state financial burdens.

After acknowledgment of the president's and Congress's discord on a national health reform program, in 1995, congressional attention sharply focused on stemming the tide of Medicare cost growth and how to achieve broader choices for Medicare beneficiaries through managed care plans, which were providing models of cost-containment and consumer satisfaction.[73] Additional reform measures were needed to ensure that Medicare would meet the needs of the baby-boom generation with the same benefits as their predecessors.[73]

During the presidential and congressional campaigns of 1996, public knowledge of the health care issues was brought to light during debate on the National Health Security Act, and emerging consumer concerns about managed care coalesced into the rapid formulation and passage of the Health Insurance Portability and Accountability Act of 1996, also called the Kassenbaum-Kennedy Bill. Among its important health insurance features, the act included prohibiting insurance companies from denying coverage because of preexisting medical conditions or denying the sale of personal insurance policies to individuals who were previously covered in group plans. It also established a pilot program to enable workers to save tax-free dollars for future medical expenses through medical savings accounts.[74] Although the act accomplished some beneficial outcomes, it by no means addressed the pervasive problems of the health care system in general or the Medicare and Medicaid programs in particular.

The 1998 federal budget process reflected pressures to produce a balanced budget and to respond meaningfully to national health issues from both the consumer and cost-containment perspectives. The resulting Balanced Budget Act (BBA) created major new policy directions for Medicare and Medicaid and took important incremental steps toward universal coverage through an initiative to insure uninsured children through a $23 billion allocation for a new State Children's Health Insurance Program (SCHIP).[75]

The act was characterized as containing "some of the most sweeping and significant changes to Medicare and Medicaid since their inception in 1965."[75] Overall, the BBA proposed to reduce growth in Medicare and Medicaid spending by $125.2 billion in 5 years through regulatory changes and payment changes to hospitals, physicians, postacute-care services and MCOs. It increased premiums for Medicare Part B. It required new prospective payment systems for hospital outpatient services, skilled nursing facilities, home health agencies, and rehabilitation hospitals. It reduced allowances for indirect medical education expenses of teaching hospitals and funded incentives to hospitals for voluntarily reducing the numbers of medical residents. As the largest Medicare spender, the BBA targeted hospitals for more than one-third of total anticipated savings (Figure 7-7).

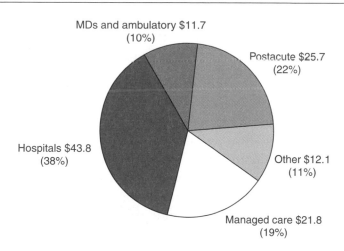

FIGURE 7-7 Sources, Percent, and Dollar Amount in Billions, of Contributions toward Balanced Budget Act Savings.
Source: Congressional Budget Office.

Decreased Medicare spending growth in the period 1998–2002 demonstrated the immediate impact of the BBA. After growing at an average annual rate of 11.1% for the 15 years before 1997, the average annual rate of spending growth between 1998 and 2000 dropped to 1.7%, resulting in approximately $68 billion in savings.[76]

Among the most significant policy shifts of the BBA was opening the Medicare program to private insurers through the Medicare + Choice Program. For the first time, this allowed sharing of financial risk for the Medicare program with the private sector. The participation of private insurers was intended to increase both the impact of competitive market forces on the program and consumer awareness of alternatives to the fee-for-service system.

The BBA constituted federal commissions to carry out monitoring and recommendation functions during implementation, including the Medicare Payment Advisory Commission and an independent National Bipartisan Commission on the Future of Medicare whose functions entailed the following:[77]

- Reviewing and analyzing Medicare's financial condition over time
- Formulating recommendations on
  - Ways to ensure the future financial viability of the Hospital Insurance Trust Fund
  - The scope and types of coverage to be included under the Medicare umbrella
  - The level of beneficiary premium contribution
  - Age eligibility
  - Contributions to medical education

Implementation of the Medicare BBA provisions experienced delays, widespread controversy, and many revisions. Significant changes to the Medicare and Medicaid program structure, payment methods, and amounts all drew fire from industry advocacy groups, professional organizations, and consumers. In the testimony of the U.S. Comptroller General before the U.S. Senate Special Committee on Aging in early 1999, "The outcry from providers to undo BBA reforms aimed at savings and efficiency was intense. In response, Congress made refinements."[78] Just before the date when several of the BBA's provisions were to take effect, President Clinton signed the Consolidated Appropriations Act for Fiscal Year 2000, providing $17 billion in additional allocations for health care providers negatively impacted by the BBA and outlining later implementation schedules for many of the BBA's original mandates. The initial impact of BBA reimbursement reductions along with other factors occurring in 1998 appeared to slow the actual rate of Medicare spending growth further than anticipated by the BBA alone. Other factors affecting the rate of Medicare spending growth in 1999 were widespread publication of initiatives to curtail Medicare fraud and abuse and a dramatic rise in the average time for processing claims as a result of more stringent criteria for claims review.[79]

By 1999, only 6.5 million, approximately 16% of beneficiaries had opted for Medicare + Choice.[80] The Medicare managed care enrollment initiative experienced serious challenges. Because of reduced Medicare reimbursement, costs of working with federal bureaucracy, and market shifts reducing profitability, MCOs lost their early enthusiasm for participation in the program. Plan withdrawals affected about 2.2 million beneficiaries in the first few years of Medicare + Choice operation.[81] To stimulate and maintain MCO participation in Medicare + Choice, Congress enacted the Balanced Budget Refinement Act of 1999 (BBRA) to slow payment reductions, provide bonuses for establishing plans in new geographic areas, and provide exemptions from quality assurance requirements for PPOs. In addition, the Benefits Protection and Improvement Act of 2000 enacted provisions to increase MCO and provider payments.[82]

The Medicare Prescription Drug, Improvement, and Modernization Act of 2003

The MMA of 2003 renamed the Medicare + Choice managed care program "Medicare Advantage," established several new plan options and created a prescription drug program for all Medicare beneficiaries. In part, the MMA responded to the lessons learned from professional, political, economic, and popular responses to the Medicare + Choice program. The MMA has been cited as enacting the most far-reaching changes in the Medicare program since its inception and as "one of the most complex pieces of health care legislation to pass Congress."[83,84]

In 2007, 80% of Medicare beneficiaries received benefits through the traditional Medicare fee-for-service program, and 20% received benefits through Medicare Advantage private health plans. Since the introduction of Medicare Advantage, the number of enrollees in private plans has increased significantly, from 5.3 million in 2003 to 8.7 million in 2007 (Figure 7-8).[85]

A key feature of the MMA was the establishment of the Part D prescription drug plan to provide financial relief from prescription costs, especially for low-income individuals. The MMA replaces Medicaid as the primary source of drug coverage for low income and disabled individuals who receive both Medicare and Medicaid benefits. The MMA also provides financial incentives for employers continuing retiree drug benefits with the intent of stabilizing the eroding trend of retiree drug benefits that began in the late 80s.[86] The drug benefit is offered through two types of private plans: stand alone plans that supplement fee-for-service Medicare, and Medicare Advantage plans such as HMOs or PPOs that cover drugs and other Medicare benefits. In 2006, the MMA began paying for outpatient prescription drugs through private plans available to

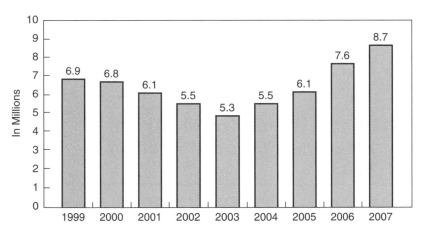

Note: Includes local HMOs, PSOs, and PPOs, regional PPOs, PFFS plans, Cost contracts, Demonstrations, HCPP, and PACE contracts.

FIGURE 7-8 Total Medicare Private Health Plan Enrollment, 1999–2007. *Source:* Medicare Advantage Fact Sheet (#2052-10). The Henry J. Kaiser Family Foundation, June 2007. *This information was reprinted with permission from the Henry J. Kaiser Family Foundation. The Kaiser Family Foundation, based in Menlo Park, California, is a nonprofit, private operating foundation focusing on the major health care issues facing the nation and is not associated with Kaiser Permanente or Kaiser Industries.*

Medicare Advantage enrollees and those who chose to remain in the traditional Medicare program. Under the standard drug benefit in 2007, beneficiaries paid[87]

- The first $265 in drug costs (deductible)
- 25% up to total drug costs of $2,400 (co-insurance)
- 100% of drug costs up to $3,850 out of pocket ("the doughnut hole")
- 5% co-insurance after reaching the $3,850 out-of-pocket limit

The MMA provides additional payment assistance to beneficiaries with very low incomes or limited assets.

When Congress passed the MMA, the prescription drug benefit cost was estimated at $400 billion for the 10 years after inception. In 2005, President Bush's federal budget estimates placed the 10-year cost at $720 billion, igniting a storm of responses from members of Congress.[88] Current projections place the program cost over the period 2008–2016 at $933 billion.[87] MMA legislation prohibits Medicare from negotiating directly with drug companies for discounts. There is no such prohibition for private plans administering Part D, and it is anticipated that private plan price negotiations will assist in holding down costs.[87] The MMA also provides several demonstration projects to test potential future improvements in Medicare coverage, expenditure controls, and quality of care.[89]

Ongoing Cost Reduction and Quality Improvement Initiatives

In 2001, the Department of Health and Human Services and Centers for Medicare and Medicaid Services inaugurated the "Quality Initiative," encompassing every dimension of the health care delivery system. Launched nationally in 2002, the Quality Initiative includes nursing homes, hospitals, home health care agencies, physicians, and other facilities.[90] The program collects and analyzes data from each participant group to monitor conformance with standards of care and performance. In addition to the Quality Initiative, the Medicare Quality Monitoring System "processes, analyzes, interprets and disseminates health-related data to monitor the quality of care delivered to Medicare fee-for-service beneficiaries."[91] The Medicare administration also is experimenting with hospital pay-for-performance plans designed to improve quality and avoid unnecessary costs.[92] With the goal of providing public, credible, valid, and user-friendly information about hospital quality, in 2005, Medicare launched the website, "Hospital Compare," encompassing four common conditions and 20 criteria that assess individual hospitals' consistency of conformance with evidence-based practice.[93] In 2007, the Medicare administration announced that beginning in 2008 it will no longer pay for procedures resulting from hospital-acquired infections. This is the first step in an aggressive initiative to identify quality standards as a basis for public reporting and payment. In consultation with the Hospital Quality Forum and many other expert organizations, Medicare has identified a list of seven categories of untoward hospital events for which it is investigating hospital payment reductions for resulting treatment.[94,95]

Medicaid

In 1965, Medicaid legislation was enacted as Title XIX of the Social Security Act. Medicaid is administered by the Centers for Medicare and Medicaid Services and is a mandatory joint federal–state program in which federal and state support is shared based on the state's per capita income. Prior to Medicaid's implementation, health care services for the economically needed were provided through a patchwork of programs sponsored by state and local governments, charitable organizations, and community hospitals.

Today, Medicaid finances health care and long-term care services for 45.6 million low-income Americans.[96] The program represents a major source of health care system funding, accounting for approximately one-fifth of $1.7 billion in personal health services spending and almost 45% of spending for nursing home care in 2005 (Figure 7-9).[97]

The federal government establishes broad guidelines for the program, but program requirements are the prerogative of state governments. Medicaid requires states to cover certain types of individuals or groups under their plans and states may include others at their discretion. The program provides three types of coverage:[98]

- Health insurance for low-income families with children
- Long-term care for older Americans and individuals with disabilities

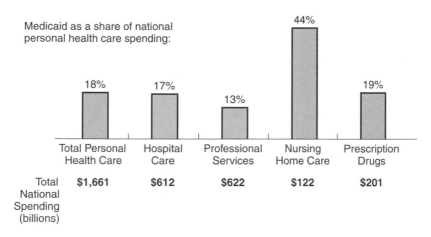

FIGURE 7-9 Medicaid in the Health System, 2005.
Source: Centers for Medicare and Medicaid Services, National Health Care Expenditure Data, 2005.

- Supplemental coverage for low-income Medicare beneficiaries for services not covered by Medicare, including Medicare premiums, deductibles, and co-insurance

Until the enactment of Medicare Part D, the third type of coverage also paid for prescription drugs.

Medicaid federal guidelines established a mandated core of basic medical services that must be available in each state program. Included were inpatient and outpatient hospital services, physician services, diagnostic services, and nursing home care for adults. Later Medicaid amendments expanded mandated benefits to include home health care, preventive health screening services, family planning services, and assistance to recipients of Supplemental Security Income. State Medicaid programs currently must extend benefits to all pregnant women who meet federal income level guidelines and children whose family incomes fall below specified federal income guidelines. Individual states have broad discretion to include additional services in their Medicaid programs, and many have elected extended benefits well beyond the core of mandated benefits.

The sources of funds for Medicaid are distinct from those for Medicare. Medicare, funded from contributions of payroll taxes matched by employers, is an entitlement because individuals have contributed to their cost of coverage. Medicaid, which is funded by personal income and corporate and excise taxes, is a transfer payment representing funds transferred from more economically affluent individuals to those in need.[99]

Unlike Medicare, which reimburses providers through intermediaries such as Blue Cross, Medicaid reimburses service providers directly. Rate-setting formulas, procedures, and policies vary widely among states. Because of the variations in benefits and reimbursement policies, Medicaid has been described as "50 different programs."[99]

Throughout the 1980s, as costs grew rapidly, states tested various prepaid, managed care approaches and some implemented prospective payment systems modeled on DRG reimbursement. Several states experimented with voluntary Medicaid managed care enrollment, contracting with HMOs to provide some or all of their Medicaid benefits under federally approved demonstration projects. Today, all 50 states offer some type of Medicaid managed care plans. Through a provision of the BBA, the federal government allows states to mandate managed care enrollment for their Medicaid beneficiaries without prior approval.

Over 65% of Medicaid beneficiaries are enrolled in managed care plans.[96] The number and proportion of Medicaid enrollees in managed care continue to increase as states seek ways to control costs and ensure access (Table 7-1 and Figure 7-10). All states are struggling with the burden of rising Medicaid costs; however, experience suggests that most view Medicaid managed care as preferable to the fee-for-service system and will likely make the necessary accommodations to ensure that they do not relinquish the value managed care has brought to beneficiaries and purchasers, regardless of the reforms that may be undertaken to curtail increasing costs.[100]

The Balanced Budget Act: Medicaid and the State Children's Health Insurance Program

Provisions of the BBA intended to reduce the growth of federal Medicaid outlays by $10.1 billion over 5 years. Sources of anticipated savings included reduced payments to hospitals serving a disproportionate share of low-income patients, reduced federal cost sharing for "dual eligibles" entitled to both Medicare and Medicaid benefits, and enforcement of new fraud and abuse provisions.

Table 7-1 Medicaid Managed Care Trends, 1997–2006

Year	Total Medicaid Population	Managed Care Population	Other Population	% Managed Care Enrollment
2006	45,652,642	29,830,406	15,822,236	65.34%
2005	45,392,325	28,575,585	16,816,740	62.95%
2004	44,355,955	26,913,570	17,442,385	60.68%
2003	42,740,719	25,262,873	17,477,846	59.11%
2002	40,147,539	23,117,668	17,029,871	57.58%
2001	36,562,567	20,773,813	15,788,754	56.82%
2000	33,690,364	18,786,137	14,904,227	55.76%
1999	31,940,188	17,756,603	14,183,585	55.59%
1998	30,896,635	16,573,996	14,322,639	53.64%
1997	32,092,380	15,345,502	16,746,878	47.82%

These figures represent point-in-point enrollment as of June 30th for each reporting year. The **unduplicated** managed care enrollment figures include enrollees receiving comprehensive benefits and limited benefits. This table also provides **unduplicated** national figures for the Total Medicaid population and Other population. The statistics also include individuals enrolled in State health care reform programs that expand eligibility beyond traditional Medicaid eligibility standards.

Source: Centers for Medicare and Medicaid Services, 2006 Medicaid Managed Care Enrollment report, Summary Statistics as of June 30, 2006.

The BBA contained a major child health initiative to build on the Medicaid program by targeting uninsured children whose family income was too high to qualify for Medicaid and too low to afford private health insurance. SCHIP targeted enrollment of 5 million children with $24 billion in federal matching funds for states over the 10-year period of 1998 to 2007.[101] The BBA granted states federal block grant funds and provided authority to use any of three vehicles, singly or in combination, for establishing their programs to provide coverage for uninsured children. Methods included increased Medicaid funding, state health insurance programs, or direct payment for services using up to 15% of block grants.

By 1999, all 50 states were receiving federal support from BBA allocations under the SCHIP. By 2006, 10 years after passage of the authorizing legislation, 6.6 million children had been enrolled in the program (Figure 7-11).[101] Currently, about half of the 33.2 million low-income children receive health care coverage from public programs, whereas 29% have private coverage (Figure 7-12). Twenty-eight million children are enrolled in the Medicaid program, in addition to the 6.6 million enrolled in SCHIPs.[102] Nine million children remain uninsured.

Because of reauthorization in 2007, a revised SCHIP was proposed with broad bipartisan support for a $60 billion allocation over 5 years to

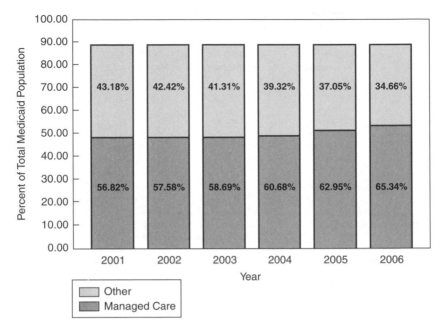

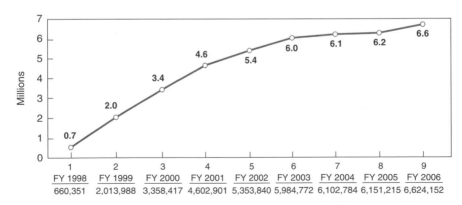

FIGURE 7-10 Total Annual Medicaid Population Distribution by Year: Managed Care versus Other As of June 30, 2006.
Source: Centers for Medicare and Medicaid Services, 2006 Medicaid Managed Care Enrollment Report, Summary Statistics as of June 30, 2006.

FIGURE 7-11 Numbers ever enrolled in the State Children's Health Insurance Program by Year, 1998–2006.
Source: Centers for Medicare and Medicaid Services.

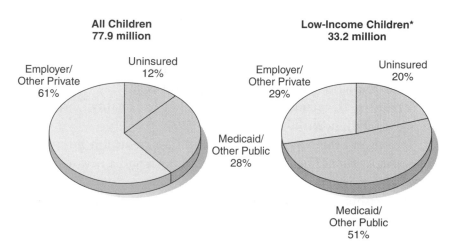

All Children
77.9 million

Low-Income Children*
33.2 million

*Below 200% of the federal poverty level, or $39,942 for a family of four in 2005 (according to the U.S. Census Bureau's poverty thresholds). Data may not total 100% due to rounding.

FIGURE 7-12 Health Insurance Coverage of Children by Income, 2005. *Source:* Health Coverage for Low-Income Children. (#2144-05). The Henry J. Kaiser Family Foundation, June 2007. *This information was reprinted with permission from the Henry J. Kaiser Family Foundation. The Kaiser Family Foundation, based in Menlo Park, California, is a nonprofit, private operating foundation focusing on the major health care issues facing the nation and is not associated with Kaiser Permanente or Kaiser Industries.*

continue coverage for current enrollees and to cover 4 million additional children. Both houses of Congress support passage, but President Bush pledges a veto based on the cost and because the program constitutes "an incremental step toward the goal of government-run health care."[103] The reauthorization outcome awaits final action by Congress and the President.

Medicaid Quality Initiatives

The Center for Medicaid and State Operations has the principle responsibility for developing and carrying out Medicaid and SCHIP quality initiatives through working partnerships with the respective state's programs. The center's statement of purpose cites working "in partnership to achieve safe, effective, efficient, patient-centered, timely and equitable care."[104]

The Center for Medicaid and State Operations articulates a quality strategy encompassing six key elements:

- Evidence-based care and quality measurement: achieve consistency in performance measurement through consensus
- Pay-for-performance: promote payment for quality, access, efficiency, and successful outcomes
- Health information technology: build a new health information infrastructure using electronic health records and a new network to link records nationwide
- Partnerships: engage internal and external expert organizations
- Information dissemination and technical assistance: share best practices, innovative models, and other information of value to stakeholders
- Health care disparities: engage in collaborations and incorporate a health disparities component into quality initiatives

A recently created Division of Quality, Evaluation, and Health Outcomes will focus on providing technical assistance to states in their quality improvement initiatives.

On the Horizon

In a Henry J. Kaiser Family Foundation health tracking poll conducted in summer of 2007 that focused on the 2008 presidential election, participants named health care as the top domestic issue they wanted presidential candidates to address, trailing only the Iraq war in priority. Nearly 6 in 10 people did not know or could not name a candidate who best represents their own views on health.[105] Given voter interest, candidates are speaking about their plans for health care system reforms, but if the poll is an indicator, they are not yet articulating with sufficient clarity.

With virtually no federal action in recent years to address rising costs and declining access, states are leading with experimentation to meet their health care challenges. Proposed in 2005 and passed in 2006, Massachusetts has enacted a model that is very close to universal coverage. The plan uses a mandate of personal responsibility to purchase health insurance combined with government subsidies to ensure affordability.[106] In addition to the individual mandate, the plan requires all but the smallest employers to provide health insurance coverage or pay a per-employee "fair-share" annual contribution. Employers also must offer a plan allowing workers to purchase health care with pretax dollars or pay a "free rider" surcharge if employees make excessive use of uncompensated care. The plan makes approved, affordable, quality insurance products available to individuals and small businesses through a "connector" and through a special fund provides government subsidies to assist low-income individuals with premiums. It also expands the state's Medicaid program by raising adult and children's income eligibility caps. The plan also converts the existing uncompensated care pool into a new Health Safety Net Trust Fund to combine with other Medicaid and hospital disproportionate share funds anticipating that as uncompensated care drops, funds will be shifted into the health insurance subsidy program. Finally, mergers with the individual and small-group insurance markets will be combined, resulting in a minor increase in business premiums and a major decrease in individual premiums. In just 1 year after passage, over 100,000 previously uninsured individuals had gained coverage, Medicaid enrollment increased by 53,000, and 80,000 individuals had enrolled in the subsidized insurance program.

In an analysis of the Massachusetts plan, the Kaiser Commission on Medicaid and the Uninsured cites important considerations for future reform proposals. Considerations include the value of the Medicaid system as a foundation, the importance of adequate subsidies and benefits to encourage a critical mass of early enrollment, and the creativity of combining different strategies across the political spectrum to gain support from key stakeholders.[106]

Also in 2006, Vermont enacted a plan with over 35 special initiatives targeted to increase access, contain costs, and improve quality.[107] The plan includes a new health insurance product for the uninsured that provides premium assistance. It also provides for employer-sponsored premium assistance, employer contributions, and a statewide plan for preventing and managing chronic conditions.

Citing billions of dollars in "hidden taxes" in the forms of higher premiums, co-pays, and deductibles to absorb the costs of treating the state's 6.5 million uninsured, in 2007, California's Governor Schwarzenegger proposed a health care reform plan.[108] Primary tenets of the plan would be coverage for all residents, prevention and health promotion, affordability, and cost-containment. The plan would:

- Require all residents to have health insurance
- Require insurers to guarantee coverage with affordable products
- Encourage healthy lifestyles through incentives and rewards
- Expand access to the Medicaid program
- Assist low-income workers with premium subsidy from a new, state-administered purchasing pool
- Increase Medicaid rates to encourage more provider participation
- Increase efficiency by requiring HMOs, insurers, and hospitals to spend 85% of each premium dollar on patient care
- Enhance tax advantages for individuals and employers for the purchase of insurance
- Assess a "coverage dividend" of 2% on physicians and 4% on hospitals to cover increased Medicaid rates, in recognition of the financial benefits of increased Medicaid rates and eliminating the uninsured
- Assess an "in lieu fee" of 4% on employers of 10 or more who do not provide coverage

As these experiments demonstrate, the allocation of finite resources in a manner acceptable to political, professional, economic, and consumer interests defines the challenge of health care financing. Continued complacency about America's return on its health care investment is becoming more of a moral than economic issue as U.S. health status indicators lag seriously behind other developed countries while our nation spends multiple times more than its peers and leaves 16% of its population disenfranchised from the health care system.

Current and future policy makers have a daunting array of health care issues before them whose solutions will demand unprecedented creativity and courage to make meaningful changes. Paying for required changes may be considerably easier than breaking loose from old philosophies, value systems, and politics that have brought the U.S. health care system to its present paradoxical state of superior technology embedded in an antiquated system available on an increasingly selective basis.

References

1. Catlin A, Cowan C, Heffler S, et al. National health spending in 2005: the slowdown continues. *Health Affairs.* 2007;26:142–146.
2. Levit K, Lazenby H, Braden H, et al. National health expenditures, 1996. *Health Care Financing Rev.* 1997;19:162.

3. Levit K, Smith C, Cowan C, et al. Inflation spurs health spending in 2000. *Health Affairs.* 2002; 21:179.

4. U.S. Department of Health and Human Services, Administration on the Aging. A statistical profile of older americans aged 65+. Available from http://www.aoa.dhhs.gov/press/fact/pdf/ss_stat_profile.pdf. Accessed July 16, 2007.

5. Coile RC Jr, Trusko BE. Healthcare 2020: challenges of the millennium. *Health Care Manage Technol.* 1999;20:37.

6. DeFrances CJ, Hall MJ. 2005 national hospital discharge survey. *Advance Data* no. 385, Hyattsville, MD: national Center for Health Statistics. Available from http://www.cdc.gov/nchs/data/ad/ad385.pdf. Accessed July 31, 2007.

7. Smith S, Heffler S, Freeland M, et al. The next decade of health care spending: A new outlook. *Health Affairs.* 1999;18:89–90.

8. U.S. Department of Labor, Bureau of Labor Statistics. *Occupational outlook handbook 2006–07 edition.* Available from http://www.stats.bls.gov/oco/ocos074.htm#training. Accessed July 22, 2007.

9. Karen Davis The Commonwealth Fund. Census data on growing number of uninsured make clear: national health care strategy is needed. Available from http://www.commonwealthfund.org/General/General_show.htm?doc_id 519979. Accessed August 30, 2007.

10. Kaiser Commission on Medicaid and the Uninsured. Key facts about americans without health insurance. Available from http://www.illinois covered.com/assets/cover_7451.pdf. Accessed August 9, 2007.

11. American College of Physicians-American Society of Internal Medicine, No health insurance: it's enough to make you sick. Available from: http://www.acponline.org/uninsured. Accessed July 22, 2007.

12. U.S. Department of Labor, Bureau of Labor Statistics. Career guide to industries, 2006–2007 edition. Available from http://www.bls.gov/oco/cg/cgs035.htm#outlook. Accessed August 10, 2007.

13. Centers for Medicare and Medicaid Services. The nation's health dollar, calendar year 2005: where it went. Available from http://www.cms.hhs.gov/NationalHealthExpendData/downloads/PieChartSourcesExpenditures2005.pdf. Accessed July 12, 2007.

14. Centers for Medicare and Medicaid Services. National health expenditures aggregate amounts and average annual percent change, by type of expenditure: selected calendar years 1960–2005, Table 2. Available from http://www.cms.hhs.gov/NationalHealthExpendData/downloads/tables.pdf. Accessed July 12, 2007.

15. Centers for Medicare and Medicaid Services. The nation's health dollar, calendar year 2005: where it came from. Available from http://www.cms.hhs.gov/NationalHealthExpendData/downloads/PieChartSourcesExpenditures2005.pdf. Accessed July 12, 2007.

16. Stevens R. *In Sickness and in Wealth: American Hospitals in the Twentieth Century.* New York, NY: Basic Books; 1989:183.

17. Centers for Medicare and Medicaid Services. National health expenditures aggregate amounts and average annual percent change, by type of expenditure: selected calendar years 1960–2005, Table 2. Available from http://www.cms.hhs.gov/NationalHealthExpendData/downloads/tables.pdf. Accessed July 12, 2007

18. Wilson F, Neuhauser D. *Health services in the United States.* 2nd ed. Cambridge, MA: Ballinger Publishing Co; 1982.

19. Kovner A. *Jonas' Health Care Delivery in the United States.* 5th ed. New York, NY: Springer Publishing Co; 1995:275.

20. Stevens R. *In Sickness and in Wealth: American Hospitals in the Twentieth Century.* New York, NY: Basic Books; 1989:183.

21. Stevens R. *In Sickness and in Wealth: American Hospitals in the Twentieth Century.* New York, NY: Basic Books; 1989:190.

22. Stevens R. *In Sickness and in Wealth: American Hospitals in the Twentieth Century.* New York, NY: Basic Books; 1989:193.

23. Stevens R. *In Sickness and in Wealth: American Hospitals in the Twentieth Century.* New York, NY: Basic Books; 1989:260–261.

24. Kongstvedt PR. *The Managed Health Care Handbook.* Gaithersburg, MD: Aspen Publishers; 1989:17.

25. Kongstvedt PR. *The Managed Health Care Handbook.* Gaithersburg, MD: Aspen Publishers; 1989:12.

26. Miller R, Luft H. Managed care plans: characteristics, growth and premium performance. *Ann Rev Public Health.* 1994;15:439.

27. Claxton G, Gabel J, DiJulio B, et al. Health benefits in 2007: premium increases fall to an eight-year low, while offer rates and enrollment remain stable. *Health Affairs.* 2007;26:1407–1416.

28. The Henry J. Kaiser Family Foundation and Health Research and Educational Trust. Employee health benefits 2005 annual survey exhibit 5.1. Available from http://www.kff.org/insurance/7672. Accessed September 13, 2007.

29. Trespacz KL. Staff-model HMOs: don't blink or you'll miss them. *Managed Care Magazine.* Available from http://www.managedcaremag.com/archives/9907/9907.staffmodel.html. Accessed September 9, 2007.

30. U.S. Congressional Budget Office. Projections of national health expenditures: 1997–2008, the economic and budget outlook: fiscal years 1999-2008. Available from http://www.cbo.gov/showdoc.cfm?index=316&sequence=13. Accessed March 21, 2007.

31. Levit K, Cowan C, Lazenby H, et al. Health spending in 1998: signals of change. *Health Affairs* 2000;19:131.

32. The Henry J. Kaiser Family Foundation and Health Research and Educational Trust. Health insurance premiums rise 6.1 percent in 2007, less rapidly than recent years but still faster than wages and inflation. Available from http://www.kff.org/insurance/ehbs091107nr.cfm?RenderforPrint=1. Accessed September 13, 2007.

33. National Coalition on Health Care. Health insurance cost. Available from http://www.nchc.org/cost.html. Accessed August 19, 2007.

34. Centers for Medicare and Medicaid Services. Health care industry market update, managed care. Available from http://www.dmaa.org/pdf/CMSMkt UpdateManagedCare03.24.03.pdf. Accessed August 9, 2007.

35. Chernew M, Cutler D, Keenan P, et al. University of Michigan, Economic Research Institute on the Uninsured. Increasing health insurance costs and the decline in insurance coverage. Available from http://eriu.sph.umich.edu/pdf/wp8.pdf. Accessed September 4, 2007.

36. Blendon RJ, Brodie M, Benson J, et al. Understanding the managed care backlash. *Health Affairs*. 1998;17:80.

37. White House Backgrounder. President Clinton Releases report documenting actions federal government is taking to implement a patients' bill of rights. Available from http://www.hhs.gov/news/press/1998pres/981102.html. Accessed August 11, 2007.

38. National Conference of State Legislatures. Managed care state laws and regulations including consumer and provider protections. Available from http://www.ncsl.org/programs/health/hmolaws.htm. Accessed July 11, 2007.

39. Gabel JR, Pickreign JD, Witmore HH, et al. Behind the slow growth of employer-based consumer-driven health plans. Available from http://www.hschange.com/CONTENT/900/?topic=topic01#ib1. Accessed August 18, 2007.

40. Miller RH, Luft HS. HMO plan performance update: analysis of the literature, 1997–2001. *Health Affairs* 2002;21:81.

41. Iglehart JK. The National Committee for Quality Assurance. *N Engl J Med*. 1996;335:995.

42. National Committee on Quality Assurance. NCQA news release (July 30, 2007). Available from http://www.ncqa.org/tabod/522/default.aspx. Accessed September 14, 2007.

43. National Committee on Quality Assurance. Programs. Available from http://www.web.ncqa.org/tabid/58/default.aspx. Accessed September 11, 2007.

44. Pawlson L, O'Kane M. Professionalism, regulation, and the market: impact on accountability for quality of care. *Health Affairs*. 2002;21:202.

45. Epstein M. The role of quality measurement in a competitive marketplace. In: Altman SH, Reinhardt UE, eds. Strategic choices for a changing health care system. Chicago, IL: Health Administration Press; 1996:217.

46. National Committee on Quality Assurance. HEDIS and quality compass (2007 measures list). Available from: http://web.ncqa.org/Default.aspx?tabid=187. Accessed September 16, 2007.

47. National Committee on Quality Assurance. Helping people make informed decisions. Available from http://web.ncqa.org/tabid/67/default. aspx. Accessed September 16, 2007.

48. National Committee on Quality Assurance. Report cards. Available from http://hprc.ncqa.org/. Accessed September 16, 2007.

49. National Committee on Quality Assurance. The state of health care quality 2006: executive summary. Available from http://web.ncqa.org/Default.aspx?tabid=447. Accessed September 16, 2007.

50. National Committee on Quality Assurance. The state of health care quality 2006. Available from http://web.ncqa.org/Default.aspx?tabid=447. Accessed September 16, 2007.

51. National Committee on Quality Assurance. The state of health care quality 2004. Available from http://web.ncqa.org/tabid/447/Default.aspx. Accessed September 16, 2007.

52. Fireman B, Bartlett, J, Selby J, et al. Can disease management reduce health care costs by improving quality? *Health Affairs*. 2004;23:63–64

53. Butler PA. ERISA update: the Supreme Court Texas decision and other recent developments. *Academy Health*. 2004;5. Available from http://www.statecoverage.net/pdf/issuebrief804.pdf. Accessed August 9, 2007.

54. The Henry J. Kaiser Family Foundation. Medicare at a glance. Available from http://www.kff.org/medicare/upload/1066-10.pdf. Accessed August 17, 2007.

55. Stevens R. *In Sickness and in Wealth: American Hospitals in the Twentieth Century*. New York, NY: Basic Books; 1989:281–282.

56. Stevens R. *In Sickness and in Wealth: American Hospitals in the Twentieth Century*. New York, NY: Basic Books; 1989:286–287.

57. The Henry J. Kaiser Family Foundation. Insurance to supplement Medicare. Available from http://www.kff.org/medicare/7076/med_supplement.cfm. Accessed July 9, 2007.

58. U.S. Code: Title 42,246. Comprehensive health planning and services. Available from http://www.law.cornell.edu/uscode/html/uscode42/usc_sec_42_00000246-.html. Accessed August 9, 2007.

59. National Conference of State Legislatures. Certificate of need: state health laws and programs. Available from http://www.ncsl.org/programs/health/cert-need.htm. Accessed July 11, 2007.

60. Congressional Budget Office. Testimony on the professional standards review organizations program. Available from http://www.cbo.gov/ftpdoc.cfm?index=5226&type=0. Accessed July 7, 2007.

61. Compilation of the Social Security laws: Social Security online. Available from http://www.ssa.gov/OP_Home/ssact/title11/1154.htm. Accessed July 9, 2007.

62. Mistichelli J. National Reference Center for Bioethics Literature. Diagnosis-related groups and the prospective payment system: forecasting social implications. Available from http://bioethics.georgetown.edu/publications/scopenotes/sn4.pdf. Accessed August 14, 2007.

63. Thorpe KE. Health care cost containment: results and lessons from the past 20 years. In: Shortell SM, Reinhardt UE, eds. *Improving Health Policy and Management*. Ann Arbor, MI: Health Administration Press; 1992:241.

64. Thorpe KE. Health care cost containment: results and lessons from the past 20 years. In: Shortell SM, Reinhardt UE, eds. *Improving Health Policy and Management.* Ann Arbor, MI: Health Administration Press; 1992:246.

65. Thorpe KE. Health care cost containment: results and lessons from the past 20 years. In: Shortell SM, Reinhardt UE, eds. *Improving Health Policy and Management.* Ann Arbor, MI: Health Administration Press; 1992:240.

66. Centers for Medicare and Medicaid Services. EMTALA overview. Available from http://www.cms.hhs.gov/EMTALA. Accessed July 9, 2007.

67. Thorpe KE. Health care cost containment: results and lessons from the past 20 years. In: Shortell SM, Reinhardt UE, eds. *Improving Health Policy and Management.* Ann Arbor, MI: Health Administration Press, 1992:244.

68. Kovner A, *Jonas' Health Care Delivery in the United States.* 5th ed. New York, NY: Springer Publishing Co; 1995:316.

69. Thorpe KE. Health care cost containment: results and lessons from the past 20 years. In: Shortell SM, Reinhardt UE, eds. *Improving Health Policy and Management.* Ann Arbor, MI: Health Administration Press, 1992:249.

70. The American Medical Association. Overview of RBRVS. Available from http://www.ama-assn.org/ama/pub/category/16392.html. Accessed August 14, 2007.

71. Board of Trustees, Federal Hospital Insurance Trust Fund. *1995 Annual Report of the Board of Trustees of the Hospital Insurance Trust Fund.* Washington, DC: U.S. Government Printing Office; 1995.

72. Reischauer RD. Medicare: beyond 2002, preparing for the baby-boomers. *Brookings Rev.* 1997;15:24.

73. Reischauer RD. Medicare: beyond 2002, preparing for the baby-boomers. *Brookings Rev.* 1997;15:318.

74. U.S. Department of Labor-Health Plans-Portability of Health Coverage. Available from http://www.dol.gov/ebsa/newsroom/fshipaa.html. Accessed August 12, 2007.

75. *The Balanced Budget Act of 1997, Public Law 105-33, Medicare and Medicaid Changes.* Washington, DC: Deloitte & Touche LLP and Deloitte & Touche Consulting Group LLC; 1997:1.

76. Medicare Payment Advisory Commission. Report to the Congress: Medicare payment policy (March 2003), chapter 1, context for Medicare spending. Available from http://www.medpac.gov/publications/congressional_reports/Mar03_Entire_report.pdf. Accessed August 16, 2007.

77. National Bipartisan Commission on the Future of Medicare-Task Forces. Available from http://medicare.commission.gov/medicare/task.html. Accessed July 19, 2007.

78. U.S. Senate Special Committee on Aging. Medicare: program reform and modernization are needed but entail considerable challenges. 106th Congress, 1st session, February 8, 2000:13.

79.   U.S. Congressional Budget Office, U.S. Senate Committee on Finance. The impact of the Balanced Budget Act on the Medicare Fee-for-Service Program. June 10, 1999, by Paul N. Van de Water, Assistant Director for Budget Analysis, 2. Washington, DC: U.S. Congressional Budget Office.

80.   Health Care Financing Administration. First Medicare + Choice private fee-for-service plan approved. Available from *Medicare News*. http://www. hcfa.gov. Accessed July 13, 2007.

81.   Berenson RA. Medicare + Choice: doubling or disappearing? *Health Affairs* Web Exclusives 2001:W66; November 28, 2001. Available from http:// content.healthaffairs.org/cgi/reprint/hlthaff.w1.65v1?maxtoshow=&HITS= 10&hits=10&RESULTFORMAT=&author1=Berenson&fulltext=Medicare +%2BChoice&andorexactfulltext=and&searchid=1&FIRSTINDEX=0& resourcetype=HWCIT. Accessed July 13, 2007.

82.   Ross MN. Paying Medicare + Choice plans: the view from MedPac. Health Affairs Web Exclusive (2001). Available from http://content.healthaffairs. org/cgi/reprint/hlthaff.w1.90v1?maxtoshow=&HITS=10&hits=10& RESULTFORMAT=&author1=M.N.+Ross&fulltext=Medicare+%2B Choice&andorexactfulltext=and&searchid=1&FIRSTINDEX=0& resourcetype=HWCIT. Accessed September 16, 2007.

83.   Biles B, Dallek G, Nicholas LM, et al. Medicare advantage: déjà vu all over again? Health Affairs Web Exclusive. December 15, 2004:1, 4–5. Available from http://content.healthaffairs.org/cgi/reprint/hlthaff.w4.586v1?maxto show=&HITS=10&hits=10&RESULTFORMAT=&author1=Biles& fulltext=Deja+Vu&andorexactfulltext=and&searchid=1&FIRSTINDEX= 0&resourcetype=HWCIT. Accessed July 14, 2007.

84.   The Henry J. Kaiser Family Foundation. Consumer protection issues raised by the Medicare Prescription Drug, Improvement and Moderni- zation Act of 2003. Available from http://www.kff.org/medicare/7130. cfm. Accessed August 8, 2007.

85.   The Henry J. Kaiser Family Foundation. Medicare Advantage. Available from http://www.kff.org/medicare/upload/2052-10.pdf. Accessed September 9, 2007.

86.   American Association of Retired Persons. Will the new medicare law encour- age employers to drop or keep their retiree drug plans? Available from *AARP Bulletin* 2005; 46:14. Available from http://www.aarp.org/bulletin/medicare/ medicare_anxiety.html. Accessed August 19, 2007.

87.   The Henry J. Kaiser Family Foundation. The Medicare prescription drug benefit. Available from http://www.kff.org/medicare/7044.cfm. Accessed September 1, 2007.

88.   Pear R. New White House estimate lifts drug benefit cost to $720 billion. *New York Times*, February 9, 2005. Available from http://www.nytimes.com /2005/02/09/national/09medicare.html. Accessed September 12, 2007.

89.   Centers for Medicare and Medicaid Services. CMS demonstration projects under the Medicare Modernization Act (MMA). Available from http://

www.cms.hhs.gov/researchers/demos/MMAdemolist.asp. Accessed September 12, 2007.

90. Centers for Medicare and Medicaid Services. Quality initiatives-general information. Available from http://www.cms.hhs.gov/QualityInitiativesGen Info/. Accessed September 12, 2007.

91. Centers for Medicare and Medicaid Services. About MQMS. Available from http://www.cms.hhs.gov/qualityinitiativesgeninfo/downloads/quality aboutmqms.pdf. Accessed September 11, 2007.

92. Centers for Medicare and Medicaid Services. Developing the Medicare hospital pay-for-performance plan. Available from http://www.cms.hhs.gov/ MLNGenInfo/downloads/Hospital_Pay-for-Performance_plan.pdf. Accessed September 11, 2007.

93. Centers for Medicare and Medicaid Services. Hospital quality initiative overview. Available from http://www.cms.hhs.gov/HospitalQualityInits/ downloads/HospitalOverview200512.pdf. Accessed September 14, 2007.

94. Pear R. Medicare won't cover hospital errors. *New York Times.* Available from http://www.nytimes.com/2007/08/19/washington/19hospital.html. Accessed September 12, 2007.

95. Centers for Medicare and Medicaid Services. Eliminating serious, preventable, and costly medical errors-never events. Available from http://www.cms. hhs.gov/media/press/release.asp?counter=1863. Accessed September 14, 2007.

96. Centers for Medicare and Medicaid Services. 2006 Medicaid managed care enrollment report, summary statistics as of June 30, 2006. Available from http://www.cms.hhs.gov/MedicaidDataSourcesGenInfo/Downloads/mmc er06.pdf. Accessed September 17, 2007.

97. Henry J. Kaiser Family Foundation. The Kaiser Commission on Medicaid and the Uninsured. Medicaid at a glance. Available from http://www.kff. org/medicaid/upload/7235-02.pdf. Accessed August 19, 2007.

98. Almanac of Policy Issues. Medicaid. Available from http://www.policy almanac.org/health/medicaid.shtml. Accessed September 11, 2007.

99. Koch AL. Financing health care services. In: Williams SJ, Torrens PK, eds. *Introduction to Health Care Services.* 4th ed. Albany, NY: Delmar Publishers; 1993:309.

100. Hurley R, Somers SA. Medicaid and managed care: a lasting relationship? *Health Affairs.* 2003;25:86.

101. Centers for Medicare and Medicaid Services. National SCHIP policy overview. Available from http://www.cms.hhs.gov/NationalSCHIPPolicy/ 01_Overview.asp#TopOfPage. Accessed September 13, 2007.

102. The Henry J. Kaiser Family Foundation. Health coverage for low-income children. Available from http://www.kff.org/uninsured/upload/2144-05.pdf. Accessed September 18, 2007.

103. Pear R, Hulse C. Congress set for veto fight on child health care. *New York Times.* Available from http://www.nytimes.com/2007/09/25/washington /25health.html?fta=y. Accessed September 26, 2007.

104. Centers for Medicare and Medicaid Services. Center for Medicaid and state operations. Available from http://www.cms.hhs.gov/medicaidschipqualprac/downloads/qualitystrategy.pdf. Accessed September 13, 2007.

105. The Henry J. Kaiser Family Foundation. Health08.org. Available from http://www.kff.org/kaiserpolls/h08_pomr083007pkg.cfm. Accessed September 17, 2007.

106. The Henry J. Kaiser Family Foundation. Massachusetts Health Care Reform Plan: update. Available from http://www.kff.org/uninsured/upload/7494-02.pdf. Accessed September 4, 2007.

107. State of Vermont, Agency of Administration. Vermont's health care reform of 2006. Available from http://hcr.vermont.gov. Accessed September 4, 2007.

108. California Office of the Governor. Governor Schwarzenegger tackles California's broken health care system, proposes comprehensive plan to help all Californians. Available from http://gov.ca.gov/index.php?/press-release/5057. Accessed September 4, 2007.

Long-Term Care

The number of Americans requiring long-term care services is increasing. Advances in medical care have made a longer life span possible, even in the presence of chronic disease and disability. This chapter provides an overview of some of the diverse array of long-term care services presently provided in institutional, community, and home-based settings. The long-term care needs of older adults are given particular attention because they are the fastest growing proportion of the population in the United States today and are the major consumers of long-term care services.

Each individual life span, from birth to death, can be seen as a connected flow of events—a continuum. The unrelenting progression of time is the one constant that expresses the diverse range of life's possibilities. An infant may be born with a birth defect, a young adult may suffer a head injury from an automobile accident, or an older adult may have a stroke. Such unanticipated events as these have a profound long-term impact on an individual's capacity to develop or to maintain abilities for self-care and independence. These individuals may require very different kinds and intensities of personal care assistance, health care services, and/or psychosocial and housing services over an extended segment of their life span.

The age, diagnosis, and ability to perform personal self-care and the sites of care delivery vary widely for recipients of long-term care. Thus, long-term care requires diversified, yet coordinated, services and flexibility within the service system to respond to recipients' changing needs over time.

The ideal health care delivery system provides participants with comprehensive personal, social, and medical care services. This ideal delivery system requires mechanisms that continually guide and track individual clients over time through the array of services at all levels and intensity of care that they require.[1] Because it generates a continuous flow of high costs over an extended period, long-term care has a particular need to use what the American Hospital Association calls a seamless continuum of care[2] that will promote the highest quality of life but still respond to growing public concerns about cost-effectiveness.[3] The particular package of services provided to each person should be tailored to meet his or her needs. Service needs vary from assistance with personal care and basic needs for food and safe shelter to rehabilitation when possible and socialization opportunities. Additionally, the type and extent of physical disability and the intensity of services required determine the location of long-term care. For example, an older individual with paralysis following a stroke may be able to remain at home with services that dovetail with family caregivers in the home. Another with a similar disability may require nursing home placement because that environment best meets the particular requirements of the situation. Configuring a package of services that will promote independence and maintain lifestyle quality as far as is possible within personal, community, and national resources makes the variety of long-term care services complex and sometimes confusing. Concern about cost-effectiveness and the desire to accommodate personal and family desires, finances, and reimbursement eligibility results in the need for both the availability of an array of services and coordination of those services to meet individual needs in the most effective way.

Within the last 50 years, extensive changes in demographics and the types and availability of health care services have occurred in the United States. The economic ramifications of a rapidly increasing population of older Americans, advances in medicine that have made many heretofore unknown life-sustaining measures available to health care professionals, and an emphasis on preventive care and healthy lifestyle all have had an impact on the continued growth of the population, who presently require or potentially will require long-term care services. Older adults represent the largest population group requiring long-term care services. Current estimates place the population 65 years of age and older at 36.3 million, or about one of every eight Americans. The number of persons aged 65 years or older, 71.5 million, is expected to comprise 20% of the population by 2030.[4] The population 85 years of age and older is expected to grow to 18.9 million by 2050, making this group the fastest growing pop-

ulation segment over the next four decades (Figures 8-1 and 8-2).[4,5]
Many will grow old alone because of smaller family size and divorce. The
increasing economic need for family members to delay retirement and
work outside the home also reduces the availability of family caregivers to
participate in the informal family caregiving system.

Development of Long-Term Care Services

The colonists who emigrated from Europe to the New World brought
with them many of the social values and institutional models of their
native countries. One of these, the almshouse, was a place where the people who were sick or disabled or older adults who lacked adequate family
or financial support could be cared for in a communal setting. Charitable
community members purchased private homes and converted them to
almshouses that operated as communal residences. Municipal and county
governments also created homes and "infirmaries" to care for impoverished
older adults. These early models were the basis for "homes for the elderly,"
which existed until the economic upheavals of the Great Depression and
the restructuring of the social welfare system after World War II.

The economic devastation experienced during the Great Depression
affected the availability of long-term care services, especially homes for

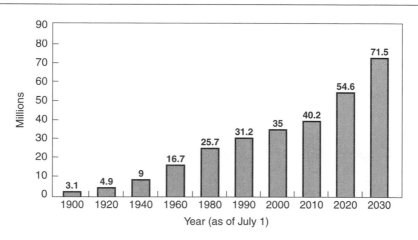

FIGURE 8-1 Number of Persons 65+, 1900–2030.
Source: U.S. Bureau of the Census.

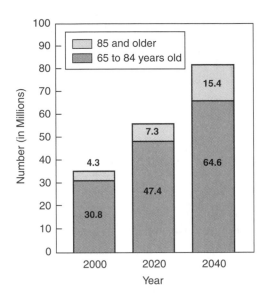

FIGURE 8-2 Elderly Population, 2000–2040.
Source: U.S. Bureau of the Census.

older adults, in several ways. Operating small private nursing homes became attractive to people in financial danger of losing their homes to mortgage foreclosure because taking in outsiders and providing care generated a new source of income. After the Great Depression, many local charitable agencies could no longer afford to provide care based on the almshouse tradition, and the federal government became more involved in developing, overseeing, and paying for long-term care services as part of the social welfare reforms, such as the 1935 Social Security Act.[6] The Social Security Act provided financial assistance for particular categories of older Americans and people with disabilities. Additionally, the Social Security Act established a form of old age and survivors insurance that allowed workers and their employers to contribute to a fund that could supplement retirement income. This form of income security reduced the extent of indigence frequently found in the older population and increased the amount of secure income that older Americans could spend on services and care in later years. Government lending programs available to not-for-profit organizations beginning in the 1950s spurred the development of nursing homes in this sector; major growth in the proprietary sector did not occur until after the passage of Medicare and

Medicaid in 1965. Today, over 60% of nursing homes are operated on a proprietary or for-profit basis, and 31% operate as not-for-profit organizations (Figure 8-3).[7]

Public and private homes for older adults often varied in the adequacy of care and the kinds of services provided. Nursing homes often were thought of as homes where minimal custodial care required to meet the basic needs of food, clothing, and shelter was provided, sometimes in very unhygienic and inhumane environments. Nursing homes often were places where older and frail adults, some of society's most vulnerable members, were taken to die, rather than seen as a residence option where they could receive needed care to prolong or enhance the quality of their lives. Physical care often was substandard, and emotional, spiritual, and social needs were ignored. Because many frail, older people suffer from perceptual and cognitive disabilities in addition to physical disabilities, their behavior in a group setting was often considered by nursing home staff to be a problem, and sometimes it led to the overuse of physical and chemical restraints such as sedatives and mood-altering drugs.

The provision of home nursing care also has a long tradition in the United States as an alternative to institutional care provided in hospitals and nursing homes. Family members traditionally have provided home care to their own relatives. An interest in providing formal professional

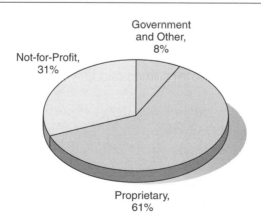

FIGURE 8-3 Percent Distribution of Nursing Home Facilities by Ownership.
Source: National Center for Health Statistics, "Nursing Home Facilities, December 2005."

home care services began in the late 19th century as a social response to the unhealthy living conditions of immigrants residing in urban tenements. Such crowded and unsanitary conditions became a public health concern because they were frequently implicated in the spread of contagious diseases, such as tuberculosis, typhoid, and smallpox. Agencies such as the Visiting Nurses Association were established to provide trained nurses to tend to the sick in their homes. Their role quickly expanded to include preventive education regarding hygiene, nutrition, and coordination of social welfare intervention, especially in caring for society's most vulnerable populations of people with illnesses, low incomes, or disabilities.[8]

The passage of Medicare and Medicaid legislation in 1965 provided more stable sources of reimbursement than were previously available through private pay and charitable funding and promoted expansion of the long-term care industry. Medicare and Medicaid have affected the long-term care industry in several overt ways. They established minimal standards of care and services required for recipients to qualify for reimbursement, as well as funding sources for older Americans, people with disabilities, and those lacking the means to pay. This funding simultaneously attracted both the scrupulous and the unscrupulous into the long-term care industry, as it quickly became apparent that being a provider of long-term care could be very profitable.

The long-term care industry came under increasing scrutiny in the early 1970s during congressional hearings on the nursing home industry, after several hundred exposés published in newspapers and additional publications such as the Nader Report and Mary Adelaide Mendelson's book, *Tender Loving Greed*.[9] The litany of nursing home corruption and abuses that were exposed during that period includes:[10,11]

- Care that did not recognize the right to human dignity
- A lack of activities for residents
- Untrained and inadequate staff, including untrained administrators
- Unsanitary conditions
- Theft of residents' belongings
- Inadequate safety precautions (especially fire protection)
- Unauthorized and unnecessary use of restraints
- Both overmedication and undermedication of patients
- Failure to act in a timely manner on complaints and reprisals against those who complained

- Discrimination against patients who were members of minority groups
- A lack of dental and psychiatric care
- Negligence leading to injury and death
- Ineffective inspections and nonenforcement of laws that were meant to regulate the nursing home industry
- Reimbursement fraud

These congressional hearings and simultaneous public outcry resulted in more strict enforcement of Medicare and Medicaid guidelines and credentialing, increased establishment and enforcement of nursing home and home care licensure, more active accreditation procedures by the Joint Commission on Accreditation of Healthcare Organizations, laws related to elder abuse reporting, federal guidelines regulating the use of physical restraints, and establishment of ombudsman programs. All of these measures have led to a much more regulated and responsive long-term care industry. More vocal and astute consumers also have provided economic and social mandates for high-quality standards of care—which had previously not been adhered to in any meaningful, organized quality assurance process—to be maintained in the long-term care industry overall. The Omnibus Budget Reconciliation Act of 1987 (OBRA) legislated new guidelines and restrictions on the use of physical and chemical restraints, established a nursing home resident bill of rights, mandated quality assurance standards, established a standard survey process, and mandated training and educational requirements.[12]

Modes of Long-Term Care Service Delivery

The site of care delivery categorizes long-term care programs. Institution-based services are those long-term care services provided within an institution such as a nursing home, hospital with inpatient extended care or rehabilitation facility, or inpatient hospice. Community-based services coordinate, manage, and deliver long-term care services such as adult day care programs or care in the recipient's home.

Nursing home facilities and assisted living facilities are two examples of institutional-based long-term care settings. Both provide a place of extended residence, and as such, care recipients are called residents, not patients. The major difference between skilled nursing facilities (SNFs) and assisted-living facilities lies in the intensity of care provided. A SNF that is Medicare and Medicaid certified is defined as "a facility, or distinct part of one, primarily engaged in providing skilled nursing care and related services for people requiring medical or nursing care, or rehabilitation services."[13] Skilled nursing care is provided by or under the direct supervision of licensed nursing personnel, such as registered nurses and licensed practical nurses, and emphasis is on the provision of 24-hour nursing care and the availability of other types of services.

Skilled Nursing Care

Current estimates are that 1.5 million Americans reside in 16,100 SNFs. Average annual costs per resident for private-pay residents for a single room are $70,912; average annual costs per resident for a semi-private room total $62,532.[14] Annual national expenditures for nursing home care in 2005 totaled $121.9 billion. Medicare, Medicaid, and other public funds pay the largest portion, 62%; 38% is funded by out-of-pocket, private insurance and other private funds (Table 8-1).[15] The nursing home industry remains the dominant sector of the long-term care industry, with expenditures greater than double those for home care.[15]

Despite the burgeoning numbers of older Americans, national nursing home bed occupancy rates are declining.[16] Many factors are believed to be contributing to the decline. Today's older adults are healthier, delaying the need for skilled nursing services. The vastly increased availability of assisted-living facilities and the availability of other community-based

Table 8-1 Sources of Payment for Nursing Home Care, 2005

Source of Payment	Amount in Billions	Percent
Total	121.9	100
Medicare	19.2	15.7
Medicaid (Federal and State)	53.5	43.9
Other Public	3.3	2.7
Private (out-of-pocket and other private funds)	36.8	30.2
Private Insurance	9.1	7.5

Source: Centers for Medicare and Medicaid Services.

assistance through day care and home care are also playing roles in delaying the need for skilled, institutional care.

Nursing home residents can be of any age, although most are adults in their later years. The typical nursing home resident is an older female with cognitive impairment who was living alone on a limited income before nursing home placement. The decreased ability to function independently and a lack of family caregivers are additional factors associated with an increased risk of nursing home admission.

Typical staffing in SNFs includes a physician medical director, a nursing home administrator, a director of nursing, at least one registered nurse on the day and evening shifts, and either a registered nurse or a licensed practical nurse on the night shift. Additional registered nurses and licensed practical nurses are employed as needed to distribute medications and carry out medical treatments. Nursing assistants provide direct custodial care under the supervision of licensed nursing personnel. Ancillary professional staff includes physical therapists, occupational therapists, pharmacists, nutritionists, recreational therapists, and social workers. Support staff, including kitchen, laundry, housekeeping, and maintenance workers, complete the employee complement. The exact number and staffing pattern also are based on the level of skilled nursing care required by the residents of any particular nursing home. The licensed nursing home administrator, along with the owner/operator, is responsible for carrying out the regulatory mandates regarding the mix and ratio of licensed and unlicensed personnel and the availability of licensed nursing personnel on an around-the-clock basis to provide skilled care and supervision.

Nursing homes are highly regulated by both state licensure and federal certification. The 1987 OBRA increased government involvement in nursing home industry regulation by[12]

- Mandating regularly scheduled comprehensive assessments of the functional capacity of residents in nursing homes
- Establishing training standards for nursing home aides
- Placing restrictions on the use of physical restraints and psychoactive drugs
- Establishing a nursing home resident bill of rights
- Setting guidelines for the role of the medical director, including continuing education, involvement, and responsibility

States license nursing home administrators. Individual states set criteria for licensure in relationship to minimum age, educational requirements, passing examination scores, and continuing education requirements. In 2006, the National Association of Boards of Examiners of Long-Term Care Administrators announced endorsement of a uniform set of "principles of interstate licensure" that will allow reciprocity between and among states' licensing requirements. This new interstate licensure endorsement intends to assist mobility of administrators across states while ensuring maintenance of the highest entry-level standards in the profession.[17] A lack of nursing home compliance with state and federal mandates can lead to penalties such as direct fines, exclusion from Medicare and Medicaid certification, and withdrawal of nursing home licensure. Accreditation through the Joint Commission provides an additional quality check. Although highly desirable, Joint Commission accreditation remains voluntary.

Assisted-Living Facilities

Assisted-living facilities are appropriate for long-term care for individuals who do not require skilled nursing services and whose needs lie more in the custodial and supportive realm. The Assisted Living Federation of America defines an assisted-living residence as "a special combination of housing, personalized supportive services and health care designed to meet needs—both scheduled and unscheduled—of those who need help with activities of daily living."[18] Current estimates place the number of assisted-living facilities at 20,000, housing over 1 million people.[19] The assisted-living population is expected to grow to over 2 million individuals by 2025 (Figure 8-4). Assisted-living facilities vary significantly in size, ranging from just a few residents to several hundred. They may take the form of small to large homes with just a few residents or large multiunit apartment complexes with several hundred residents. Available services also vary, but generally include, in addition to housing, congregate meals, 24-hour monitoring for emergencies, medication supervision, and assistance with one or more activities of daily living such as bathing, dressing, and personal grooming. Assisted-living facilities also typically provide scheduled activities, including communal recreation and group transportation for medical appointments and for social and cultural events.

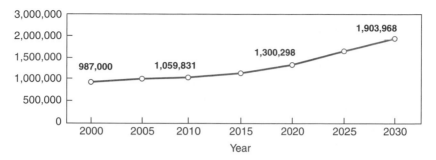

FIGURE 8-4 Projected Growth of Assisted Living Beds Based on Population Growth for Those 75 years and Older.
Source: National Center for Assisted Living, reprinted with permission.

Many assisted-living facilities contract with home health agencies to provide skilled nursing care and with hospice service providers. States carry out oversight and regulation of assisted-living facilities at varying levels. These variations in laws and regulations create a diverse operating environment, as well as a wide range of terminology and available services for consumers.[19] The quality of facilities, care, and services, therefore, may be an exclusive function of the policies of the owner organization or a combination of owner and organization policies coupled with state regulatory oversight. Costs of assisted living are borne largely from private resources, although in certain circumstances, Supplemental Social Security Income, private health insurance, long-term care insurance (LTCI), or special government rent subsidies for low-income older adults may apply. Estimates place the average monthly cost at $2,350, but costs can range across a broad continuum, depending on the level of amenities desired in a facility and the types of services required (Figure 8-5).[19]

Residential institutions such as adult homes, board and care homes, and centers for people with mental or developmental disabilities also represent assisted living arrangements. Care provided in adult homes has been available only to people who are for the most part healthy but limited in their ability to do their own housekeeping, household maintenance, and cooking. Residents must be able, for the most part, to meet their own personal care needs for dressing, eating, bathing, toileting, and ambulation, unassisted. Oversight of residents may include services such as supervision of medications to the extent of reminding residents to take their medication or providing some assistance with bathing, grooming,

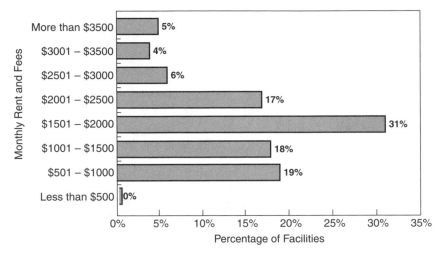

FIGURE 8-5 Monthly Rent and Fees in Assisted Living Facilities.
Source: National Center for Assisted Living, reprinted with permission.

transportation, laundry, and simple housekeeping. If provided at all, direct nursing care can be provided only in the case of minor illness of a temporary nature. Staffing levels in adult homes are state defined, with the ratio determined by the number of beds.

Home Care

Home care is community-based care provided to patients, more often referred to as "clients," in their own residences. The vast majority of home care recipients are over the age of 65 years. Home care can be either a long-term provision of supportive care and services to chronically ill clients to avoid institutionalization, or short-term intermittent care of clients after acute illness and hospitalization until the clients are able to return to an independent level of functioning. Home care may be provided through the formal system of paid professional home care providers, such as registered nurses, licensed practical nurses, home health aides, physical therapists, speech-language pathologists, social workers, and homemakers who make home visits. An informal system also provides home care through caregivers consisting of family, neighbors, and friends of people in need of health care support services. Very often, a combination of both formal and informal systems delivers care most expeditiously; other instances may use only one or the other exclusively.

Professional home care services originated in social welfare initiatives in the early 20th century in public response to the horrific living conditions of immigrants in U.S. industrialized cities. Public health concerns also gained impetus at that time as the germ theory of disease became accepted, and the control of contagious disease using preventive measures of hygiene and sanitation became a public health concern and mandate of local, state, and national health departments and agencies.

Formal home care continues to play an important role in the provision of care to those requiring long-term care services. Changes in Medicare reimbursement and regulation beginning in the late 1990s resulted in significant downward shifts in both expenditures and the number of Medicare certified home health agencies.[20] Since 2003, the number of Medicare-certified home health agencies has grown to 8,100 agencies, serving 2.4 million individuals.[21] Medicare remains the largest payer for home health care services, accounting for approximately 38% of total annual home care expenditures (Table 8-2).[15]

The home care industry expanded its scope of services in response to demographic, economic, and legislative changes that include:

- An increase in the number of older persons and their expressed desire to remain in their own homes for care whenever possible
- Decreased numbers of informal caregivers that are available to provide in-home care to their relatives
- Increased innovations in high-technology home care that have redefined and expanded the categories of diseases and chronic conditions that can be cared for efficaciously in the home care setting

Table 8-2 Sources of Payment for Home Care in 2005

Source of Payment	Amount in Billions	Percent
Total	47.5	100
Medicare	17.9	37.7
Medicaid (Federal and State)	15.5	32.6
Other Public	2.1	4.4
Private (out-of-pocket and insurance)	12.0[a]	25.3

[a]less than 50 million private insurance

Source: Centers for Medicare and Medicaid Services.

- Medicare and Medicaid reimbursement that allowed expanded coverage
- The 1999 Olmstead decision of the Supreme Court upholding the right of citizens to receive care in the community

Home care's material cost-effectiveness, when compared with institutional care, is pronounced (Figure 8-6). Research published between 1999 and 2004 in the *Journal of the American Medical Association*, the *New England Journal of Medicine*, the *Journal of the American Geriatrics Society*, and other sources notes that as compared with institutional care[22]

- Homecare reduces costs by 37% for heart failure patients.
- One year of long-term oxygen therapy at home costs less than 1 day in the hospital.
- The cost of home intravenous antibiotic treatment was 15% of the same care provided in the hospital and 23% of the cost of the same care provided in a SNF.

The initial growth spurt in the home care industry dates from the enactment of Medicare and Medicaid in the 1960s, which ensured a stable source of income available to certified agencies. The Medicare pro-

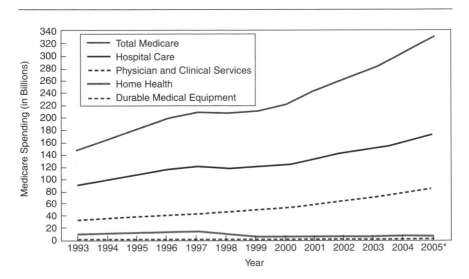

FIGURE 8-6 Comparative Medicare Spending 1993–2005.
Sources: Centers for Medicare and Medicaid Services and Congressional Budget Office.

gram made home health care much more accessible to older adults. Medicare Part A benefits cover skilled nursing care, physical, occupational, and speech therapies, and medical social services delivered in the home care setting. Eligibility criteria included four basic mandatory features:

1. Home care must include the provision of skilled nursing care; physical, occupational, and speech therapies; and medical social services as warranted by the patient's condition.
2. The person must be confined to the home.
3. A physician must order that home care services are required.
4. The home care agency must meet the minimum quality standards as outlined by Medicare and be Medicare certified.

In 2006, the Centers for Medicare and Medicaid Services recommended a "post-acute care reform plan" that emphasizes a consumer-centered approach to services. The plan outlined goals of [23]

- Increasing consumer choice and control of post-acute care services by patients, family members and caregivers
- Providing high quality services in the most appropriate settings
- Developing effective measures to drive the system toward delivery of the highest possible quality
- Providing a seamless continuum of care through improved coordination of acute care, post-acute care, and long-term care services, including better management of transitions between care settings

Beginning in 1982, growth in the number of private proprietary agencies was stimulated when Medicare reimbursement opened to the for-profit sector. Today, proprietary home health agencies comprise 62% of all Medicare-certified agencies.[24]

State licensing is required for Medicare certification.[25] Most states issue a license for 1 year and require that an application be resubmitted and an annual state reinspection be performed by a survey team. The state licensing agency has the right to investigate complaints and to conduct periodic reviews of all licensure requirements. Those few agencies that treat only private pay or private insurance patients may not require a license; however, most home health care agencies want to participate in Medicare and Medicaid reimbursement and actively seek to meet the guidelines established by Medicare and Medicaid for certification. Participation in voluntary accreditation indicates that home care agencies have a commitment to continuous improvement in quality and accomplishment. Organizations that are actively engaged in the accreditation process for home health care agencies include the Community Health Accreditation Program, an independent, consumer-based subsidiary of the National League for Nursing, the Joint Commission on Accreditation of Health Care Organizations and the National Association for Home Care and Hospice.

Professional caregivers are trained health care workers, such as registered nurses, licensed practical nurses, personal care aides, nursing assistants, homemakers, licensed occupational, physical, and respiratory therapists, and social workers, who provide necessary health care services within their areas of expertise to clients in their homes. The client's physician directs all care. Most home care workers provide care under the auspices of proprietary home care agencies or through programs provided by not-for-profit agencies and are employees of those agencies or organizations. A considerably smaller number are self-employed health care workers who contract privately with clients.

Until the proliferation of social programs in the 1960s and 1970s, individuals requiring long-term health care were almost always handled within the family, at the family home, and by family members or friends. This informal care system provided a valuable social service at little or no cost to the public. This arrangement is still the most used system of long-term care—family members care for about 80% of older adults needing some level of assistance. The informal care system offers a significant savings to the public; however, the potential for caregivers to suffer physical and emotional burnout and the growing inability of family caregivers to handle care completely without partial or total outside assistance have begun to diminish these savings.

Recent estimates place the number of family caregivers at over 50 million, of whom 60% are women.[26] Because women are an integral part of the workforce, the available pool of caregivers for family members needing care at home is much smaller than in the past. Now, family caregivers are frequently required to make major compromises in their finances, lifestyles, and personal freedom in order to care for another. The costs can be high. Stresses experienced by the caregiver can lead to exhaustion, illness, and depression.[27] In addition, with greater longevity of the population, middle-aged individuals often find themselves caring for children and aged parents simultaneously. Dubbed the "sandwich generation," these caregivers suffer even more stress from this dual role. Employers also experience losses because of the demands of caregiving on their employees. One study estimates the annual costs of lost productivity for U.S. businesses due to caregiving at $34 billion.[28] Employer costs are associated with worker replacement, absenteeism, workday interruptions, elder care crises, and supervisory time.[27,28] Some employers are responding with flexible scheduling and other considerations to help accommodate their employees' caregiving responsibilities.[28]

Estimates place the market value of long-term care delivered by unpaid family members and friends at over $306 billion per year, more than double the annual national health care expenditures for nursing home and home care combined[29] (Figure 8-7). Both the economic and personal contributions of the informal caregiving system form the bedrock of the nation's chronic care system and require more policy-level attention and support. The federal government took an important first step to assist family caregivers through the Family Medical Leave Act (FMLA) of 1993. The FMLA provides up to 12 months unpaid leave per year for the birth of a child or adoption of a child, or for employees to care for themselves or a sick family member while ensuring

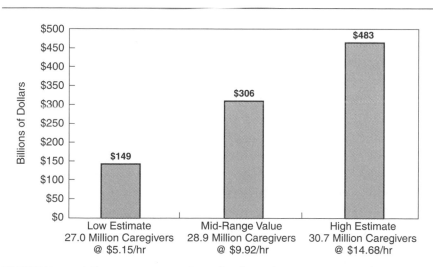

FIGURE 8-7 The Economic Value of Informal Caregiving, US, 2004. *Source:* Veterans Administration Caregiving Forum, Peter S. Arno handout.

continuation of health benefits and job security. The FMLA has serious shortcomings, however. It provides only for unpaid leave, a condition that makes its use financially unfeasible for many individuals. Also, the FMLA does not cover workers in companies of 50 or fewer employees, effectively excluding approximately half of America's workers.[30] States have responded with programs to assist caregivers by expanding paid leave provisions. California was a leader in this regard when it enacted The Paid Family Leave Law in 2002, allowing workers up to 6 weeks of partially paid leave to bond with a new biological, adopted, or foster child or to care for a seriously ill family member.[30] Fifteen additional states have enacted paid leave legislation or regulations for private sector employees, and several additional states have such legislation under consideration. Similar provisions now exist for public employees in at least 40 states.[30]

In the 1990s, President Clinton and the Congress responded to dramatic increases in service use and spending in home health care. These concerns also encompassed issues about service quality and the fiscal integrity of Medicare- and Medicaid-supported home health and other services.[31] One major response was the initiation of a 2-year antifraud and abuse pilot project, Operation Restore Trust (ORT), which concentrated on investigations of home health agencies, nursing homes, hospice, and medical equipment and supplies in five states with the highest rates of use. In 1997, ORT was expanded to selected home health care agencies in 12 states and included training for agency surveyors in identifying care improperly billed to Medicare.[32]

The Balanced Budget Act (BBA) of 1997 also contained several provisions to enable the Health Care Financing Administration to control costs and address service quality issues more effectively in Medicare-funded home health agencies. Provisions targeted reducing unnecessary and inappropriate services and included dividing Medicare home health services funding into separate streams for posthospital and chronic health problems. Other provisions of the BBA changed Medicare reimbursement from a retrospective to prospective basis, and several measures were introduced to thwart fraudulent practices by home health clients and agencies.[32] The Clinton administration also proposed revisions in the federal standards that home health care agencies must meet to continue participation in the Medicare program. Revisions included the following:[32]

- Requiring criminal background checks of home health aides as a condition of employment
- Expanding home health aide qualifications to include appropriate nurse aide training or competency evaluation requirements
- Requiring home health agencies to provide their staffs with continuous feedback on qualifications and performance as part of their continuous improvement programs
- Requiring home health agencies to discuss with patients the expected outcomes of care so that patients can be more involved in planning their own care
- Requiring home health agencies to coordinate all care prescribed by physicians for their patients to assure quality for patients being served by several agencies

In 1997 the Department of Health and Human Services promulgated additional regulations to require home health agencies to implement a standardized reporting system, the Outcomes and Assessment Information Set, which is designed to monitor patients' conditions and satisfaction with services. It also required the completion of standardized assessments of new patients within 48 hours of admission to a home health care agency and continuous updates of the admitting information, which include documentation of changes in condition and patient and family satisfaction. The Medicare prospective payment system for home health care services links with Outcomes and Assessment Information Set data.[33]

Home health care services are an integral component of the health care delivery system's continuum, which can provide an effective, safe, and humane alternative to institutional care for the medical treatment and personal care of individuals of all ages. Ideally, lessons learned from ORT and industry responses will help assure that home health care will be a beneficiary-centered service that safeguards both payers and recipients from fraud and abuse while ensuring adherence to appropriate standards of quality care.

Hospice Care

Hospice is a philosophy supporting a coordinated program of care available to the terminally ill. The most common criterion for admission into hospice is that the applicant has a diagnosis of a terminal illness with a limited life expectancy, usually anticipated to be of 6-months' duration or less. Aggressive medical treatment of the patient's disease may no longer be medically feasible or personally desirable. The disease may have progressed despite available medical treatments, making continuance of curative treatment futile or intolerable, or the patient may elect to discontinue such treatment for a variety of personal reasons, such as continued deterioration of quality of life relating to side effects of the treatment.

The term palliative care often is used synonymously with hospice care. Palliative care is care or treatment given to relieve the symptoms of a disease rather than attempting to cure the disease. Pain, nausea, malaise, and emotional distress caused by feelings of fear and isolation are only some of the difficulties that patients encounter during the final stages of a terminal illness. Hospice treatment is directed toward maintaining the comfort of the patient and enhancing the patient's quality of life and sense of independence for however long is possible.

Hospice has its historical roots in medieval Europe. Hospices were originally way stations where travelers on religious pilgrimages received food and rest. Over time, the concept evolved into sanctuaries where impoverished people or those who were sick or dying received care. The word "hospice" derives from the same Latin root that forms the words "hospital" and "hospitality."

English physician Dame Cicely Saunders established St. Christopher's, a hospice located in a London suburb, in 1967, and it became a model for the modern hospice. Here, terminally ill patients received intensive symptom management, modern techniques of pain control, and psychological and emotional support. She brought the founding concepts of modern hospice to the United States in a lecture tour in the late 1960s, during which she emphasized that dying patients were also on a kind of pilgrimage and needed a more responsive environment than could be provided in high-technology, impersonal, cure-oriented hospitals.

The U.S. hospice movement began as a consumer-based grassroots movement supported by volunteer and professional members of the community. Today, over two thirds of hospice organizations continue operating as not-for-profit entities (Figure 8-8).[34] The U.S. founders shared the belief that the hospice concept was a more humanized alternative to the care of the dying than was being provided in hospitals, which focused most intently on medical cure. Because the medical system can view

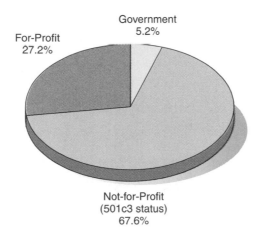

For-Profit
27.2%

Government
5.2%

Not-for-Profit
(501c3 status)
67.6%

FIGURE 8-8 Hospice Organization Auspices.
Source: National Hospice and Palliative Care Organization, reprinted with permission.

choosing to discontinue aggressive medical treatment, based on the recognition that the treatment is not altering the course of the disease, as a failure, terminally ill patients can feel depersonalized and isolated inside a traditional hospital setting. Ideally, the physician, the patient, and the patient's family jointly recognize the need to refer the patient to hospice when deciding to stop aggressive curative treatment.

The first U.S. hospice was established in New Haven, Connecticut in 1974. The number of hospices has increased steadily every year, with over 4,100 hospices now serving over 1.2 million individuals annually (Figures 8-9 and 8-10).[34] Major growth in the availability of hospice care followed the enactment of 1982 legislation that extended Medicare coverage to hospice services, allowing the movement to escape its prior dependency on grant support and philanthropy. A 73-fold increase in the number of hospice providers occurred between 1984 and 1998. In 2005, approximately one-third of all U.S. deaths occurred in hospice care.[34]

Consistent with the hospice philosophy, a multidisciplinary team of nurses, social workers, counselors, physicians, and therapists provides services. Hospices also provide drug therapies and medical appliances and supplies. Bereavement services for surviving family members continues for a year or longer after the patient's death. Most hospice organizations also provide bereavement services for the larger community.[34]

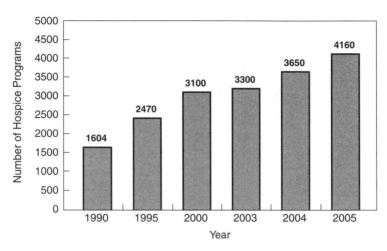

FIGURE 8-9 Number of Hospice Programs 1990–2005.
Source: National Hospice and Palliative Care Organization, reprinted with permission.

A variety of different settings accommodate hospice care, including the home, hospitals, SNFs, assisted-living facilities, or hospice inpatient facilities or residences. The most important unifying concept about hospice is that no matter where the care is delivered, a specialized multidisciplinary team of health care professionals works together to manage the patient's care. A physician directs the team, coordinated by a nurse. The team members can include physicians, nurses, respiratory and physical therapists, pharmacists, pastoral care providers, social workers, psychologists, home health aides, and homemakers. Each team member contributes his or her particular skills and expertise to assist in managing pain, alleviating emotional distress, promoting comfort, and maintaining the independence of the hospice patient. Hospice care also encompasses the patient's family and routinely includes counseling (including bereavement counseling), spiritual support, and respite care for family members.

The hospice philosophy emphasizes volunteerism, and in 2005, the movement estimated that 400,000 volunteers are assisting hospice organizations.[34] Volunteers from the community are actively encouraged to participate in a wide range of hospice activities, from fundraising to direct patient contact and family caregiver support.

Hospice care has demonstrated its cost savings in care for the terminally ill. The unique blend of care provided by a specialized team, use of

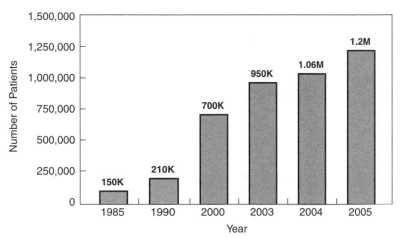

FIGURE 8-10 Number of Hospice Patients Served, 1985–2005.
Source: National Hospice and Palliative Care Organization, reprinted with permission.

volunteers, and frequent use of family members as primary caregivers in the home all decrease the expense involved. The focus on palliative care rather than on more technological, cure-oriented care also decreases the cost. A number of research studies have examined the savings involved in the use of hospice care. Hospice care continues to represent only about 2.5% of total Medicare spending (Table 8-3).[35] Similar to Medicare, annual Medicaid expenditures for hospice care represent only a small fraction of total expenditures.[35]

Managed care organizations and traditional health insurers have recognized both the humane and economic benefits of hospice care and typically include hospice in their benefit packages. Insurers may have their own team of hospice-type providers within their respective networks or may contract with community hospice organizations to provide hospice care. Medicare-eligible subscribers of Medicare-participating managed care organizations are automatically eligible for hospice care, and services must be provided through a Medicare-certified hospice organization. The patient is not required to obtain a referral from their managed care organization and is not required to disenroll from their managed care contract in order to receive hospice care.

A basic tenet of the hospice philosophy is that hospice care is based on a need for care, rather than on the patient's ability to pay. In instances

Table 8-3 Comparison of Hospital, Skilled Nursing Facility, and Hospice Medicare Charges, 1998–2005

	1998	1999	2000	2001	2002	2003	2004	2005
Hospital inpatient charges per day	$2,177	$2,583	$2,762	$3,069	$3,574	$4,117	$4,559	$4,787
Skilled nursing facility charges per day	482	424	413	422	475	487	493	521
Hospice charges per covered day of care	113	113	118	120	125	126	129	131

Sources: Social Security Administration, U.S. Bureau of Labor Statistics, Health Care Financing Administration.

where the patient does not have health insurance and cannot qualify for Medicare or Medicaid, hospice services may still be available. A hospice may offer a sliding payment scale to the patient, with the hospice drawing on internal funds garnered through its fundraising activities or bequests to supplement available patient payments.

Ongoing quality assurance to monitor the quality of care is an inherent concept in the provision of hospice care. Three standards used most frequently are licensure, certification, and accreditation. Licensure is based on state-imposed statutes as part of the consumer protection code of a state. Not all states have such licensing statutes. States that do have licensing statutes require that all hospices within their jurisdiction meet the standards set forth in the law. Certification means that hospices have been examined on the federal level and have been found to at least minimally meet mandated requirements for Medicare and Medicaid reimbursement. Certification status is important, particularly for those patients whose hospice care reimbursement source is Medicare or Medicaid. A hospice program that is not certified may still operate legally but is ineligible to bill Medicare or Medicaid for its services.

Accreditation indicates that hospices meet voluntary standards of quality established by nongovernmental, independent monitoring organizations. Until recently, the Joint Commission on Accreditation of Health Care Organizations offered a program of hospice accreditation. Another organization that continues to offer accreditation is a subsidiary of the National League of Nurses Community Health Accreditation Program. Many hospices decline participation in voluntary accreditation programs because of stringent requirements and the lack of financial or other resources necessary to meet accreditation requirements.

Respite Care

The informal caregiving system of family members and friends traditionally provided the majority of in-home, long-term care services to children and adults in the community who are frail or have chronic physical or mental disabilities. Family caregivers have been a key factor in keeping many long-term care recipients in their communities rather than using institutions. Providing care up to 24 hours a day can place enormous physical and emotional stress on family caregivers.

Respite care is temporary surrogate care given to a patient when that patient's primary caregiver must be absent. In the 1970s, formal respite-care programs originated to meet the increasing need for assistance after the rapid deinstitutionalization of individuals who had developmental disabilities or mental illness. Since then, the respite-care model has expanded to include any family-managed care program that helps to avoid or forestall the placement of a patient in a full-time institutionalized environment by providing planned, intermittent caregiver relief. Respite care offers an organized, reliable system in which both patient and primary caregiver are the beneficiaries.

Respite care may be offered in a variety of settings: the home, a day care situation, or at institutions with overnight care, such as hospitals or nursing homes. Respite-care auspices may include private, public, and voluntary not-for-profit agencies. The length of respite care varies, but it is intended to be short term and intermittent.

Respite-care services are highly differentiated. Some are very structured and self-contained; others are highly flexible and exist in a more casual support capacity. A number of services are oriented to treating only patients with a particular ailment, but for many, the only criterion the patient must meet for admission is that he or she requires supervised medical treatment and nursing care, provided by family or friends as principal caregivers. Respite models include:

- Alzheimer's disease care on an inpatient basis with admissions lasting for several weeks
- Community-based, adult day care centers that offer nursing, therapeutic, and social services
- In-home aides, where visiting aides supply services
- Temporary patient furloughs to a hospital or nursing home at regular intervals

Respite-care program staffing varies widely, deploying both professionals and/or nonprofessionals. For example, respite care could be as informal as having a member from the caregiver's church come into the home for a few hours while the caregiver goes out or as professional as a specialized dementia day care program where nurses, aides, and recreational and physical therapists are specifically educated to care for dementia patients in a structured, caregiving environment. When respite care entails overnight care in an institutional setting, such as a nursing home or hospital, the staff providing care will be the same staff employed by the institution to provide care to their regular patients in the institution.

Formal respite programs in the United States that are financially accessible to all in need have remained sparse. One of the greatest barriers limiting the expanded use of respite care is cost. Family caregivers accustomed to operating on a limited budget may have difficulty finding funds to compensate a health care professional who supplies respite care. Although some respite providers offer care on a sliding scale, there are cases in which almost any standard fee exceeds the financial means of the family caregiver. In these situations, not-for-profit organizations may assist by providing home aides for respite care at a tolerable cost for patients who meet certain financial or medical parameters.

Historically, there have been few provisions in the Medicare and Medicaid programs to support formal respite care. Medicare contains no allowances for respite. Medicaid has stringent requirements regarding the specific type and length of care provided, as well as financial eligibility for services. Some states are attempting to provide wage income subsidy for respite in the cases of citizens over age 60 with very low incomes.

Available respite programs offered by voluntary agencies as the result of federal grants often provide service for only specific medical conditions, such as Alzheimer's disease. Both proprietary and not-for-profit organizations are developing specialized dementia and connected respite-care programs in response to recent federal legislation. Many specialized dementia respite-care programs currently are being developed and marketed to private pay customers, but such programs often are beyond the financial capability of many families.

One of the major barriers to responsive changes in reimbursement for respite care has been that funding mechanisms have viewed respite care as meeting a social need but not an acute medical care need. In addition, community systems of respite care can be difficult to organize because the level of need is intermittent and unpredictable. Family caregivers often are viewed as the most direct beneficiaries of respite care, rather than the patients who actually receive the health care. With the indisputable conclusion that respite-care programs offer society value and cost savings through postponement or avoidance of costly institutionalization, bipartisan federal legislation was developed in 2003 to address respite care issues. Entitled The Lifespan Respite Care Act, over 200 national, state, and local organizations advocated its passage, culminating in its signing into law late in 2006.[36] The new law authorizes $289 million over 5 years for state grants to develop respite programs. The act defines respite programs as "coordinated systems of accessible, community-based respite care services for family caregivers of children and adults with special needs."[36] Passage of this legislation is a landmark, as it provides a nationwide acknowledgment of the inherent economic value of the informal family-provided care system. In addition, as a major thrust of federal initiatives, the U.S. Administration on Aging continues to pilot several different types of demonstration programs targeted at determining the cost-effectiveness and consumer acceptability of various combinations of community-based services that support older persons' ability to continue living independently. In its 2006 passage of the Older Americans Act Amendments, Congress emphasized the federal government's role in assisting older Americans to remain independent members of their communities.[37]

Adult Day Care

An adult day care center may provide a supervised program of social activities and custodial care (social model), medical and rehabilitative care through skilled nursing (medical model), or specialized services for patients with Alzheimer's disease or other forms of dementia. An adult day care center operates during the day in a protective group setting outside the home. The primary intent of adult day care is to prevent the premature and inappropriate institutionalization of older adults by providing socialization, health care, or both. Older adults maintain their mental and physical well-being longer and at a higher level when they continue to reside in their homes and communities. Furthermore, for those who depend on the services of a regular family caregiver, an adult day care center can provide respite for the caregiver and therapeutic social contacts for the care recipient.[38]

The concept of adult day care grew out of social concern for the quality of life and care of older adults based on the work of Lionel Cousins, who in the 1960s, established the first adult day care center in the United States to "prepare patients for discharge by teaching and promoting independent living skills."[39] Originally, development and growth in such programs were slow because there was no national policy to support the idea, nor a permanent funding base, as the prototype Medicare and Medicaid programs supported and encouraged institutionalization; however, as the cost of institutionalization, the inhumanity of many nursing homes, and the burden placed on family caregivers were recognized, the focus of long-term care has been redirected toward support of community-based care as a preferred alternative to institutionalization whenever possible. Since then, growth in the number of adult day care programs has been rapid. The first adult day care center in this country was opened in 1947, but by 1981, only 15 were active.[40] Today, estimates place the number of licensed and unlicensed centers in operation at over 4,000, with many more needed to meet demand. Not-for-profit organizations operate 80% of adult day care centers.[41]

The services that adult day care centers offer are similar, but the emphasis varies with the model they follow. Most adult day care centers offer a variety of medical, psychiatric, and nursing assessments, counseling, physical exercises, social services, crafts, and rehabilitation in activities of daily living skills. Special-purpose adult day care centers serve particular populations of clients, such as veterans, older persons with mental health problems, the blind, people with Alzheimer's disease, or people with cerebral palsy.

Staffing patterns of adult day care programs vary from program to program and are directly related to the type of program and specific services being offered. The ratio of staff to patients also is diverse but is in the range of 1 staff member to every 3 to 12 clients. The mix of unskilled to skilled employees also depends on the kinds of services being offered. For example, programs based on the medical model are more likely to employ more registered nurses, occupational therapists, and physical therapists to provide skilled assessment, direct care, and rehabilitative therapies than in a social model, where aides may perform most of the custodial care and a recreational therapist may be employed to plan and deliver recreational and socialization activities. The number of clients enrolled in a day care program varies according to the staffing pattern and facility size. The cost of care may vary widely depending on the range and scope of services provided. Medicare generally does not provide reimbursement for day care services. Medicaid may provide reimbursement for services in a medical model day care program, but this practice varies from state to state. Often, services are paid for through private fees or through programs supported by grant funds or by charitable or religious organizations.

A substantial proportion of adult day care centers are regulated by state licensure laws, although licensing is not mandatory in all states. Most also are certified by the particular community agency that is funding the day care center. Licensure and credentialing ensure that the day care center meets minimum standards and guidelines set by the overseeing funding agency in order for the community agency to meet criteria for obtaining underlying federal government grants. In 1999, the Commission on Accreditation of Rehabilitation Facilities, along with the National Adult Day Services Association, published adult day care standards, which include organizational measurement and quality, and information systems and outcomes quality. The new standards provided an enhanced level of quality guidance to adult day care management, as well as more recognition of the value of adult day care services in the overall continuum of long-term care.[42]

Innovations in Long-Term Care

Innovative long-term care services that meet the diverse medical needs, personal desires, and lifestyle choices of older Americans have made important strides. The continuum of care model recognizes the complex configuration of individual needs and encourages the implementation of programs and services of adequate variety, intensity, and scope to provide the best configuration of care to any individual. Concepts such as aging in place, life care communities, naturally occurring retirement communities, and high-technology home care are some of the changes that offer enriched alternatives to long-term care recipients.

Aging in Place

Moving to a nursing home or dependent care facility is seen by many as a change in lifestyle to be steadfastly avoided for as long as possible. Most people prefer to remain actively engaged in their own support and care, in their own residence, and within the context of their own family. Research indicates enhanced quality of life and longevity when older adults are able to remain in their own residences. The term "aging in place," in the context of older and frail persons, refers to at least partial fulfillment of this desire. An aging-in-place health care system allows older adults to maintain their health while living as independently as possible in their own homes, without a costly, and in many cases traumatic, move to an institutional setting. The proportion of older people in our society is increasing, and government resources to assist them have come under increasing scrutiny in an effort to control escalating long-term care costs. At the federal, state, and local governmental levels, as evidenced by recent legislation, and at the grassroots level, an increasingly favorable light is shining on the well-documented cost-effectiveness of health care programs that encourage the aging-in-place concept and the concurrent maintenance of independent living.

A number of aging-in-place programs have been developed that guarantee participants a lifetime health care plan and support services. In these models, institutionalization occurs only if it becomes medically imperative because necessary care is unavailable in the home setting. Services that participants receive may vary slightly, but most frequently include

- Nursing services provided by registered and licensed nurses
- Home care aide assistance
- Homemaker services to assist with meals and housekeeping
- 24-hour emergency response system
- Home-delivered groceries
- Adult day care

Participants continue to have the full financial responsibility of home maintenance and upkeep because direct assistance with these tasks is limited to a list of names of prequalified tradesmen and mechanics.

In 1972, a model of aging-in-place service delivery called On Lok Senior Health Services was established as a demonstration project to provide health services to a selected population of frail older people in San Francisco. The term "On-Lok" derives from the Chinese language, meaning "peaceful and happy abode."[43] Participants in the On Lok program live in their own residences with an interdisciplinary team of health care professionals managing their health care. When institutional care is required (either in a nursing home or hospital) or ancillary diagnostic or specialty physician services are needed, they are provided through contractual arrangements with outside providers. The prototype program was so successful that Congress mandated replication of this model by establishment of demonstration programs, called the "Program for All-Inclusive

Care for the Elderly" (PACE), in other parts of the country. The early success of PACE was evidenced by the fact that, although its clients were certified eligible for nursing home placement, only 6% were placed in nursing homes; the rest were able to remain in their homes.[43] Also impressive was the low hospitalization rate of participants when compared with typical Medicare beneficiaries with similar health status. Through provisions of the BBA, PACE earned permanent status as a Medicare-approved benefit.[44]

Continuing Care Retirement and Life Care Communities

Continuing care retirement communities (CCRCs) are available for those Americans who do not wish to stay in their own homes as they get older, yet are essentially well enough to avoid institutionalization. Current estimates place the number of CCRCs at over 2,200, accommodating approximately 750,000 older Americans.[45] CCRCs provide residences on a retirement campus, typically in apartment complexes designed for functional older adults. Unlike ordinary retirement communities that offer only specialized housing, CCRCs offer a comprehensive program of social services, meals, and access to contractual medical services in addition to housing. Religious or not-for-profit organizations sponsor most CCRCs.

A continuing life care community (CLCC) is a type of CCRC, but health care services are prepaid and can be guaranteed for life. A CLCC typically provides services ranging from independent living accommodations to skilled nursing care. Cost varies widely, and such programs are expensive; however, as advocates for this lifestyle point out, many Americans approaching their retirement years have sufficient equity in their homes and investment income to pay the required entrance and monthly maintenance fees.

CLCCs achieve financial viability by using an insurance-based model and as such are regulated by state insurance departments, as well as other regulatory agencies to which their services may be subject in their respective states. The program administrators establish eligibility criteria for participants using actuarial data from the insurance industry. The future lifetime medical costs of participants are anticipated, and rates and charges are set accordingly. Prospective CLCC residents are provided a contract outlining what the CLCC will provide in terms of home accommodations, social activities, services and amenities, and access to onsite levels of health care. Most CLCCs require a one-time entrance fee and a monthly fee. There are many variations to the types of contracts offered.[46] In general, services may include:

- Meals
- Scheduled transportation
- Housekeeping services
- Housing unit maintenance
- Linen and personal laundry
- Health monitoring
- Wellness programs
- Some utilities
- Social activities
- Home health care
- Skilled nursing care

A life care community offers more comprehensive benefits and support systems for the older persons than any other option available today in the United States. Less than 1% of older citizens have taken advantage of this option, in great part because of the expense and requirement of an extended commitment.

Naturally Occurring Retirement Communities

A "naturally occurring retirement community" (NORC) is a term coined by Professor Michael Hunt of the University of Wisconsin-Madison in the 1980s to describe apartment buildings where the majority of residents were 60 years of age or older.[47] Now, the NORC acronym is widely used to describe apartment complexes, neighborhoods, or sections of communities where residents have opted to remain in their homes as they age. Today, numerous communities throughout the United States formally recognize NORCs.

The U.S. Administration on Aging recognized NORCs through the development of a competitive grant awards program for demonstration projects designed to test and evaluate methods to assist older Americans in their desire to age in place. Community centers and other not-for-profit organizations could compete for grant funding, and demonstration projects were enacted in several states.[47] NORC programs use a combination of services such as case management, nursing, social and recreational activities, health education, transportation, nutrition, and referral linkages to enhance quality of life and safety for older adults who wish to remain in their homes during their aging process. NORCs appear to hold much potential as a positive alternative to institutionalization and possible cost savings for individuals and government.[47]

High-Technology Home Care: Hospitals Without Walls

Traditionally, home health care has focused on providing supportive care to persons with long-term disability and chronic disease. Changes in reimbursement mechanisms to a prospective payment system based on diagnosis-related groups have led to the more rapid discharge of all patients from hospitals following episodes of hospitalization for acute illness, exacerbation of chronic disease, progression of disability, or surgery. Patients frequently are discharged home while they still require advanced intensive therapeutic treatments and rely on complex, high-technology services such as ventilators, kidney dialysis, intravenous antibiotic therapy, parenteral nutrition, and cancer chemotherapy.

The delivery of high-technology home care is not only more cost-effective than hospitalization or institutionalization in a nursing home, but also allows the client to move from the more dependent patient role to the more autonomous role as a client in their own residence. Home health care agencies have accommodated this trend toward provision of advanced high-technology therapy in the home setting through innovations in the type and organization of the specialty services they provide. Improvements and innovations have taken place in the portability, mobility, reliability, and cost of medical devices such as intravenous therapy pumps, long-term venous access devices, continuous ambulatory peritoneal dialysis equipment, and ventilators. Innovative teams of skilled practitioners in specialized areas such as intravenous therapy and kidney dialysis and the concurrent development of innovative support teams of pharmacists and specialty technicians who prepare and deliver necessary intravenous, parenteral nutrition, and dialysis solutions and medications have made the home setting an appropriate environment for the delivery of high-technology therapies.

Long-Term Care Insurance

Long-term care insurance (LTCI) is a financing option for long-term care. In 1986, there were only 30 companies that offered this type of coverage. The number of companies has increased many fold since then.[48] In 2007, the American Association for Long-Term Care Insurance estimated that 8 million Americans owned LTCI policies.[49] Individuals purchase the majority of policies, but an increasing number of employers are now offering coverage through group purchase plans. The Federal government encourages the purchase of long-term care policies by offering tax deductions to employers and many states now offer incentives for individuals who purchase tax-qualified long-term care policies.[50]

The benefits of LTCI policies vary across a broad spectrum. The most desirable policies cover services across the continuum of potential long-term care needs, with maximum subscriber flexibility. Specialists counsel buyers to be wary of limitations relative to inflationary factors in the costs of coverage, renewability clauses, limits on payments for various modes of long-term care, requirements for prior hospitalization for eligibility for home care, cancellation features of policies, and lifetime benefit limits. As with life insurance, the premium cost reflects age at purchase of the policy. LTCI companies also use underwriting criteria and may reject applicants or increase premiums for individuals with preexisting conditions that render them at high risk for future long-term care services.

Insurance industry advocates and other analysts contend that individuals and society will benefit in the future from the proliferation of LTCI. In this view, public dependency, especially on Medicaid, to fund long-term care needs would decrease, and individuals would have the ability to access the highest quality long-term care services without risk of impoverishment.[51]

The decision to invest in an LTCI product is very personal and depends on many factors, primarily on the level of assets the individual has, or expects to have at risk if long-term care is required. Other alternatives to LTCI, such as transferring assets to children to become financially eligible for Medicaid, using the equity in a home, selecting special living arrangements, and using personal savings, are not universally applicable. All of these options must be carefully assessed against the cost of LTCI in order to make viable and appropriate future plans.

The Future of Long-Term Care

The United States will need more and diverse long-term care programs in the future to serve increasing needs, especially of older adults. Some of the causes underlying the intensifying need for diverse long-term care service options are

- Changes in the demographics of the U.S. population
- Social and economic changes in families
- Increasingly sophisticated medical technology
- Greater consumer sophistication
- Increasing scrutiny of federal and state government financial involvement in support of long-term health care

The final configuration of the long-term care service delivery system is difficult to predict with certainty, although an analysis of current trends suggests certain directions.

Long-term care services have become increasingly diversified and specialized, which allows programs and providers to focus on becoming experts in meeting specific needs of specialized populations such as people with Alzheimer's disease or AIDS. To be avoided is one danger in allowing specialization to lead to fragmentation, duplication of services, and pressure to categorize participants into narrow service niches. Services such as subacute care and the provision of transitional health care after acute-care hospitalization for medically complex long-term care patients, are responding as the drive to discharge patients from hospitals quickly results in a greater need for more intense supportive care environments beyond hospital walls. Service delivery systems that function within the managed care environment are becoming increasingly common, and the bundling of posthospitalization care with hospitalization into one episode of care provided through one integrated service provider is occurring more frequently. Whether such trends will contribute to a seamless continuity of care will remain under scrutiny.

Demonstrated cost-effectiveness and expressed client preferences for community-based care will continue to increase the demand for home health services. Federal and state administrations are increasingly recognizing consumer preferences, exemplified by legislation emphasizing community-based care over institutionalized care.

Long-term caregivers traditionally have been paid less and given less status than workers in the acute-care health services. The long-term care industry is enduring an employment crisis with an inadequate number and quality of applicants to fill vacancies in the direct caregiver positions across all industry sectors. Factors contributing to the long-term care employment crisis include:[52]

- The growing need for services
- Competition among employers
- Workload and working conditions
- Employee turnover
- Wages and benefits constrained by reimbursement policies
- A lack of social supports for workers, including childcare and transportation
- A lack of opportunities for education and career mobility

Staffing shortages directly and seriously affect the quality of long-term care services. The industry's ability to develop innovative approaches to attracting and retaining staff will have particularly important implications as service demands swell with aging of the baby-boom generation. Supported by major philanthropies such as the Robert Wood Johnson Foundation, identifying solutions to the staffing crises in long-term care is the subject of ongoing research and demonstration projects at a number of academic and policy development institutions throughout the country.[53]

Until recently, the needs of the informal caregiver system were virtually ignored. Significant legislative action at the federal and state levels only recently begins to recognize these needs in terms of employer allowances and other programmatic and economic considerations at the federal and state levels.

An undercurrent of concern runs beneath all aspects of long-term health care delivery, especially with regard to the development of responsive, patient-centered, quality-driven, accessible, affordable, and cost-effective health care services for all citizens—including society's most vulnerable, people with chronic disabilities and frail older adults. Many

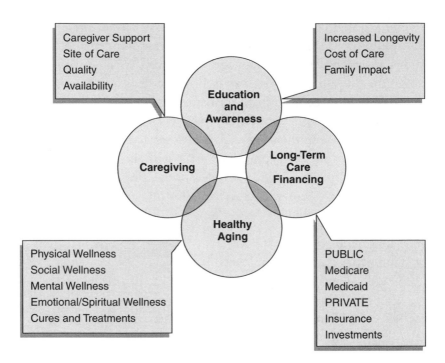

FIGURE 8-11 Components of a National Long-Term Care Strategy. *Source:* Genworth Financial, reprinted with permission.

concerns related to future long-term care will remain open ended, and the part that long-term care services will play within any restructuring of the U.S. health care system is undetermined, although it undoubtedly will be of major concern to the increasingly large portion of older adults in our society. Insurance industry experts suggest the need for a national long-term care strategy that incorporates four primary components of education and awareness, caregiving, healthy aging, and long-term care financing (Figure 8-11).[54] Given the industry's current unmet needs and rising demands, the ensuing years will be a period of experimentation, innovation, and change in the long-term health care system.

References

1. Evashwick CJ. Strategic management of a continuum of care. *J Long-Term Care Admin.* 1993;21:13–24.

2. Shortell SM. *Transforming Health Care Delivery: Seamless Continuum of Care.* Chicago, IL: American Hospital Publishing; 1994:1–7.

3. Jack CM, Paone DL. *Toward Creating a Seamless Continuum of Care: Addressing Chronic Care Needs.* Chicago, IL: Section for Aging and Long-Term Care Services of the American Hospital Association; 1994:3–5.

4. U.S. Department of Health and Human Services, Administration on Aging. Profile of older Americans: 2005. Available from http://www.aoa.gov/prof/statistics/profile/2005/2005profile.pdf. Accessed January 16, 2007.

5. U.S. General Accounting Office. Long-term care financing, growing demand and cost of services are straining federal and state budgets. Available from http://www.gao.gov/new.items/d05564t.pdf. Accessed January 9, 2007.

6. Shore HH. History of long-term care. In: Goldsmith SB, ed. *Essentials of Long-Term Care Administration.* Gaithersburg, MD: Aspen Publishers; 1994: 5–6.

7. National Center for Health Statistics. Number and percent distribution of nursing homes by selected facility characteristics, according to number of beds per nursing home and occupancy rate, 2004. Available from http://www.cdc.gov/nchs/data/nnsd/nursinghomefacilities2006.pdf. Accessed January 9, 2007.

8. Pavri JM. Overview: One hundred years of public health nursing: visions of a better world. *Imprint.* 41 1994;4:43–48.

9. Glasscote RM, et al. *Old Folks at Homes: A Field Study of Nursing and Board and Care Homes.* Washington, DC: American Psychiatric Association; 1976:3.

10. Moss FE, Halamandaris VJ. *Too Old, Too Sick, Too Bad.* Gaithersburg, MD: Aspen Publishers; 1977:15–37.

11. Glasscote, RM, et al. Old Folks at Homes: A Field Study of Nursing and Board and Care Homes. Washington, DC: American Psychiatric Association; 1976:3.

12. Evans JM, Fleming KC. Medical care of nursing home residents. *Mayo Clin Proc.* 1995;70:694.

13. Long Term Care Education.com. Definition of the skilled nursing facility. Available from http://www.longtermcareeducation.com/c2/c4.asp. Accessed January 8, 2007.

14. Genworth Financial. 2006 cost of care survey for nursing homes, assisted living facilities and home care providers. Available from http://www.aahsa.org/advocacy/assisted_living/reports_data/documents/Genworth_cost_study.pdf. Accessed January 9, 2007.

15. Centers for Medicare and Medicaid Services. Expenditures for health services and supplies, by type of service and sources of funds, CY 1980–2005. Available from http://www.cms.hhs.gov/NationalHealthExpendData/02_NationalHealthAccountsHistorical.asp#TopofPage. Accessed January 20, 2007.

16. Health United States, 2006, Table 116. Nursing home beds, occupancy, and residents by geographic division and state: United States, selected years 1995–2004. Available from http://www.cdc.gov/nchs/data/hys/hus06.pdf. Accessed January 9, 2007.

17. National Association of Boards of Examiners of Long Term Care Administrators. NAB urges states to approve nationwide standards for nursing home administrator licensing. Available from http://www.nabweb.org/uploaded files/endorsement%20release%203-8-06.pdf. Accessed January 12, 2007.

18. Assisted Living Federation of America. What is assisted living? Available from http://www.alfa.org/i4a/pages/index.cfm?pageid=3285. Accessed January 11, 2007.

19. Assisted Living Federation of America. Frequently asked questions about assisted living. Available from http://www.alfa.org/i4a/pages/index.cfm?pageid=3285. Accessed January 11, 2007.

20. Centers for Medicare and Medicaid Services. Health care industry market update: home health. Available from http://www.cms.gov/capmarketupdates/downloads/hcimu92203.pdf. Accessed January 11, 2007.

21. Centers for Medicare and Medicaid Services. Home health quality initiatives. Available from http://www.cms.hhs.gov./HomeHealthQualityInits/01_overview.asp. Accessed February 11, 2007.

22. Medical News Today. Medical literature shows homecare is cost-effective in Medicare, Medicaid-USA (August 21, 2005). Available from http://www.medicalnewstoday.com/printerfriendlynews.php?newsid=29446. Accessed February 11, 2007.

23. Centers for Medicare and Medicaid Services. Post acute care reform policy council document. Available from http://www.cms.hhs.gov/SNFPPS/Downloads/pzc_reform_plan_2006.pdf. Accessed February 12, 2007.

24. Centers for Medicare and Medicaid Services. 2006 CMS statistics, Table 20. Available from http://www.cms.hhs.gov/capmarketupdates/downloads/2006cmsstat.pdf. Accessed February 11, 2007.

25. Centers for Medicare and Medicaid. Home health agencies, certification and compliance, home health providers. Available from http://www.cms.hhs.gov/CertificationandComplianc/06_HHAs.asp. Accessed February 12, 2007.

26. National Family Caregivers Association. Caregiving statistics. Available from http://www.nfcacares.org/who_are_family_caregivers/care_giving_statistics.cfm. Accessed February 25, 2007.

27. National Association of Social Workers. Working family caregivers: issues and opportunities for social work practice. Available from http://www.socialworkers.org/practice/aging/aging0804.pdf. Accessed February 25, 2007.

28. MetLife Mature Market Institute and National Alliance for Caregiving. The MetLife Caregiving Cost Study: productivity losses to U.S. businesses. Available from http://www.metlife.com/WPSAssets/135517774261164052327V1Fcaregivercoststudy.pdf. Accessed February 25, 2007.

29. Arno PS. The economic cost of informal caregiving: 2004. Available from http://www.va.gov/Conferences/caregiverforum/docs/Arno-handout.pdf. Accessed February 25, 2007.

30. Family Caregiver Alliance, National Center on Caregiving. Support for working family caregivers: paid leave policies in California and beyond, issue brief, June 2006. Available from http://www.caregiver.org/caregiver/jsp/content/pdfs/op_2006_paid_leave2.pdf. Accessed February 25, 2007.

31. Centers for Medicare and Medicaid. Operation restore trust accomplishments. Fact sheet. Available from http://www.os.dhhs.gov/news/press/1997/pres/970520d.html. Accessed February 25, 2007.

32. Centers for Medicare and Medicaid. Improving quality, tightening standards. Fact sheet, 1–3. Available from http://www.cms.gov/media/press/release.asp?Counter=330. Accessed February 26, 2007.

33. Centers for Medicare and Medicaid. OASIS and outcome-based quality improvement in home health care: research and demonstration findings, policy implications, and considerations for future change. Available from http://www.cms.hhs.gov/homehealthqualityinits/downloads/HHQIOASIS ReportSummary.pdf. Accessed February 25, 2007.

34. National Hospice and Palliative Care Organization. NHPCO's facts and figures—2005 findings. Available from http://www.nhpco.org/files/public/2005-facts-and-figures.pdf. Accessed February 25, 2007.

35. National Association for Home Care, Hospice Association of America. Hospice facts & statistics, March 2006. Available from http://www.nahc.org/hospicefs06.pdf. Accessed February 25, 2007.

36. National Family Caregivers Association. President signs Critical Respite bill for family caregivers. Available from http://www.nfcacares.org/press_room/detail.cfm?num=93. Accessed March 1, 2007.

37. Administration on Aging. Older Americans Act Amendments of 2006. Available from http://www.aoa.gov/OAA2006/Main_Site/index.aspx. Accessed March 1, 2007.

38. Cefalu CA, Heuser M. Adult day care for the demented elderly. *Am Family Phys.* 1993;47:723–724.

39. Lamden RS, Tynan CM, Warnke J, et al. Adult day care. In: Goldsmith SB, ed. *Long-Term Care Administration Handbook.* Sudbury, MA: Jones and Bartlett Publishers; 1993:395–396.

40. Kirwin PM. *Adult Day Care: The Relationship of Formal and Informal Systems of Care.* New York, NY: Garland Publishing; 1991:48.

41. National Respite Network and Resource Center. Fact sheet number 54. Adult day care: one form of respite for older adults. Available from http://www.archrespite.org/archfs54.htm. Accessed March 3, 2007.

42. MacDonnell C. CARF accredits adult day care. *Nursing Homes.* 1999;48:53.

43. Miller JA. *Community-Based Long-Term Care.* New York: Sage Publications; 1991:203.

44. Deloitte & Touche, LLP, and Deloitte & Touche Consulting Group, LLC. *The Balanced Budget Act of 1997, Public Law 105-33 Medicare and Medicaid Changes.* Washington, DC: Deloitte & Touche, LLP, 1997:4.

45. American Association of Homes and Services for the Aging. Aging services: the facts. Available from http://www.aahsa.org/aging_services/default.asp. Accessed March 1, 2007.

46. Senior Resource for Continuing Care Retirement Communities. Continuing care retirement communities (CCRCs) and life care. Available from http://www.seniorresource.com/hccrc.htm, 1. Accessed March 11, 2007.

47. U.S. Department of Health and Human Services, Office of Disability, Aging and Long Term Care Policy and the Urban Institute. Supportive services programs in naturally occurring retirement communities. Available from http://aspe.hhs.gov/daltcp/reports/NORC ssp.htm. Accessed March 11, 2007.

48. Snowe OJ. *Long-Term Care Improvement Act. Congressional Record: 1472.* Washington, DC: U.S. Congress; 1994.

49. American Association for Long-Term Care Insurance. Long-term care insurance policies paid $3.3 billion in claims in 2006—one third allocated to home care. Available from http://www.aaltci.org/subpages/media_room/story_pages/media020107.html. Accessed March 12, 2007.

50. American Association for Long-Term Care Insurance. 2007 tax deductible limits for LTCI announced. Available from http://www.aaltci.org/subpages/media_room/story_pages/media110906.html. Accessed March 12, 2007.

51. Merlis M. *Financing Long Term Care in the Twenty-first Century: The Public and Private Roles. Institute for Health Policy Solutions.* New York, NY: The Commonwealth Fund; September 1999:20.

52. New York State Association of Homes and Services for the Aging. The Staffing Crisis in New York's Continuing Care System, A Comprehensive Analysis and Recommendations. (March 2000): Albany, NY: New York State Association of Homes and Services for the Aging; 1.

53. Medical News Today. Solutions to impending U.S. long term care facility staffing crisis. Available from http://www.medicalnewstoday.com/medical news.php?newsid=7520. Accessed March 14, 2007.

54. Genworth Financial. Long-term care insurance overview, thought leadership. Available from http://longtermcare.genworth.com/overview/thought_leader ship.jsp. Accessed March 14, 2007.

CHAPTER 9

Mental Health Services

Susan V. McLeer, MD, MS

This chapter describes the clinical characteristics of people who receive mental health services. Historic trends and forces affecting the distribution and kinds of care are examined and compared with epidemiologic data regarding the prevalence of psychiatric disorders to hypothesize whether national needs for mental health care are being met. Evolution in the science and technology available for the treatment of psychiatric disorders is reviewed briefly. Opportunities for improvement and evidence of the impact of managed care on effective mental health service delivery are examined.

Historical Overview

In the early years of our nation, the mentally ill were confined at home, in jails, or in almshouses, where they suffered severely. It was not until the early 19th century that sensitivity to the special needs of the mentally ill emerged through the Quaker emphasis on mental illness as being treatable. This approach, established earlier in Europe and known as "moral treatment," was tried in a few mental hospitals where patients received kind, but firm, treatment while participating in work, educational activities, and recreation.[1] Effective biological treatments were nonexistent, and the majority of patients did not have access to moral treatment; rather, they were confined under the most adverse circumstances. Hospitals became overcrowded custodial facilities, not only for the mentally ill, but also for criminals, alcoholics, and low-income, homeless people.

Awareness of the needs of the mentally ill became more focused after World War I with the return of thousands of men with disabilities and suffering from "war neurosis," also known as "shell shock," a condition synonymous with current criteria for posttraumatic stress disorder. In the 1930s, the first effective biological treatments emerged in the forms of insulin coma, drug-induced convulsions, and electroconvulsive therapy. Psychosurgery emerged briefly as an area of potential benefit to psychiatric patients. With the advent of World War II, the federal government became active in the mental health field, passing the National Mental Health Act in 1946, which resulted in the establishment of the National Institute of Mental Health (NIMH). Federal, state, and county dollars were allocated for training, research, and service in mental health. The Department of Veterans Affairs recognized the need for increased mental health services and established psychiatric hospitals and ambulatory clinics.

Psychiatric care still remained focused on inpatient services, with the number of people placed in inpatient facilities expanding to a new maximum by the mid-1950s, when over half a million patients were hospitalized in state or county mental hospitals. Fortuitously, this corresponded with the development of the first psychoactive medications specifically targeted for treating psychiatric disorders. These agents included chlorpromazine (Thorazine) and reserpine, used for the treatment of schizophrenia and other psychotic disorders. These advances profoundly changed patterns of care, reducing the need for convulsive therapies and psychosurgery and providing patients with effective interventions that allowed them to live outside of a mental hospital. Ambulatory services were intensified with the addition of partial hospitalization programs, intensive after-care programs, and the development of nonhospital transitional residential facilities, or halfway houses, for the mentally ill.

By 1955, the U.S. Congress established the Joint Commission on Mental Illness and Health. The commission attacked the quality of care and patient access to care in the large state and county mental hospitals. This was the first time a federal body had considered the allocation of resources for the mentally ill. The commission's report began a substantial shift in sites for the provision of mental health services from the inpatient state and county mental hospitals to outpatient facilities. The commission's recommendations fell on fertile ground and were reiterated by President Kennedy in his first message to Congress.

By the early 1960s, the winds of change had been whipped up not only by the commission, but also by the development of new, effective psychotropic medications and psychosocial treatments that could provide positive intervention for many disorders outside the hospital. Congress passed the Mental Retardation Facilities and Community Mental Health Centers Construction Act, resulting in considerable federal support for community-based services. Large entitlement programs became accessible to the mentally ill, mainly Medicaid, Medicare, Supplemental Security Income (SSI), Social Security and Disability Insurance, and housing subsidies, among others.

Throughout the 1960s and 1970s, the federal government became more involved in financing mental health care. Community mental health centers developed and expanded, and more health professionals entered the mental health field. Federal and state money, originally targeted for severely mentally ill patients, was shunted through the community mental health systems to provide services for those with less severe illness.[2,3] This shift in service was based on two untested assumptions that provided the underpinnings for changes in program planning in community mental health centers. These assumptions were (1) mental disorders lie on a quantitative continuum, with severe mental illness not differing qualitatively from lesser forms of mental distress, and (2) early intervention can prevent the development of major psychiatric disorders. Neither assumption has been demonstrated to be valid. Nonetheless, based on these assumptions, much money was invested and services provided to people with mild to moderate dysfunction and "problems in living," with the hope that the incidence of severe mental illness would be reduced through primary prevention.[4]

Treatment of less severe problems was handled through psychosocial interventions without proven efficacy and without systematic and standardized evaluations of outcome. In addition, payment for mental health services with public dollars was allocated on the basis of units of service provided; therefore, there was no incentive for limiting the duration of treatment, and patients were provided nonspecific, psychosocial interventions for years. From 1955 to 1980, the number of patient care episodes provided in organized mental health settings increased fourfold, from 1.7 million to 7 million.[5] Few of these patients were severely mentally ill.[6]

Simultaneously with the institution of these programmatic changes in community mental health centers, many severely mentally ill patients who formerly had been warehoused in large state or county mental hospitals were discharged to community boarding houses and nursing homes.

The deinstitutionalization movement was presented as being important to the rehabilitation of those with severe mental illness. Emphasis was placed on the necessity of providing services in community settings. In actuality, the states, through Medicaid, were receiving major financial incentives to move patients from inpatient mental hospitals to nursing homes. This transfer, coupled with the changes in the staffing and programs at community mental health centers, resulted in many severely mentally ill patients finding limited access to care. Treatments provided at the mental health centers no longer targeted the vulnerable group of people with severe disabilities. Advocacy groups such as the National Alliance for the Mentally Ill (NAMI) emerged, directing their efforts to have public dollars reallocated to include the funding of biomedical research that targeted severe and persistent psychiatric disorders. Advocates maintained that the pivotal issue was the treatment of psychiatric illness, not the maintenance of mental health. Through their efforts, those of NIMH, and clinical researchers across the United States, the assumptions fueling the staffing and programming of mental health centers during the 1970s and early 1980s were proved erroneous. Psychiatric disorders are not on a quantitative continuum, but are discontinuous in development. They are biologically based illnesses, frequently precipitated and exacerbated by psychosocial stressors. These disorders and their symptoms require specific, targeted treatments.

By the late 1970s, health care costs had soared, and the federal government became concerned with identifying mechanisms for restraining health-related spending. President Carter, recognizing that new research findings presented opportunities for improving care to the mentally ill, appointed a Presidential Commission on Mental Health. Because of fiscal constraints and political infighting both in Washington and in the field of psychiatry itself, the majority of the commission's findings and recommendations were not put into operation; however, the commission's work quietly filtered down to the Department of Health and Human Services, resulting in substantial changes of great importance to those with severe mental illness. Psychosocial rehabilitation programs were expanded under Medicaid. Medicaid payment for outpatient mental health care was expanded; co-payment requirements for case management services were reduced. Patients with severe and persistent mental illness became eligible for SSI funding. These changes meant a substantial shift in quality-of-life issues for this population; however, by the mid-1980s, programs became sharply curtailed again, with cutbacks in housing subsidies, social services, and increased exclusion of people with mental illness from SSI benefits.

By 1990, although controversy still raged over which services should be delivered to whom, the locus of mental health care in the United States had shifted from inpatient to outpatient settings. Of the 1.7 million episodes of mental health services delivered in 1955, 77% were in inpatient settings and 23% in outpatient programs. By 1990, 67% of the 8.6 million episodes of mental health services delivered were provided in outpatient programs, 7% in partial hospitalization settings (not 24-hour facilities), and 21% in inpatient services.[7]

Over the past decade, because of constant and rigorous pressure placed on Congress and legislative bodies by advocacy groups such as NAMI and psychiatric researchers, the focus on severe mental illness has returned. Through block grants, state departments of mental health have refocused their energies and reallocated resources to ensure the provision of services to the most vulnerable population—those afflicted with severe and persistent mental illness. Federal money has been reallocated for research and training, with efforts focused on treatment, not prevention. The results of these shifts have been considerable. Now, in the 21st century, the chances of people with severe mental illness receiving significant benefit through effective treatments have never been better. Yet few people access these treatments.

Recipients of Mental Health Services

The recipients of mental health services in the United States constitute a small subpopulation of those individuals afflicted with a mental illness. Access to mental health services is and has been controlled by a variety of factors, including, but not limited to, persistent myths regarding the nature and treatability of mental illness, nonparity in insurance coverage for mental illness, and political decisions regarding the distribution of resources in our communities.

Mental illness is enormously painful and debilitating, both for those directly afflicted and for their families. Well-designed epidemiologic studies, conducted by the Epidemiologic Catchment Area (ECA) Program and the National Co-Morbidity Study, have reported that as many as 20% to 29% of the U.S. population will have a mental disorder during a

1-year period;[8] however, many of these disorders are temporary and have minimal effects on individual function. Less than 7% of adults in the United States have mental disorders that persist for 1 year or more,[9] and approximately 9% of the population have reported significant disability associated with a mental disorder.[10] A total of about 15% of the adult U.S. population uses mental health services in any given year (Table 9-1).[11] However, over the course of a year, less than one-third of adults with diagnosable mental disorders receive treatment.[12] Factors recognized as contributing to barriers to care access include financial limitations, social stigmatization, misunderstandings about the treatability of conditions, personal and provider attitudes, cultural issues, and an insensitive delivery system organization.[13]

In contrast to widely held assumptions, mental disorders can now be diagnosed and treated as effectively as physical disorders. They are classified according to criteria that provide predictability regarding the natural history of the illness and its responsiveness to specific, disorder-targeted treatments. Seventeen diagnostic categories are described in the *American Psychiatric Association's Diagnostic and Statistical Manual of Mental Disorders*, and within these categories, the specific diagnostic criteria for over 450 conditions are delineated.[14] The criteria for specific diagnoses in each of these categories have been subjected to extensive field testing for diagnostic reliability and validity.

Although these diagnostic categories are useful for obtaining precise diagnoses and prescribing specific treatment plans for mentally ill patients, they have not been used extensively by those who set policy and

Table 9-1 Proportion of Adult Population Using Mental/Addictive Disorder Services in One Year

Type of Service	Percentage of Population
Total health sector services	11%*
Specialty mental health	6%
General medical	6%
Human services professionals	5%
Voluntary support network	3%
Any of above services	15%

*Subtotals do not add to total due to overlap.

Source: Reprinted from U.S. Department of Health and Human Services Publication No. SMA-96-3098.

distribute resources nationally. Rather, the concept of "severe mental illness" has evolved, and those with mental disorders that fall into this broad category have been targeted to receive services. This group represents approximately 3% of the U.S. population.[15,16]

According to the National Advisory Mental Health Council,[17] severe mental illness encompasses a group of discrete mental disorders that differ in cause, course, and treatment. This population encompasses people afflicted with schizophrenia, schizoaffective disorders, autism, affective disorders (bipolar, formerly called manic-depressive disorder and severe depression), other psychotic disorders, as well as some of the anxiety disorders (severe panic disorders and obsessive-compulsive disorders). In addition to carrying a primary psychiatric diagnosis, people with severe mental illness are highly likely to have additional problems with substance abuse, as well as developmental disorders that are neurologically based (e.g., mental retardation or specific learning disabilities). These conditions further compromise patients' abilities to function.

The coexistence of two diagnoses is called "comorbidity." According to the ECA Study, in 1 year, people with substance use disorders made 56.3 million visits to ambulatory mental health/addiction services. Of these, 62% were visits made by those with comorbid substance use and mental disorders.[17] In further ECA studies, in both clinical and nonclinical settings, the prevalence of substance abuse comorbidity has been determined for specific psychiatric disordered patients. These findings indicated a range in prevalence of 23% to 80%, depending on diagnosis.[18]

Substantial comorbidity also has been documented among people with mental retardation. In studies of clinical populations of people with mental retardation, 30% to 67% have been found to have comorbid psychiatric disorders.[19] The importance of these epidemiologic studies cannot be overemphasized because research on service provision to subpopulations with substantial comorbidity has demonstrated that comorbidity adds significantly to the complexity of providing adequate and effective treatments. The implications to resource allocation are considerable.

Only a little over half of the people who are most vulnerable and have severe mental illness use mental health services; however, the use of services does not imply adequate access or use of effective services. Although some of these individuals have severe disabilities, are treatment resistant, and hence, require lifelong supervision of living arrangements, the vast majority are people who, with accurate diagnosis and access to effective treatment and rehabilitative services, can lead productive and fulfilling lives in the community. Yet many of these individuals go undiagnosed or untreated.

Children and Adolescents

Data on service use by children and adolescents with diagnoses of mental disorder and at least minimal impairment only recently have become available from a NIMH survey of children and adolescents between 9 and 17 years of age. Approximately 9% of the entire child/adolescent sample (less than one-half of those affected) received some mental health services in the general medical and specialty mental health delivery sectors, although the largest provider of services to this population group was the school system.[20]

Clinical research targeted toward determining effective treatments for children and adolescents suffering from mental illness has lagged considerably behind that for adults. Although diagnostic techniques have been highly refined through standardized diagnostic interviews and symptom rating scales that facilitate the accurate identification of those in need of service, research funding for treatment of mental illness in childhood and adolescence has not kept pace. The effects of a mental disorder on the developmental process of children are only beginning to be appreciated, but they clearly interfere with emotional, social, and cognitive growth and development. The need for early intervention that provides treatment and rehabilitation is urgent. Nevertheless, few practitioners have access to research findings regarding treatment efficacy, and few well-trained child and adolescent psychiatrists are available to the population at risk. Although some progress has been made, much more research is urgently needed. The results of newer research on effective treatments of specific disorders need widespread dissemination, with improved training and skills of those providing services for children and adolescents.

Older Adults

Although many advances have been made in the treatment of mental disorders, a crisis looms in providing mental health services to the older population. By the year 2020, the "baby boomers" will reach age 65, with the result that almost 55 million Americans will be classified as "elderly."[21] In addition to sheer volume, epidemiologic studies have indicated that baby-boomer cohorts have high prevalence rates for depression, suicide, anxiety, and alcohol and drug abuse.[22,23] The implications of these findings on future resource allocation decisions are enormous.

Older adults suffer from many of the same mental disorders suffered by their younger counterparts; however, assessment and diagnosis may be more difficult and complicated because of accompanying medical conditions that mimic or mask mental disorders and patients' reluctance to accurately report symptoms. Patients tend to emphasize physical complaints and minimize complaints about their mental status. In addition, stereotypes about aging, leading older adults to believe that mental changes are to be expected, can make assessment and diagnosis particularly challenging.[24]

Primary care providers carry much of the burden of diagnosing mental disorders in older adults, and the rates at which they recognize and properly identify disorders are low. In addition, primary care providers may be reluctant to communicate a diagnosis of mental disorder to their patients and have strikingly low confidence rates in diagnosing and prescribing treatments for these disorders. Researchers estimate that up to 63% of older adults with mental disorders may not be receiving treatment.[24]

More research is needed on the treatment of some of the anxiety disorders and substance use disorders in older adults. Coordination of health care with monitoring of medications and their interactions is critical because older patients are frequently on several prescribed drugs that affect behavior, mood, and cognition. The treatment of psychiatric disorders in older adults differs from that for other age groups because it must take into account age-related changes in metabolism and physiologic function that affect the impact of drugs. Progressive social isolation and financial losses also clearly affect symptom formation and may have substantial effects on treatment responsiveness and outcome.

The Organization and Financing of Mental Health Services

Mental health problems and disorders are treated by an array of providers representing several disciplines working in a diverse array of public and private settings. The loose coordination of facilities and services has resulted in the mental health delivery system being referred to as a "de facto mental health service system."[9] The system is usually described as having four major components.[25]

The first component is the specialty mental health sector with mental health professionals such as psychiatrists, psychologists, psychiatric nurses, and psychiatric social workers providing the majority of care in outpatient settings, in private office practices, or in private or public clinics. Most acute hospital care is provided in psychiatric units of general hospitals or beds located throughout the hospitals. Intensive treatment for adults and children is provided in private psychiatric hospitals or residential treatment centers for children and adolescents. Public sector facilities include state and county mental hospitals and multiservice facilities that provide or coordinate a wide range of outpatient, intensive case management, partial hospitalization, or inpatient services.

The second component is the general medical/primary care sector consisting of health care professionals such as internists, pediatricians, and nurse practitioners in private office-based practices, clinics, hospitals, and nursing homes. This sector often is the initial point of contact and may be the only source of mental health services for a large proportion of mental health patients.

The third component is the human services sector, comprised of social service agencies, school-based counseling services, residential rehabilitation services, vocational rehabilitation services, criminal justice/prison-based services, and religious professional counselors.

The fourth component is the voluntary support network sector consisting of self-help groups. This is a rapidly growing component of the mental health system.

Mental health services have been funded in many ways, including private health insurance, Medicaid, Medicare, state and local services provided directly or through contracts with local agencies, Veterans Affairs hospitals and clinics, and other programs for specialized populations. Because many U.S. citizens lack basic health insurance coverage for the treatment of mental disorders, people with severe mental illness are often dependent on the welfare system for services and supports for basic living.[26–28]

In his review on the establishment of mental health priorities, D. Mechanic and D. Rochefort writes that

> *. . . mental health policy has evolved in a disjointed and nonlinear fashion, reflecting the multiplicity of decision points, prevailing ideologies, emerging technologies, and financial, and other incentives as they interact with the local political, economic, and organizational frameworks of care.*[29]

Mental disorders impose an enormous personal and financial burden on ill individuals, their families, and society as a whole. Their national toll is taken in reduced and lost productivity and the use of medical and other resources for diagnosis, treatment, and rehabilitation. The total cost of U.S. mental health services is estimated at $148 billion. In terms of lost productivity, additional indirect costs of all mental illness results in a nearly $79 billion loss to the U.S. economy.[30] The United States spends over $99 billion for the direct treatment of mental disorders, substance abuse, Alzheimer's disease, and other dementias.[31] More than two-thirds of this amount is funded from private sources (Figure 9-1).[32]

Health Insurance Coverage and Managed Behavioral Health Care

The history of health insurance coverage for mental health services has been sullied by some of the private treatment providers being driven by financial considerations rather than by clinical need, resulting in an

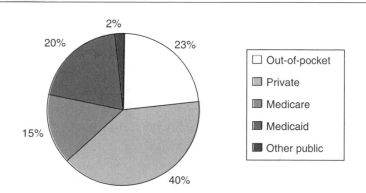

FIGURE 9-1 Distribution of Payment for Mental Health/Substance Abuse Treatment.
Source: Author-created with data from: S.H. Zuvekas, "Trends in Mental Health Services Use and Spending 1987–1996, *Health Affairs* 20, no 2.

exaggeration of the severity of clinical diagnoses in order to maximize payments. Additionally, because coverage has been so limited for ambulatory services, hospitalization was overprescribed.[33] Mary Jane England, president of the American Psychiatric Association from 1995 to 1996, stated that costs had been increased "through sophisticated marketing campaigns targeting adolescents and substance abusers, resulting in many unjustified and even harmful hospitalizations as well as sharply increased costs."[34] On the other end of the continuum, those with severe and persistent psychiatric disorders—those who truly needed intensive services—found that inpatient benefits would be used up before stabilization was gained. Less costly forms of intensive treatment, such as partial hospitalization and day hospitalization programs, frequently were not covered by insurance plans, resulting in ill patients being transferred from the private into the public sector the moment insurance coverage was depleted. This transfer resulted in interrupted treatment, changes in providers, loss of continuity, substantial financial hardship, and impoverishment.

In the public sector, insurance programs, including those of federal, state, and local government, provided payment for services based on units of service delivered, called "the deliverables." Limits were placed on the duration of inpatient treatment, particularly through Medicare, but not substantially on the duration of day treatment, partial hospitalization, or outpatient treatments. Financial incentives were solidly in place for providing increased units of service. As long as need could be documented, there were few checks and balances on the use of ambulatory services or on evaluation of treatment efficacy, as long as payment would be forthcoming.[35] Mental health professionals, particularly in ambulatory settings, were frequently psychodynamically trained and provided patients with generic outpatient care, not targeted treatments of proven efficacy for specific psychiatric disorders. Bringing new research findings to clinicians in the trenches and retraining and re-engineering service delivery are costly. Consequently, for as long as financial incentives for change were lacking, minimal effort went into ensuring that clinicians were providing state-of-the-art interventions. Incentives ensured that practitioners overused ambulatory services. Also, the private sector increased its use of inpatient services, and both sectors escalated their indicators of diagnostic severity. This not only resulted in an increase in the costs of caring for people with mental illness, but also provided support for the following assumptions held by third-party payers that[36]

- Costs of psychiatric treatment are uncontrollable and unpredictable.
- Coverage encourages unnecessary and excessive use.
- Mental health care is not cost-effective.
- Psychiatric treatment is not accountable to insurance carriers.

In fact, it appears that inadequate health insurance coverage for mental health services has paradoxically provided financial incentives for some private practitioners to abuse the system, resulting in increased use and costs without ensuring access to quality and efficacious care. Saul Feldman, chairman of the board at U.S. Behavioral Health and former director of the staff college at the NIMH, has summarized the financial incentives of the 1980s and 1990s by stating that without a structure for ensuring utilization review, the problem becomes one of "people getting too much of the wrong care, in the wrong place."[37]

In the mid-1990s, expenditures for health care hit new highs in the United States. Dramatic cost increases for mental health care paralleled those of the rest of medicine. Between 1986 and 1990, employer spending for meeting the mental health component of health care costs increased by 50%, with the most generous plans reflecting the greatest increases.[38] Feldman noted the following in his analysis of the role of the market in shaping new directions for mental health care:

> But the greatest contributors to the development of managed mental health, a development they now bemoan, have been the service providers themselves, practitioners and facilities. By not paying sufficient attention to or not caring about costs and length of treatments, they killed or at least seriously wounded the goose that laid the golden egg, a goose that for them is not likely ever to be as prolific. It is ironic that those who are most unhappy about the advent of managed mental health have done the most to bring it about![37]

As a consequence of these escalating costs, mechanisms for financing mental health services have been restructured radically. Managed care has been developed to manage costs through the provision of financial incentives that reward outcome, not service utilization. In fact, with managed care systems for people with mental illness, utilization is tightly controlled, and heavy users of mental health services are closely monitored.

Today, over 175 million Americans, more than 90% of all privately insured individuals, receive their health coverage through their employer. Employer surveys indicate that 95% of all workers covered by employer benefits are enrolled in some type of managed care plan.[39]

Under managed care contracts, mental health benefits are more limited than in other contracts. Packages typically cover a maximum of 20 outpatient visits and 30 days of hospitalization per year, far too little for those with severe and persistent mental illness. Managed care firms have frequently handled concerns about the costs associated with chronic mental illness by not incorporating coverage for these disorders in their basic contracts.[40]

Insurers have additionally protected themselves from "catastrophic" costs by setting annual or lifetime limits on benefit amounts that would be paid for mental illnesses. Nonetheless, even with these exaggerated concerns regarding costs, the growth of managed care has spawned an enormous managed behavioral health care industry with $4.4 billion in annual revenues, covering 176.8 million Americans.[41] Concerns that the "worried well" would consume a disproportionate amount of service resulted in insurers and health maintenance organizations (HMOs) instituting strict criteria for accessing reimbursement for mental health services. Utilization review mechanisms were developed to require preapproval before referral for service.[42] Concerns regarding the potential costs of caring for those with severe and persistent mental illness resulted in the majority of insurers and HMOs seeking mechanisms for offsetting financial risk through contracting with external vendors rather than providing or overseeing the provision of psychiatric care themselves.[43] Such patterns of delegation of both responsibility and financial risk to external vendors are referred to as "carve-outs."

As in managed care generally, the preoccupation with cost-containment and tight oversight of service patterns produced strict management of service utilization. Oversight is usually provided by a qualified person, usually remote from the site of service, who monitors rendered or proposed care using predetermined, protocol-driven criteria. Communication between the reviewer and provider is usually by telephone. Both positive and negative effects can be realized by such oversight. Positively, clinicians who have the skill to treat patients with concentrated, brief, but efficient treatments that limit hospitalization are rewarded. Standardization of care through the use of protocols with demonstrated efficacy is encouraged, thus potentially reducing much of the individual provider variations from medical care. Unmonitored provision of services with dubious levels of efficacy can be reduced, as can the excessive use of hospitalization. On the other hand, service authorization by remote utilization managers, who are working from protocols that may not fit individual patients and who may not know the providers' credentials, expertise, and competence, may not be in the best interest of quality patient care.

Public sector initiatives have paralleled private sector efforts to control mental health services costs. Throughout the 1990s, state governments experiencing dramatic increases in Medicaid spending sought ways to control costs of mental health services for public beneficiaries. States such as Massachusetts and Iowa began contracting with managed behavioral health care corporations (MBHCCs) in the anticipation that they would experience savings similar to private sector employers who were seeing reductions in psychiatric hospitalizations and lengths of stay.[44] For the most part, these programs provide payment for mental health services on a per capita basis. Such an approach builds on the cost-savings incentives of managed care firms, relying heavily on closely monitored use of costly services and increased reliance on measuring outcome versus the number of units of service provided. In such systems, less is better, assuming an acceptable outcome level. Preliminary data are available assessing the cost-effectiveness and outcome with managed care approaches in this publicly supported population with special needs, suggesting that there are no significant differences in outcome and that cost savings are considerable.[45–48] States continue to turn to the managed behavioral health care industry to serve Medicaid and other populations receiving publicly financed mental health benefits. By 2000, over 85% of the managed behavioral health market was controlled by 11 managed behavioral health organizations.[49] Estimates are that between 25% and 40% of combined federal and state Medicaid spending on mental health and substance abuse is funneled through MBHCCs.[50] Recent research indicates that MBHCCs and public programs are facilitating access to those in greatest need as more people with serious mental illness are now more likely to receive mental health specialty services than in the past.[51]

Advocacy to achieve parity in mental health insurance benefits as compared with general health insurance benefits is a continuing issue dating back to the 1950s.[52] "Parity" refers to requirements that insurers cover mental health care at the same level as medical care. The 1990s saw much legislative activity on parity at both the state and federal levels as discrepancies between mental health and medical care coverage grew with claims that private employers and MBHCCs cut both care and costs too drastically.[50] Medical plans typically do not limit the number of covered outpatient visits or inpatient days of care; however, a typical employer-sponsored mental health plan may carry several limits, often including outpatient-visit or hospital-day limits in addition to annual or lifetime dollar limits in coverage. Discrepancies also occur in deductibles, co-payments, and coinsurance rates.[52] The impact of parity legislation in terms of both costs and quality of care is controversial. Some argue that such mandates would be costly and would have the impact of causing employers to reduce contributions to employee benefits; however, recent empirical studies show that employers switching to managed care see dramatic drops in mental health costs even when benefits are expanded.[52] The Mental Health Parity Act of 1996 was introduced into Congress and was passed after receiving overwhelming bipartisan support. Effected in 1998, this legislation equates aggregated lifetime limits and annual limits for mental health services with aggregate lifetime and annual limits for medical care; however, the law does allow many cost-shifting mechanisms, such as adjusting limits on mental illness inpatient days, prescription drugs, outpatient visits; raising coinsurance and deductibles; and modifying the definition of medical necessity.[53] The act does not require employers to offer mental health coverage, nor does it impose any limits on coinsurance, deductibles, days, or visits. Furthermore, coverage is not required for people suffering from substance use and abuse disorders, a problem of substantial public health significance.

In 2001, the Mental Health Equitable Treatment Act, which would have expanded coverage to an additional 15 million Americans, was introduced into Congress; however, by the close of 2002, Congress had abandoned the proposed legislation.[54] The states, on the other hand, took up the cause of parity, and by 2004, 34 states had enacted some form of parity legislation.[55] Although parity legislation focuses on the removal of caps on benefits, which is an important, positive development, there still exist significant mechanisms that create financial barriers to accessing services necessary for people with severe and persistent mental illness. Both employers and insurers have a broad range of alternatives in responding to state and federal parity laws, including totally dropping mental health benefits or imposing other constraints.[52] Recent data from national employer surveys are disconcerting and indicate that mental health benefit coverage has declined. In 1991, 36% of employees in all large firms had unlimited mental health outpatient visit benefits;[56] by 2004, the figure had fallen to 19% possibly due, in part, to employer concerns over significantly increasing health insurance premiums.[57]

It is clear that people with severe and persistent mental illness should receive the services and support necessary for them to live relatively stable and high-quality lives within their communities. This population has been subjected to episodic rather than continuous care, in spite of professional community awareness that these people can be treated effectively through medication, support, and structure. Long-term impairments and disabilities require the coordination of enormous resources that cross funding streams and agency interests. In a national survey conducted by the NAMI, members of families with mentally ill members indicated the following:[58]

- 59.3% needed help with illness management
- 67.9% needed help with crisis management
- 23.1% needed help with activities of daily living, including bathing, dressing, and personal hygiene
- 74.3% needed help with community living skills, including shopping and managing money
- 64.7% needed help with establishing and maintaining friendships
- 72.8% needed help with gaining and maintaining productive activities

These issues must be addressed if individuals suffering from mental illness are to live lives not characterized by chaos, poverty, homelessness, and social ostracism.[59] According to extensive studies by the NAMHC, for an additional annual cost of about $6.5 billion, the nation could provide coverage for adults and children with severe mental disorders commensurate with coverage for other types of illness.[16] The NAMHC has presented compelling data that this investment would result in a 10% decrease in the use and costs of nonpsychiatric medical services and that this decrease, combined with reductions in indirect costs, would result in a savings of $8.7 billion—an estimated net economic benefit to the nation of $2.2 billion per year. The United States has the scientific, technical, and financial resources necessary to serve this special population suffering severe disabilities. Barriers need to be removed, services re-engineered, and access to efficacious treatments ensured.

Barriers to Accessing Services

If so many people require mental health services but do not seek them out or receive them, what is preventing them from gaining access to necessary services?

The mentally ill still suffer from stigmatization. A person is much more likely in casual conversation to mention that he or she is going to an appointment with the family doctor or gynecologist than mention an appointment with a psychiatrist. A poignant reminder of the stigmatization of the mentally ill is that in one of the New England states, mental health services were bureaucratically placed in the State Department of Corrections, an action that might be interpreted as mental illness being perceived as a criminal problem. In spite of the past 10 years being the "Decade of the Brain," with enormous advances in delineating the neurobiologic basis and treatment of many psychiatric disorders, many people still feel that having a psychiatric disorder is shameful and in some way reflective of personal failure.[60]

Consumer and advocacy groups working with professional societies have done much to dispel the myths fueling these societal misunderstandings. Nonetheless, they continue to exist and provide both direct and indirect barriers to service. Directly, an undetermined number of people may not seek needed care because of personal and familial shame and embarrassment. The indirect consequences are even more significant. Those determining public policy and establishing guidelines for health insurance traditionally have viewed mental illness as being poorly defined, with diagnostic uncertainty and ineffective treatments. A major consequence of this misinformation is that health insurance coverage for psychiatric disorders continues to lag considerably behind coverage for other medical conditions.[61-65] The surgeon general's report on mental health emphasizes that dispelling the myths that contribute to stigmatization must be made a major national priority.[66]

Priorities for Mental Health Services

The NIMH National Plan delineates five essential areas that should be addressed in developing a comprehensive national plan for mental health services. These include:[67,68]

1. *Epidemiology.* Accurate and current epidemiologic databases are available and need to be used to delineate the characteristics of those seeking mental health services, their demographics, risk factors, and cultural and family issues. Services need to be designed in

accord with actual need and geographic distribution of need. Services need to be provided by mental health professionals who have the appropriate training in treatments of proven efficacy and the commitment to provide care with sensitivity and respect for factors associated with cultural and familial diversity.

2. *Assessment.* Assessment techniques used throughout various programs providing services for citizens with mental disorders vary tremendously in comprehensiveness, usability, sensitivity, and selectivity. Accurate, standardized assessment tools have been developed. The best need wide dispersion, and mental health professionals need training to achieve complete, accurate assessment.

3. *Treatment.* The gap between empirical research findings on the efficacy of specific pharmacological and psychosocial treatments and the use of these treatments in clinical settings is enormous. Treatment plans need to be rescued from the ideology of the past, the conventional wisdom of what works best. Effective treatments need to be made available to those in need. This means that dollars must be allocated for training and retraining mental health professionals in these newer techniques. Third-party payers need to evaluate which treatments being prescribed for specific disorders are actually effective before approval of payment. Such action will facilitate the move away from the traditions of the past and increase the likelihood of interventions resulting in functional improvement.

4. *Rehabilitation and habilitation.* Treatment goals must extend beyond the remission or reduction of acute symptoms. The onset of severe mental illness is likely to occur at critical times in a person's development, resulting in impairments in educational, vocational, and social achievement. Quality-of-life issues are critical if patients with severe and persistent mental illness are to lead fulfilling and productive lives. Studies comparing patients with and without access to rehabilitative services have demonstrated that those with access have lower hospitalization rates, increased independent living, employment, and social capabilities, and greater satisfaction with life.[16] In brief, the indirect social costs of mental illness decrease substantially with the utilization of rehabilitative services.

5. *Outcome.* Payment systems for mental health services are rapidly moving away from providing incentives for increasing the units of service provided. Fiscal incentives are being developed within

managed care firms and capitated systems that provide financial rewards based on outcome. Mental health services need to be evaluated systematically across four outcome domains: (1) clinical symptoms, (2) social and vocational functioning, (3) sense of well-being for the consumer and his or her family, and (4) public welfare benefits (indirect social costs).

Payment systems dependent on outcome criteria may do much to hasten the application of recent scientific advances to the care of mental illness. Managed care systems can supply an incentive for emphasizing quality over quantity in mental health care; however, the unique needs of these patients must be recognized, and the services to them designed sensitively and realistically.

Caring for the mentally ill is costly, but the money and expertise are there for providing a rational and effective system, as long as these resources are channeled wisely. Unfortunately, some recent cases have come to light where chief executive officers and shareholders of for-profit managed care firms have diverted money needed for patient care to such self-serving purposes as seven- and eight-figure compensation packages and private planes. To the extent that our society allows such practices to persist, a portion of our population suffering from severe and chronic mental illness will be denied services and continue to experience homelessness and other dehumanizing conditions.

As the stages of organization of behavioral health care provisions evolve, the critical question will be whether the management of health care money will benefit those in need of care through an outcome-driven behavioral system or whether it will simply be redistributed among the insurers, HMOs, MBHCCs, and providers without substantial benefit to patient care. The need to retrain behavioral health providers to ensure that they possess the knowledge base and skills emerging from cutting-edge research is critical. Ensuring that scarce health care dollars benefit the patients who need mental health services will require creativity and the collaborative work of patient advocates, providers, business, and government if the interests of those suffering from mental illness are to be safeguarded.

Need for Further Research

Over the past two decades, health systems research has increased markedly.[67–71] However, there remain strong needs for well-designed studies that examine the effects of patterns and modalities of care on both mental and physical outcome.

A variety of systems has evolved to provide mental health services. These systems differ widely in what services are provided, for whom, by whom, and in what setting. Decisions regarding resource allocation rarely are made on the basis of documented need and the distribution of psychiatric illness in U.S. communities. Instead, they are made in our nation's capital or in state assemblies or legislatures. Choices of specific services are based on beliefs held by generations of psychiatrists and other mental health professionals rather than on demonstrated efficacy. The gap between research and practice continues to be considerable. Although cost-containment efforts through managed care have increased the use of effective psychopharmacologic agents for treating people with psychiatric disorders, the use of psychosocial interventions with demonstrated efficacy that goes beyond that of pharmacologic agents has been minimal.[72]

The 1999 U.S. Surgeon General's report on mental health called for continued efforts to "build the science base" in mental health and illness. Citing developments in the neurosciences and molecular genetics that can offer promising opportunities for research and future treatment applications, the report also highlighted the research challenges inherent in new clinical and health services interventions posed by the evolution of new pharmacologic agents and psychotherapies.[66] Today, scientific research into mental health and illness is referred to as "bottom-up" and "top-down." "Bottom up" refers to research that examines the most fundamental levels of brain functioning such as neurochemical activity and genetics and their interactions with environmental influences. "Top-down" research refers to research into the broader behavioral context of the brain's cellular and molecular activity and how individual cells communicate to perform mental functions. New, highly sophisticated laboratory methods as well as computer-aided technologies such as magnetic resonance imaging and positron emission tomography are aiding in advanced research. A major challenge in the near future will be to facilitate transfer of new, evidence-based treatments into diverse service delivery settings and systems, while trying to assure better coordination among the elements of the existing delivery system.[73] Given the complex and fragmented nature of the current system, additional research is needed to enlighten policy makers and administrators on the most effective methods of carrying out this transfer in a patient-centered manner.

With the advent of managed care, accusations have been made that financial incentives are driving the market and that decisions are being based on economic considerations, not patient need. This is a simplistic analysis of a complicated issue. The delivery of mental health care has been driven for years in part by financial incentives that differ from those present under managed care. More research is needed to identify the impact of changing reimbursement systems on the access, quality, and cost benefit of various types of service arrangements in order to inform policy makers, payers, clinicians, and advocates more accurately. In addition, new methods of measuring functional status can make it possible to determine the impact of treatment on the mental health of the general public, with the potential to develop mechanisms to monitor indicators of mental health on a nationally representative sample, similar to studies done for physical illnesses.[8] Additional research on measurement methods and their transfer to the mental health field will be central to accomplishing this goal.

Addendum by Co-Authors, Sultz and Young

By an executive order issued in 2002, President Bush established the Freedom Commission on Mental Health, whose mission was to conduct a comprehensive review of the mental health service delivery system and "to recommend improvements to enable adults with serious mental illness and children with serious emotional disturbances to live, work, learn, and participate fully in their communities."[74] The commission issued an interim progress report 6 months after its establishment, which stated that, "America's mental health service delivery system is in shambles." Further describing the system as severely fragmented, the report cited needless suffering, frustrated caregivers, and millions of dollars in wasted resources.[75] The Commission's final report, issued in 2003, concluded that "traditional reform measures are not enough to meet the expectations of consumers and families."[76] The report further noted that successfully transforming the mental health service delivery system must facilitate recovery and build patient resilience, not only treat symptoms. The commission summarized its findings and recommendations in six goals:[76]

Americans understand that mental health is essential to overall health.
Mental health care is consumer and family driven.
Disparities in mental health services are eliminated.

Early mental health screening, assessment, and referral to services are common practice.
Excellent mental health care is delivered, and research is accelerated.
Technology is used to access mental health care and information.

Keeping these goals high on the political agenda and incorporating them into research, bureaucratic, consumer, and policy-making decisions would have posed numerous, provocative challenges in the foreseeable future. Such was not the case, however. In the several years since the report was published, little if any progress has been noted. The reason lies with the commission's impractical and unrealistic advisories that had little or no chance for achievement.

Two of the many recommendations are illustrative of the unrealistic nature of the commission report. One recommendation calls for "eliminating the disparities in mental health services between urban centers and rural and geographically remote areas." Another recommendation calls for "addressing mental health with the same urgency as physical health." Those familiar with both the political climate and the apparent trend toward progressive decreases in Medicare, Medicaid, and private, third-party benefits for people with psychiatric illnesses, quickly recognized that the commission's goals were not likely to be achieved. Thus, the work of the commission, like that of so many other "commissions" is essentially ignored.

The lack of mental health system improvement since the 2003 report of the Freedom Commission on Mental Health was confirmed by a detailed national survey of local mental health services by the NAMI. Its "Report On America's Health Care System for Serious Mental Illness, Grading the States, 2006" lists each state's score on 39 specific criteria. The scores were then tabulated to produce an overall grade and four subcategory grades. The subcategories were infrastructure, information access, available services, and recovery supports. The national average was "D."[77]

Michael J. Fitzpatrick, Executive Director of NAMI, summarized the situation in the following words, "Simply put, treatment works, if you can get it."

References

1. Bockoven JS. *Moral Treatment in Community Mental Health*. New York, NY: Springer Publishing Co; 1972.

2. Morrissey JP, Goldman HH. Cycles of reform in the care of the chronically mentally ill. *Hospital Community Psychiatry*. 1984;35:785–789.

3. Gronfein W. Incentives and intentions in mental health policy: a comparison of the Medicaid and community mental health programs. *J Health Social Behav*. 1985;26:192–206.

4. Mechanic D. *Mental Health and Social Policy*. 3rd ed. Englewood Cliffs, NJ: Prentice Hall; 1989:27–46.

5. Klerman GL. The psychiatric revolution of the past 25 years. In: Gove WR, ed. *Deviance and Mental Illness*. Newbury Park, CA: Sage Publishing; 1982:180.

6. Mechanic D. Establishing mental health priorities. *Milbank Q*. 1994;72: 501–514.

7. Redick RW, Witkin MJ, Atay JE, et al. The Evolution and Expansion of Mental Health Care in the United States Between 1955 and 1990. In: *Mental Health Statistical Note 210*. Washington, DC: U.S. Department of Health and Human Services; 1994.

8. Norquist G, Hyman SE. Advances in understanding and treating mental illness: implications for policy. *Health Affairs*. 1999;18:36–37.

9. Regier DA, Narrow WE, Rae DS, et al. The de facto U.S. mental and addictive disorders service system: epidemiological catchment area prospective 1-year prevalence rate of disorders and services. *Arch Gen Psychiatry*. 1995; 50:85–94.

10. Regier DA, Burke JR, Manderscheid RW, et al. The chronically mentally ill in primary care. *Psychol Med*. 1995;15:265–273.

11. Kessler RC, Berglund PA, Zhao S, et al. The 12-month prevalence and correlates of serious mental illness (SMI). In: Manderscheid RW, Sonnenschein MA, eds. *Center for Mental Health Services, Mental Health United States, 1996* (DHHS Publication No. SMA 96-3098). Washington, DC: Superintendent of Documents, U.S. Government Printing Office; 1998:59–70.

12. U.S. Department of Health and Human Services. *Mental Health: A Report of the Surgeon General*—Chapter 6. Rockville, MD: U.S. Department of Health and Human Services, Substance and Mental Health Services Administration, Center for Mental Health Services, National Institutes of Health, National Institute of Mental Health; 1999:408.

13. U.S. Department of Health and Human Services. *Mental Health: A Report of the Surgeon General*—Chapter 6. Rockville, MD: U.S. Department of Health and Human Services, Substance and Mental Health Services Administration, Center for Mental Health Services, National Institutes of Health, National Institute of Mental Health; 1999:72–73.

14. American Psychiatric Association. *Diagnostic and Statistical Manual*. 4th ed. Washington, DC: American Psychiatric Press; 1994.

15. Barker PR, Manderscheid RW, Hendershot GE, et al. *Serious Mental Illness and Disability in the Adult Household Population: Data From Vital and Health Statistics, no. 218*. Hyattsville, MD: National Center for Health Statistics; 1992.

16. National Advisory Mental Health Council. Health care reform for Americans with severe mental illnesses: report of the National Advisory Mental Health Council. *Am J Psychiatry.* 1993;150:1447–1465.

17. Narrow WE, Regier DA, Rae DS, et al. Use of services by persons with mental and addictive disorders. *Arch Gen Psychiatry.* 1993;50:95–107.

18. Regier DA, Farmer ME, Rae DS, et al. Comorbidity of mental disorders with alcohol and other drug abuse: results from the Epidemiological Catchment Area (ECA) Study. *JAMA.* 1991;264:2511–2518.

19. Campbell M, Malone RP. Mental retardation and psychiatric disorders. *Hosp Commun Psychiatry.* 1991;42:374–379.

20. U.S. Department of Health and Human Services. *Mental Health: A Report of the Surgeon General*—Chapter 6. Rockville, MD: U.S. Department of Health and Human Services, Substance and Mental Health Services Administration, Center for Mental Health Services, National Institutes of Health, National Institute of Mental Health; 1999:409.

21. U.S. Senate Special Subcommittee on Aging. *Aging America: Trends and Projections.* Washington, DC: U.S. Department of Health and Human Services; 1988.

22. Regier DA, Boyd JH, Burke JD Jr, et al. One month prevalence of mental disorders in the United States: based on five epidemiological catchment area sites. *Arch Gen Psychiatry.* 1988;45:977–986.

23. Klerman GL, Weissman MM. Increasing rates of depression. *JAMA.* 1989; 261:2229–2235.

24. U.S. Department of Health and Human Services. *Mental Health: A Report of the Surgeon General*—Chapter 6. Rockville, MD: U.S. Department of Health and Human Services, Substance and Mental Health Services Administration, Center for Mental Health Services, National Institutes of Health, National Institute of Mental Health; 1999:340–341.

25. U.S. Department of Health and Human Services. *Mental Health: A Report of the Surgeon General*—Chapter 6. Rockville, MD: U.S. Department of Health and Human Services, Substance and Mental Health Services Administration, Center for Mental Health Services, National Institutes of Health, National Institute of Mental Health; 1999:406–407.

26. Rowland D, Garfield R, Elias R. Accomplishments and challenges in Medicaid mental health. *Health Affairs.* 2003;22:73–76.

27. Lave JR, Goldman HH. Medicare financing for mental health care. *Health Affairs.* 1990;9:9–30.

28. Rupp A. Under insurance for severe mental illness. *Schizophrenia Bull.* 1991; 17:401–405.

29. Mechanic D, Rochefort D. Deinstitutionalization: an appraisal of reform. *Ann Rev Sociol.* 1990;16:301–327.

30. National Alliance for the Mentally Ill. Facts and figures about mental illness. Available from http://www.nami.org. Accessed January 3, 2003.

31. U.S. Department of Health and Human Services. *Mental Health: A Report of the Surgeon General*—Chapter 6. Rockville, MD: U.S. Department of Health and Human Services, Substance and Mental Health Services Administration, Center for Mental Health Services, National Institutes of Health, National Institute of Mental Health; 1999:412.

32. Zuvekas SH. Trends in mental health services use and spending: 1987–1996. *Health Affairs*. 2001;20:218.

33. Strumwassen I, Paranjpe NV, Udow M, et al. Appropriateness of psychiatric and substance abuse hospitalizations. *Med Care*. 1991;29:AS77–AS89.

34. England MJ, Goff VV. Health reform and organized systems of care. In: England MJ, Goff VV, eds. *New Directions for Mental Health Services*. San Francisco, CA: Jossey-Bass Publishers; 1993:5–12.

35. Frank PG, Lave J. Economics of managed mental health. In: Feldman S, ed. *Managed Mental Health Services*. Springfield, IL: Charles C Thomas; 1992: 83–99.

36. Sharfstein SS, Magnas HL, Taube CA, et al. Mental health services. In: Kovner A, ed. *Health Care Delivery in the United States*. 5th ed. New York: Springer Publishing Co; 1995:232–266.

37. Feldman S. *Managed Mental Health Services*. Springfield, IL: Charles C Thomas; 1992:xiv.

38. Gabel J. Job-based health benefits in 2002: some important trends. *Health Affairs*. 2002;21:143.

39. Kaiser Family Foundation and Health Research and Educational Trust. 2002 survey of employer-sponsored health benefits, Chart 11 (Fall 2002). Available from http://www.kff.org/content/2002/20020905a. Accessed September 10, 2002.

40. Iglehart JK. Health policy report: managed care and mental health. *N Engl J Med*. 1996;334:131–135.

41. Findlay S. Managed behavioral health care in 1999: an industry at a cross-roads. *Health Affairs*. 1999;5:117.

42. Boyle PJ, Callahan D. Managed care in mental health: the ethical issues. *Health Affairs*. 1995;14(suppl 3):7–22.

43. Hodgkin D, Horgan CM, Garnick CW. Make or buy: HMOs' contracting arrangements for mental health care. *Admin Policy Mental Health*. 1997;24: 359–376.

44. Bailit MH, Burgess LL. Competing interests: public-sector managed behavioral health care. *Health Affairs*. 1999;18:112–113.

45. Davidson H, Schlesinger M, Dowart RA, et al. State purchase of mental health care: models and motivations for monitoring accountability. *Int J Law Psychiatry*. 1991;14:387–403.

46. Brotman A. Privatization of mental health services: the Massachusetts experiment. *J Health Politics Policy Law*. 1992;17:541–551.

47. Johnson RE, McFarland BH. Treated prevalence rate of severe mental illness among HMO members. *Hospital Community Psychiatry*. 1994;45:919–924.

48. Lurie N, Finch M, Christianson J. Does capitation affect the health of the chronically mentally ill? Results from a randomized trial. *JAMA*. 1992; 267:3300–3304.

49. Center for Mental Health Services. Mental Health, United States, 2000. Manderscheid RW, Henderson MJ, eds. DHHS Pub No. (SMA) 01-3537 Washington, DC: Superintendent of Documents, U.S. Government Printing Office; 2001. Available from http://www.mentalhealth.org/publications/allpubs/SMA01-3537/acknowledgements.asp. Accessed July 11, 2007.

50. Findlay S. Managed behavioral health care in 1999: an industry at a cross-roads. *Health Affairs*. 1999;18:118.

51. Mechanic D, Bilder S. Treatment of people with mental illness: a decade-long perspective. *Health Affairs*. 2004;23:93.

52. Sturm R, Liccardo Pacula R. State mental health parity laws: cause or consequence of differences in use? *Health Affairs*. 1999;18:182–183.

53. National Alliance for the Mentally Ill. The Mental Health Parity Act of 1996. Available from http://www.laami.nami.org/update/parity96.html. Accessed August 19, 2000.

54. National Alliance for the Mentally Ill. The President, Congress, and the Mental Health Parity Amendment: let's hold leaders who killed it accountable. Available from http://www.nami.org/pressroom/20011218.html. Accessed January 3, 2003.

55. National Association for the Mentally Ill. Senate action on parity legislation expected soon. Available from http://www.nami.org/Content/Content Groups/Policy/Issues_Spotlights/Senate_Action_on_Parity_Legislation_ Expected_Soon.htm. Accessed February 2, 2005.

56. The Kaiser Family Foundation and Health Research and Educational Trust. Employer Health Benefits Survey 1999. Available from http://www.kff.org/content/1999/1538/KFFexecsum.pdf. Accessed June 18, 2000.

57. The Kaiser Family Foundation and Health Resource and Educational Trust. Employer Health Benefits Annual Survey 2004, Section 9. Prescription Drug and Mental Health Benefits. 113. Available from http://www.kff.org/insurance/7148/sections/ehbs04-sec9-1.cfm. Accessed February 2, 2005.

58. Steinwachs DM, Kasper JD, Skinner EA, et al. Data watch: patterns of use and costs among severely mentally ill people. *Health Affairs*. 1992;11:178–185.

59. Bridges K, Huxley P, Oliver J. Psychiatric rehabilitation: redefined for the 1990s. *Int J Social Psychiatry*. 1994;40:1–16.

60. National Institutes of Health. *Basic Behavioral Science Research for Mental Health: A National Investment: A Report of the National Advisory Mental Health Council*. Washington, DC: National Institutes of Health; 1995.

61. Blostin AP. Mental health benefits financed by employers. *Monthly Labor Review*. 1987;110:23–27.

62. U.S. Department of Labor, Employee Benefits Security Administration. Mental Health Parity Act, 1. Available from http://www.do.gov/ebsa/newsroom/fsmhparity.html. Accessed March 29, 2005.

63. Taube CA, Goldman HH, Salkever D, et al. Medicaid coverage for mental illness: balancing access and costs. *Health Affairs.* 1990;9:5–18.

64. Mark TL, Coffey RM, Vandivort-Warren R, et al. U.S. Spending for Mental Health. Schizophrenia Bulletin and Substance Abuse Treatment. 1999–2001. Health Affairs Web Exclusive March 29, 2005. Available from http://content/healthaffairs.org/cgi/reprint ./hlthaff.w5.133v1.html. Accessed March 29, 2005.

65. Rupp A. Underinsurance for severe mental illness. *Schizophrenia Bull.* 1991; 17:401–405.

66. U.S. Department of Health and Human Services. *Mental Health: A Report of the Surgeon General*—Chapter 6. Rockville, MD: U.S. Department of Health and Human Services, Substance and Mental Health Services Administration, Center for Mental Health Services, National Institutes of Health, National Institute of Mental Health; 1999:2.

67. Taube CA, Mechanic D, Hohmann AA, et al. Caring for People with Severe Mental Disorders: A National Plan of Research to Improve Services. DHHS Publication no. ADM 91-1762. Washington, DC: National Institute of Mental Health), U.S. Government Printing Office: 1991.

68. Lalley TL, Hohmann AA, Windel CD, et al. Caring for people with severe mental disorders: a national plan to improve services. *Schizophrenia Bull.* 1992;18:559–700.

69. National Institute of Mental Health. *The Future of Mental Health Services Research.* Washington, DC: U.S. Department of Health and Human Services; 1989.

70. Newman FL, Howard KI. Introduction to the special section on seeking new methods in mental health services research. *J Consulting Clin Psychol.* 1994; 61:667–669.

71. Stein II, Hollingsworth EJ. *Maturing Mental Health Systems: New Challenges and Opportunities.* San Francisco, CA: Jossey-Bass Publishers; 1995.

72. Side Effects: Managed Care Focus on Psychiatric Drugs—Alarming Many Doctors. *Wall Street Journal.* December 1, 1995:B1.

73. U.S. Department of Health and Human Services. *Mental Health: A Report of the Surgeon General*—Chapter 6. Rockville, MD: U.S. Department of Health and Human Services, Substance and Mental Health Services Administration, Center for Mental Health Services, National Institutes of Health, National Institute of Mental Health; 1999:100.

74. White House Office of the Press Secretary. President's New Freedom Commission on Mental Health. Available from http://www.whitehouse.gov/news/releases/2002/04/20020429-2.html. Accessed December 28, 2002.

75. U.S. Substance Abuse and Mental Health Services Administration. Interim Report of the President's New Freedom Commission on Mental Health. Available from http://www.mentalhealth.org/publications/allpubs/NMH02-0144/default.asp. Accessed January 4, 2003.

76. President's New Freedom Commission on Mental Health, Achieving the Promise: Transforming Mental Health Care in America, Executive Summary, 3-4. Available from http://www.mentalhealthcommission.gov/reports/FinalReport/FullReport.htm. Accessed January 23, 2007.

77. National Alliance for the Mentally Ill. A Report on America's Health Care System for Serious Mental Illness, Grading the States, 2006. Available from http://www.nami.org/. Accessed January 29, 2007.

CHAPTER 10

Public Health and the Role of Government in Health Care

This chapter presents the history of governmental efforts to prevent or control the problems of health and disease. Efforts to protect the public's health, begun in early European history and transferred to Colonial America, are traced, with emphasis on their purpose, motivation, and success. The rise and decline of America's once elaborate federal, state, and local partnerships in the delivery of public health services are described, as well as the efforts of private and voluntary agencies. Also discussed are the barriers to effective preventive services that result from the lack of a population perspective in the U.S health care system. The chapter concludes with a discussion of public health challenges and goals, emerging issues, and the changing role of government.

The term public health is usually defined broadly as the efforts made by communities to cope with the health problems that arise when people live in groups. Community life creates the need to control the transmission of communicable diseases, maintain a sanitary environment, provide safe water and food, and sustain people with disabilities and low-income populations.[1]

The world history of public health is a fascinating study of civilized society's attempts to deal with the biological, social, and environmental forces that have contributed to the pervasive problems of morbidity and mortality and with the unfortunate citizens who have been handicapped by illness, disability, and poverty. The following observations are presented primarily to set the stage for understanding the development of government's role in the evolution of public health in the United States.

Throughout history, public health activities have reflected the state of knowledge at the time regarding the nature and cause of the diseases that afflict mankind, the practices employed for their control or treatment, and the dominant social ideologies of political jurisdictions. From the concepts of spiritual cleanliness and community responsibility codified by the ancient Hebrews for religious reasons to the systems of personal hygiene practiced by the Greeks in an effort to achieve a perfect balance between body and mind, ancient civilizations learned patterns of individual behavior that they believed promoted health and reduced the risk of disease. It remained for the Romans, however, to develop public health as a governmental matter beyond individual practice. The feats of engineering and administrative accomplishments that provided the Romans with clean water and effective sewage and swamp drainage systems were the forerunners of politically sanctioned environmental protections of the public's health. In addition, the Roman Empire is given credit for establishing a network of infirmaries to treat illness among the disadvantaged populations. These infirmaries are considered to be the first public hospitals.

The medieval period that followed the fall of Rome was characterized by the disintegration of the cities and the return of anarchy. The overpopulated walled towns built to withstand enemy attacks crowded families together in the most unhealthy circumstances. The pest-ridden, unsanitary living conditions and the narrow, dark streets that overflowed with human waste and refuse provided fertile environments for disease epidemics that decimated large segments of those populations. Superstitious, demonic, and theological theories of epidemic disease displaced ancient concerns for personal hygiene and the quality of the environment.

The Renaissance, however, was characterized by a great revival of learning. Along with advances in art, literature, and philosophy and the rise of industry and commerce, there was a renewed interest in science and medicine. From the 16th to the 18th centuries, public health was shaped by two countervailing trends.[2] Although the administration of rudimentary medical and nursing services continued to be the responsibility of towns and other local units, the concept of the modern state was beginning to emerge. Because only a political jurisdiction that protected and cared for its citizens could reap the continuing economic benefits of production and world trade, healthy laborers and soldiers became valuable commodities. Thus, in the centralized national governments of Europe during the 16th and 17th centuries, maintaining the health of laborers and soldiers became important economic and political as well as public health concerns.

Public Health in England

Poverty, illness, and disability were common problems in the towns and parishes of England during the 16th and 17th centuries, and most communities responded with some form of publicly supported medical care provided in private homes or at public infirmaries. The Elizabethan Poor Laws of 1601 addressed the issue of the "lame, impotent, old, blind, and such other among them being poor and not able to work" without dealing directly with health matters.[3] The law was expanded subsequently to include the provision of nursing and medical care.

It was also in England that the collection and analysis of national statistics regarding industrial production and demographics began in the 17th century. The work of the father of political arithmetic, William Petty (1623–1687), and the statistical analyses of his friend, John Graunt (1620–1674), established the importance of vital statistics and led to such epidemiologic tools as population-specific and disease-specific morbidity and mortality rates, life tables, and the calculus of probability. Study of the vital statistics contained in the Bills of Mortality published weekly in London led to a better understanding of the social phenomena that were factors in the promotion of health and the occurrence of disease.

Of interest, in light of subsequent debates about the merits of national health services, was the proposal of John Bellers, a London merchant and philanthropist (1654–1725). At the turn of the century, he proposed dealing with public health problems on a national scale. In An Essay Toward Improvement of Physick, Bellers suggested that the people's health was too important to the community to be left to the uncertainty of individual initiative. He argued that the health of the people was the responsibility of the state, whose task it was to establish and maintain hospitals and laboratories, erect a national health institute, and provide medical care for the sick.

The Elizabethan Poor Laws obligated each parish in England to maintain its own disadvantaged citizens. Despite a variety of schemes to deal with the health problems of the low-income populations, including the widespread development of workhouses to teach the unemployed to support themselves, the fundamental economic and social problems that led to pervasive poverty remained unsolved. By the 19th century, the industrialization of England had made poverty and social distress more prevalent than ever. It was in that climate that the drastic Poor Law Amendment Act of 1834 was passed. The dual intent was to reduce the rates of dependency and free the labor market to spur industrialization. The law required that able-bodied people and their families be given aid in only well-regulated workhouses.

The same circumstances that supported the new industrial society, factories, and the congested dwellings of urban environments produced new health problems. As people crowded into burgeoning towns and cities, diseases flourished and spread. It was the Poor Law Commission of 1834 under the leadership of Edwin Chadwick that developed the means to address public health problems. Motivated by the belief that it would be good economy to prevent disease, Chadwick advocated the use of carefully collected data to link population characteristics, environmental conditions, and the incidence of diseases. After many investigations, political debates, and subsequent political compromises, England's Public Health Act became law in 1848, and a General Board of Health was created. Although the subsequent history of public health in England is a chronicle of social change, epidemics, and political machinations, it is evident that the growth of their sanitary reform movement and the creation of the General Board of Health in 1848 established the British as the world leaders in public health philosophy and practice. Public health in early America was heavily influenced by the medical and administrative experience of the British.[4]

Public Health and Government-Supported Services

The history of public health in the United States from the early colonial period to the end of the 19th century followed the same development pattern as that which had occurred in England. Yellow fever and cholera epidemics stimulated sanitary reforms, and the early cities and towns began to assume responsibility for the collective health of their citizens. Public medical care in the United States, however, bore the stigma of its "Poor Law" legacy. The New York Poor Law of 1788 provided that any town or city could establish an almshouse, and within a few years, most towns and cities had done so. Although there was a series of shocking exposés of terrible conditions in many of these facilities, the concept of the almshouse and town-employed physicians remained the mainstay of sick people among the low-income population until the Depression of the 1930s.

Lemuel Shattuck, a Massachusetts statistician, conducted U.S. sanitary surveys similar to those of Chadwick in England. In his Report of the Sanitary Commission, published in 1850, he documented differences in morbidity and mortality rates in different locations and related them to various environmental conditions. Consequently, he argued, the city or state had to take responsibility for the environment. Although largely ignored at the time of its release, the report has come to be considered one of the most influential documents in the evolution of public health in the United States.[5]

In 1865, emulating the Shattuck survey in Massachusetts, the New York City Council of Hygiene and Public Health published a shocking exposé of unsanitary conditions in the city. Within a year, a public health law was passed creating a city board of health. Creating an appropriate administrative structure for local public health efforts became a turning point for public health in the United States.

As in England and other countries, early federal public health initiatives were motivated more by economic and commercial concerns than humanitarian values. For instance, the Public Health Service came into being in 1798 as the Marine Hospital Service when President John Adams signed into law an act providing for the care and relief of seamen who were sick or disabled. Because healthy sailors were a valuable commercial commodity and because the seaport towns took responsibility for only their own citizens, the federal government was left to provide health services to the seamen and passengers of the important shipping industry. Additionally, it was of serious concern to the citizens of seaports that the personnel of foreign ships not transmit to them diseases contracted elsewhere.

Soon thereafter, the first Marine Hospital was set up in Boston Harbor, and seamen were receiving care in port cities along the East Coast. In 1870, the Marine Hospital Service was reorganized as a national hospital system with a central headquarters in Washington, D.C. The medical officer in charge, known at first as the supervising surgeon, was later given the title of surgeon general. It is significant in light of the commercial motivation for its creation that the Marine Hospital Service was established as a component of the Treasury Department.

In 1889, Congress established the Public Health Service Commissioned Corps. Envisioned as a mobile force of physicians to assist the nation in fighting disease and protecting health, the Corps was set up along military lines, with titles and pay corresponding to Army and Navy grades and physicians subject to duty wherever assigned.[6] In 1891, the bacteriologic laboratory of Dr. Joseph J. Kinyuon in the Staten Island Marine Hospital was moved to Washington, D.C., where it was expanded to include pathology, chemistry, and pharmacology. It was the forerunner of the National Institutes of Health, which today provides two thirds of all the federal support for biomedical research in this country.

Eleven years later, in 1902, a new law changed the Marine Hospital Service's name to the Public Health and Marine Hospital Service. In 1912, the name would be changed again to its present designation: the United States Public Health Service. From this modest start, the Public Health Service underwent a series of reorganizations and expansions until it became a major agency of the United States Department of Health and Human Services (HHS) and responsible for the largest public health program in the world.[7]

In 1933, it became apparent that state and local governments with limited tax revenues required help from the federal government to provide welfare assistance, and the Federal Emergency Relief Act was passed. It provided federal aid to the states and authorized general medical care for acute and chronic illness, obstetrical services, emergency dental extractions, bedside nursing, drugs, and medical supplies. Because participation by the states was optional, the act was not implemented in many parts of the country.[8] The passage of the Social Security Act of 1935 ended the era of makeshift federal and state programs to meet the health needs of the sick people among the low-income population. Title VI of the landmark Social Security Act of 1935 was instrumental in the expansion of the Public Health Service. The act delegated to the Public Health Service the authority to assist states, counties, health districts, and other political subdivisions to establish and maintain public health services. Title VI provided the impetus for all political jurisdictions to create public health agencies and services. After 141 years, the Public Health Service was removed from the Treasury Department to become a component of a new Federal Security Agency, created in 1939 to bring together most of the health, welfare, and educational services scattered throughout the federal government.

During World War II, the Public Health Service carried out emergency health and sanitation efforts that contributed substantially to the country's defense efforts. Immediately thereafter, a critical shortage of medical facilities prompted the passage of the National Hospital Survey and Construction Act, called Hill-Burton after its congressional sponsors. The act stimulated the growth of the health care industry by providing federal aid to the states for hospital and health center construction. Since 1946, the Public Health Service has provided national leadership in hospital planning, research, and operation. In 1946, the Federal Security Agency also was expanded to include the Children's Bureau and the Food and Drug Administration.

In 1953, the Public Health Service, with the other components of the Federal Security Agency, became part of the newly created Department of Health, Education, and Welfare (HEW). During the next decade, the health care industry faced the multiple challenges of coping with a rapidly expanding U.S. population, rising public expectations for health services, and a host of technologic advances in health care with an inadequate supply of health professionals. The HEW responded in 1963 with the Health Professions Educational Assistance Act, which provided grants to build health professional schools, and in 1964 with the Nurse Training Act, which authorized federal aid for construction and rehabilitation of nursing schools and provided loans to nursing students.

The National Institute for Occupational Health and Safety, the National Institute on Alcohol Abuse and Alcoholism, the National Health Service Corps, and major initiatives in addressing cancer and heart, lung, and blood diseases were initiated in the early 1970s. In 1979, the education component of HEW was transferred to a new Department of Education, and the HEW was renamed the Department of Health and Human Services (HHS).[9]

Now, with a proposed 2007 budget of $698 billion and close to 70,000 employees, the HHS is the federal government's principal agency concerned with health protection and promotion and provision of health and other human services to vulnerable populations. In addition to administering the Medicare and Medicaid programs, the HHS includes over 300 separate programs[10] that encompass activities such as:

- Medical and social science research
- Infectious disease prevention and control
- Assurance of food and drug safety
- Child support enforcement
- Improvement of maternal and child health
- Management of preschool education services (Head Start)
- Prevention of child abuse and domestic violence
- Substance abuse prevention and treatment
- Provision of services for older Americans

The HHS carries out these activities through the following 11 Public Health Service Operating Divisions:[10]

1. National Institutes of Health (NIH): Established first as a laboratory in 1887, the NIH is the world's premier medical research organization and includes 18 separate health institutes, the National Center for Complementary and Alternative Medicine, and the National Library of Medicine. The NIH supports over 30,000 research projects on a variety of medical conditions and has a proposed budget for 2007 of $27.8 billion. It employs over 18,600 individuals.

2. Food and Drug Administration (FDA): This agency assures the safety of foods and cosmetics and the safety and efficacy of pharmaceuticals, biological products, and medical devices. The FDA's proposed 2007 budget is almost $2 billion. It employs more than 10,000 individuals.

3. Centers for Disease Control and Prevention (CDC): Established in 1946, the CDC is the primary federal agency responsible for protecting the American public's health through monitoring disease trends, investigations of outbreaks and health and injury risks, and implementation of illness and injury control and prevention measures. The proposed 2007 budget is $8.2 billion. The agency employs more than 8,600 individuals.

4. Agency for Toxic Substances and Disease Registry: In collaboration with states and other federal agencies, the Agency for Toxic

Substances and Disease Registry focuses on preventing exposures to hazardous substances from waste sites. The agency conducts public health assessments, health studies, surveillance activities, and health education and training in communities around waste sites on the U.S. Environmental Protection Agency's National Priorities List. The agency, supervised by the CDC, employs more than 400 individuals and has a proposed 2007 budget of $75 million.

5. The Indian Health Service (IHS): The IHS operates 38 hospitals, 56 health centers, 4 school health centers, and 44 health stations. Through transfers of IHS services operating authority, tribes also administer an additional 13 hospitals, 160 health centers, 3 school health centers, 76 health stations, and 160 Alaska village clinics. Services are provided to nearly 1.5 million American Indians and Alaska Natives of 557 federally recognized tribes in Alaska and the 48 contiguous states. The service employs about 14,800 individuals and has a proposed 2007 budget of about $3 billion.

6. Health Resources and Service Administration (HRSA): Established in 1982 to provide a coordinated agency for multiple programs serving low-income, uninsured, and medically underserved populations, the HRSA provides funds for comprehensive primary and preventive services through community-based health centers at more than 3,000 sites nationwide. The HRSA also supports maternal and child health programs, programs to increase diversity and numbers of health care professionals in underserved communities, and supportive services for HIV/AIDS victims through the Ryan White Care Act. It employs more than 1,600 individuals and has a proposed 2007 budget of $6.6 billion.

7. Substance Abuse and Mental Health Services Administration: The agency works to improve the quality and availability of substance abuse prevention, addiction treatment, and mental health services through federal block grants. It provides a variety of grants to states and local communities to address emerging substance abuse trends, mental health service needs, and HIV/AIDS. The agency's proposed 2007 budget is $3.26 billion, and it employs more than 600 individuals.

8. Agency for Healthcare Research and Quality: Established in 1989, the Agency for Healthcare Research and Quality is the lead agency

for supporting research to improve the quality of health care, reduce its cost, improve patient safety, address medical errors, and broaden access to essential services. Major activities include sponsoring and conducting research to provide evidence-based information on health care outcomes with respect to quality, costs, uses, and access. With 294 employees, the agency's proposed budget for 2007 is $270 million.

9. Centers for Medicare and Medicaid Services, formerly the Health Care Financing Administration: This agency administers the Medicare and Medicaid Programs. Medicare insures over 40 million Americans, and Medicaid, a joint federal/state program, provides coverage for over 34 million low-income persons, including 18 million children, and nursing home coverage for low-income older adults. It administers the new Children's Health Insurance Program, currently covering more than 2.2 million children. The agency employs more than 4,700 individuals and for 2007 has a proposed budget of over $484 billion.

10. Administration for Children and Families (ACF): The ACF administers over 60 programs to promote the economic and social well-being of families, children, individuals, and communities. It administers the state/federal welfare program, Temporary Assistance to Needy Families, national child support enforcement, and the Head Start program. It provides funds to assist low-income families with child care expenses, supports state programs in adoption assistance and foster care, and funds child abuse and domestic violence prevention programs. The agency has more than 1,500 employees and has a proposed 2007 budget of over $47 billion.

11. Administration on Aging (AoA): The federal focal point and advocate agency for older persons, the AoA administers federal programs under the Older Americans Act. Programs assist older persons to remain in their own homes by supporting services such as Meals on Wheels. The AoA collaborates with its nationwide network of regional offices and state and area agencies to plan, coordinate, and develop community-level systems of services that meet needs of older individuals and their caregivers. The agency employs 124 individuals and has a proposed 2007 budget of almost $1.4 billion.

The HHS has been the federal government's largest grant-making agency under the aegis of its various operating divisions.[11] In recent years, however, there has been a sharp reduction in research grants, with most research and demonstration activities funded through solicited contracts. Unsolicited research proposals are unlikely to be funded.[12]

Initiated to provide care for Civil War veterans who were disabled or indigent or both, the Veteran's Health Administration system (VA) has grown to become one of the world's largest health care delivery systems. It currently operates 173 medical centers with approximately 51,000 beds, 391 outpatient and outreach clinics, 131 nursing home care units, and 39 domiciliaries, providing a broad range of medical, surgical, and rehabilitative care.[13] The system requested $34.3 billion for veterans' health care for fiscal year 2007. The almost 12% increase over the previous year's budget reflects the need to treat more devastating injuries and medical conditions.[14] On an annual basis, the VA treats nearly 1 million patients in its hospitals, 79,000 in its nursing homes, and 25,000 in its domiciliaries. The system's outpatient clinics register approximately 27.5 million visits per year.

The VA maintains major affiliations with 105 medical schools throughout the United States. VA medical centers also affiliate with 54 dental schools and 1,140 other schools throughout the United States. Each year approximately 100,000 health professionals receive training at VA medical centers.[15] The VA also conducts a broad array of world-class clinical and health services research projects.

Because the VA system usually has a life-long relationship with its patients, it has instant access to each patient's complete medical record, an advantage over private medicine that reduces both costs and medical errors. The long-term relationship also allows more preventive care, higher quality services, and greater patient satisfaction along with monetary savings.[16]

Through the Department of Defense Military Health Service program, the federal government provides both direct health care services and support for health care services for 8.1 million U.S. military personnel and their dependents, military retirees and their families, and others entitled to Department of Defense benefits.[17] The Military Health Service operates 98 hospitals and 480 clinics worldwide, primarily servicing active-duty members of the armed forces. The majority of civilian care is purchased through managed care support contracts implemented under a program entitled TRICARE. The 2007 budget for military health services programs totaled $21 billion.[17] As discussed in Chapter 3, however, both the VA budget and its services have been overwhelmed by the numbers of military personnel returning from service in Iraq with severe multiple injuries.

The states also play an important role in funding health care and health-related services. Each year, state and local governments contribute about 14% of total health care expenditures, including hospital, nursing home, or home health care services.[18] Many states also operate and fund state mental institutions, support medical schools, maintain health departments that provide direct preventive and primary care services, and support maternal and child health improvement, infectious disease monitoring and control, and other community health initiatives.

City and county government jurisdictions support and deliver general and specialty health care services through their health departments and over 100 hospitals and health systems that together comprise the infrastructure of many of America's metropolitan health systems.[19] The outpatient and inpatient services of government-supported public hospitals provide a community's "safety net" for individuals who are uninsured or underinsured and cannot access care elsewhere. Public hospitals also are often the sites of major teaching programs for an area's medical school. Frequently, they provide services that are financially unattractive to other community hospitals, such as burn care, psychiatric medicine, trauma care, and crisis response units for both natural and man-made disasters.[19] In addition, city and county health departments may provide direct patient care services in clinics or health centers, referrals for care, and other services to meet community needs of their high-risk, medically underserved populations.

Decline in Influence of the Public Health Service

Over the years, public health agencies' many accomplishments have contributed to significant improvements in both the health and life expectancy of Americans. Using population-based strategies for disease and injury prevention, public health has contributed to substantial declines in morbidity and mortality and dramatically changed the profiles of disease, injury, and death in the United States. Yet, despite the centrality of public health in providing the basis for the health of Americans, its funding has always competed with other more highly valued demands in the health sector.[20]

The several reorganizations of federal public health agencies occurred in response to continuing criticism of their failure to improve access to at least minimally adequate medical care to underserved populations. Pressures emanated from public health professionals, medical care organizations, political leaders, and the popular media. Criticism of the Public Health Service rose in the 1960s when its efforts to provide incentives to state and local agencies for more innovative approaches to meeting these demands through categorical and project grants were judged ineffective. Thus, when several new and important programs for improving access to medical care were passed, agencies other than the Public Health Service were assigned to administer them. Medicare was assigned to the Social Security Administration, Medicaid to the Social and Rehabilitation Services, Head Start and Neighborhood Health Centers to the Office of Economic Opportunity, and the Model Cities Program to Housing and Urban Development.

The end of President Johnson's term of office in 1968 marked the end of an era in federal health policy. The Nixon administration took issue with the three-tiered system of the federal Public Health Service, state health agencies, and local public health departments that was expected to combine local initiative with policy input and national standards for advancing access to adequate health services. In its place, a new policy dubbed the "New Federalism" was initiated. It involved the progressive removal of federal responsibilities for a uniform, cooperative national public health system and the transfer of those responsibilities to the states. It was the beginning, at the federal level, of the Republican strategy of converting federal program support to block grants, reducing the available funds and sending them to the states for administration. Although the effort was relatively unsuccessful during the Nixon/Ford administrations, it was revived in a new and more extreme form when Ronald Reagan was elected in 1980, and public health became the primary target. The decline of the government's organized system of public health services accelerated thereafter.[21]

Responsibilities of the Public Health Sector

In 1990, the HHS published Public Health Service: Healthy People 2000: National Health Promotion and Disease Prevention Objectives. Objective 8.14 of that document calls for 90% of the population to be served by local health departments that would effectively carry out the three core functions of public health: assessment, policy development, and quality assurance. These core health department functions are intended to put into operation, within the resource and other constraints extant in each jurisdiction, the following generally accepted health department performance responsibilities:[22]

- Focus on primary prevention: prevention that occurs before the onset of disease. Identify environmental and behavioral factors that are associated with conditions, such as lung cancer or heart disease, and educate the community or protect it from the risk.
- Protect communities from infectious and toxic agents through monitoring or surveillance. Gather information to control and, where possible, prevent health problems resulting from these agents.
- Respond to unanticipated natural and human-generated disasters. Assess health risks posed by contaminated food, water, or air and inform the public and the medical care system of sources of danger and strategies for appropriate response.
- Promote the well-being of the public through programs to notify and educate people about risks and protective measures that can be applied at the community level.
- Target hard-to-reach populations with clinical services. Create outreach programs to link high-risk populations to medical services to address individual health care needs, as well as to interrupt the spread of disease in the community.
- Maintain diagnostic laboratory services to support diverse monitoring and prevention programs. These facilities permit identification of emerging threats from infectious agents and environmental toxins. Set and enforce standards for new and existing laboratory tests conducted in medical settings.
- Collect information on health outcomes to ensure the quality of services provided through hospitals, nursing homes, and other medical care delivery institutions. Develop referral systems for high-risk

perinatal care, and plan regionalization of trauma and cardiac care. Provide aggregate information on health outcomes to inform consumers and medical care professionals about the quality of care being delivered at the community level.

It is through the fulfillment of these public health responsibilities that public health departments protect the public against preventable communicable diseases and exposure to toxic environmental pollutants, harmful products, and poor quality health care. These public health practices promote healthy personal behaviors and risk factor reduction community wide by identifying and modifying patterns of chronic disease and injury, informing and educating consumers and health care providers about appropriate use of medical services, developing and maintaining comprehensive health programs in schools and child day care facilities, providing occupational safety and health programs, and ensuring that human immunodeficiency virus (HIV) and sexually transmitted disease-prevention programs are implemented. These public health practices are the bedrock foundations of modern population-focused health care.

In 1993, however, a team of investigators from the School of Public Health at the University of Illinois at Chicago, working with representatives of the Centers for Disease Control and Prevention, surveyed 208 health departments responding from a random national sample stratified by jurisdiction and population base. The findings suggested that less than 40% of the U.S. population was served by a health department that effectively addressed the core functions of public health.[23]

Clearly, with resource support for public health continuing to decline, it was not surprising that the United States had failed to meet 85% of the challenging goals of Healthy People 2000. In a new 10-year plan, Healthy People 2010, released by the Department of Health and Human Services in January 2000, the government admitted that the nation had met only 15% of the 319 targets established in 1990. In some areas, particularly obesity, marijuana use, exercise, asthma, and diabetes, the health of Americans either stayed the same or worsened.

Nevertheless, Healthy People 2010, the third set of 10-year targets for health improvement in the United States, set two broad goals, supported by 467 objectives that are grouped into 28 focus areas. One major goal is "to increase the years and quality of health life." The other major goal is "to eliminate health disparities."[24]

These goals and their supporting objectives were developed for the new decade by Healthy People Consortium, a group of 650 national, professional, and voluntary organizations, the business community, and state and local public health agencies. Meetings began in 1996, and the first completed draft of 7,704 pages was posted on the Web for public comment in September 1998. More than 11,000 comments were received electronically. The recommendations from a series of public hearings and other Web communications were processed before publication of the final report. Given the dismal failure to meet the multitudinous objectives of the two previous Healthy People reports, one might question whether the extraordinary effort expended in these highly labor-intensive, expensive, and time-consuming exercises might be better spent in more pragmatic and potentially productive efforts.

In 1985, the Institute of Medicine, concerned about the need to protect the nation's health through an effective, organized public health sector, convened a special committee to study the status of public health in the United States. The committee reported its findings and recommendations in 1988. The report concluded, "Public health is a vital function that is in trouble."[25] In an analysis of the contributing factors, it noted the following:[26]

We have observed disorganization, weak and unstable leadership, a lessening of professional and expert competence in leadership positions, hostility to public health concepts and approaches, outdated statutes, inadequate financial support for public health activities and public health education, gaps in the data gathering and analysis that are essential to public health functions of assessment and surveillance, and lack of effective links between the public and private sectors for the accomplishment of public health objectives.

The report linked the poor public image of public health and the public's lack of knowledge and appreciation for the mission and content of public health to those deficiencies and to a number of other problems. Particular emphasis was placed on the failure of sound policy development in public health as evidenced by ambiguous responses to the AIDS epidemic, the "politicalization" of public health agencies, and the lack of clear delineation of the responsibilities between levels of government.

In 1988, the committee made organizational, educational, financial, and political recommendations for addressing these complex and interrelated problems. Unfortunately, its strategies depended on continuing strong financial support for existing public health agencies and stronger, more sharply focused leadership that could build increasingly productive links with the private and voluntary health care sectors. In the ensuing years, the required leadership has not been evident, and financial support for public health has continued to decline. Also public and political support for government public health agencies has further diminished.

Although the goals and objectives of the Healthy People reports are commendable and their definition gives the agencies involved a sense of accomplishment, it should be obvious that the lack of an effective, well-organized public health sector makes the effort an exercise in futility. Perhaps one of the weaknesses of public health is the propensity of its advocates to set arbitrary and usually unobtainable goals rather than face the much more difficult challenge of developing the leadership, expertise, and political strength to achieve them.

The September 11 terrorist attacks and the subsequent anthrax incidents revealed public health as ill prepared to provide an effective health defense system. A report of the Centers for Disease Control and Prevention called for a system of "public health armaments," including a "skilled professional workforce, robust information and data systems and strong health departments and laboratories."[27]

There are serious concerns that the inadequate numbers of skilled public health professionals, such as public health nurses, epidemiologists, laboratory workers, and others result from public-sector budget restraints and competition with other sectors of the economy. As a result, many public health employees are inadequately prepared through education and training for the jobs they perform.[28]

Relationships of Public Health and Private Medicine

Public health and clinical medicine have complementary roles in caring for the health of the American people. Although they often address the same health problems, their attention is directed at different stages of disease or injury. Clinical medicine devotes its most intensive resources to restoring health or palliating disease in relatively small numbers of individuals. Rather than targeting individuals, public health uses strategies that promote health or prevent disease in large populations.[22]

Unfortunately, the implementation of these roles has been hindered by the often contentious relationship that has existed for decades between public health leadership and the private medical practitioners and their advocacy organization, the American Medical Association. Although the need for curative medicine administered to individuals and the need for preventive measures for the protection of populations have coexisted in all societies since ancient civilizations and physicians who specialize in public health or preventive medicine have received the same basic medical education as those who pursue the diagnostic and therapeutic specialties, the ideologic differences between them have produced vigorous debate. J.G. Freymann suggests that the reasons for the persistent discord include the identification of public health by practicing physicians with governmental bureaucracy, the linking of the care of low-income populations with welfare, the focus of physicians toward individuals, and the custom of being paid only for active therapy.[29]

Historically, the different emphasis of the two types of practitioners, that is, the population-based orientation of public health professionals and the individual-centered focus of private health providers, has often divided rather than enhanced public and private health services. The scientific advances in medicine since World War II served only to emphasize the value differences between practitioners with a population perspective and those focused on individual patients. Physicians educated and socialized to a biological model of medicine that emphasized sophisticated technologies and practice specialization have shown little appreciation for the simpler organizational measures that reach out to the underserved and provide access to basic health monitoring, preventive care, and primary medical care.

Understandably, individual physicians with the daily responsibility and heavy workloads of caring for waiting rooms full of patients consider that their personal professional efforts fully meet their community or societal obligations. For the most part, they are more than willing to delegate to the public health professionals concerns for the overall health of society and for those who do not have access to their offices.

Opposition to Public Health Services

The history of public health is marked by struggles over the limits of its mandate. Just as the opponents of the several attempts to initiate programs of national health insurance described public health prejudicially as "socialized medicine," special interest groups are threatened by the perception that public health programs represent a subversive social change that constitutes an unjustified intrusion of government into the lives of private individuals.

The medical profession had both philosophical and economic reasons for voicing their concerns. Starr observed, "Doctors fought against public treatment of the sick, requirements for reporting cases of tuberculosis and venereal disease, and attempts by public health authorities to establish health centers to coordinate preventive and curative medicine."[30] Extending the boundaries of public health was regarded as the opening wedge for usurping the physicians' role. Physicians opposed disease screening and primary care services, even though they were targeted at the populations with the lowest incomes, because physicians feared that public health agencies were expanding into activities that they believed were rightfully their own.

There are, of course, many examples of the synergistic effects of private and public medicine. The immunization of children and adults against a variety of preventable diseases is a good example of how public health and private medical practitioners have worked together effectively. A number of screening programs, such as those for tuberculosis, lung cancer, breast cancer, and hypertension, have linked the personal services of private medicine and the population-oriented practice of public health in productive liaisons.

Resource Priorities Favor Curative Medicine

The allocation of U.S. health resources provides persuasive evidence of the public's and the professionals' fascination with dramatic high-technology diagnostic and therapeutic medicine. Despite the centrality of public health in providing basic health programs and the effectiveness and economic advantages inherent in prevention as compared with cure, there is little funding for research or practice for public health promotion or disease prevention. This is in contrast to the large sums that finance the research in and practice of remedial medical care. Less than 1% of the almost $1 trillion spent annually for health care was allocated to government public health activities. In fact, between 1981 and 1993, there were public health imperatives on the emergence of acquired immune deficiency syndrome (AIDS); the re-emergence of tuberculosis and measles; and the escalating problems of substance abuse, violence, and teenage pregnancy. Total U.S. health expenditures increased by more than 210%, whereas funding of public health services as a proportion of the health care budget declined by 25%.[22]

The major investment in hospital neonatal intensive care units during the last 2 decades is a dramatic example of the lack of balance in the health care system. Although numerous studies have demonstrated that funds expended for prenatal care of high-risk mothers reduce the number of premature births requiring exceedingly expensive and often futile efforts to save those infants, public subsidies for prenatal care have declined, whereas more and more costly technology has been introduced to increase the ability to salvage increasingly small and premature infants. For example, the federal Special Supplemental Food Program for Women, Infants and Children (WIC), which provides supplemental food, nutrition, and health education to low-income pregnant and postpartum women, infants, and children, is estimated, after careful studies, to reduce low birth weight rates by 25% and very low birth weight rates by 45%, with Medicaid savings of $4.21 for every WIC dollar spent on pregnant women. In contrast, neonatal intensive care, although effective in reducing neonatal mortality, is the least cost-effective strategy.[31]

These questionable funding priorities will be of critical importance in determining the effectiveness of health care in the future. Just as the preference for support of costly neonatal intensive care units rather than public health programs of prenatal care contributes to the unacceptably high rates of infant mortality in the United States, the focus on remedial medicine for America's growing older population denies the reality of the changing distribution of illness and disability. The major causes of disease and disability among the increasing numbers of older adults are chronic conditions that result from multiple causes that are not usually amenable to technologic remedies.

The traditional medical model of clinical practice poorly serves many older individuals. Normal function and the absence of disease characterize the medical definition of health. Health is assumed by the absence of symptoms and signs that the human body is in some state of biological disruption. The accepted medical focus on the biomedical aspects of care with an emphasis on specific diseases and organ systems assumes that nonphysiologic malfunction, such as the inability, common to advancing age, to carry out the roles and tasks of one's usual social milieu, is not part of health. That medical model is not appropriate to guide care for most older patients, who may need a multidisciplinary approach that focuses on overall needs. Attention needs to be paid to managing chronic conditions— helping patients adjust to their limitations and maintain daily functioning within the context of their living arrangement and family and social support.

Health Care Reform and the Public Health/Medicine Relationship

Important factors in the current effort to reform the U.S. health care system give promise of a more functional future partnership between public health and private practice medicine. The drive by those paying for health care (employers, organized consumers, and governments) for improved measures of health status and system performance and the emphasis on integrated health systems that focus on health improvement for defined populations are creating pressures within the system for more cost-effective, community-driven strategies for combining the resources of public health and networks of personal care services.

Although complementary, if not integrated, systems of public health and medical care services seem like ideal models with which to address the nation's health care problems of the 21st century, the long-standing differences in philosophy, values, and assumptions between public health and organized medicine are likely to make cooperative ventures difficult. Nevertheless, in the current era of previously inconceivable health system changes, a new and functional relationship driven by mutual needs could develop between these two sectors.

Both public health leaders and clinicians would need sufficient motivation to improve preventive service rates. Strong external incentives or requirements as well as perceptive internal vision would be required to change organizational commitment. A new emphasis on prevention would have to be seen as important for organizational promotion or financial viability before providers would be galvanized to action. The history of public and preventive health services in the United States illustrates, time and again, that the prestige priorities—and profits—in its remedial medicine system lie with diagnosing and treating already existing disease.

The current medical care system fails to provide effective preventive services even when they are demonstrated to be the most cost-effective procedures available. In contrast, new treatment technologies are implemented despite serious reservations about their efficacy and cost-effectiveness. Thus, with all of its groundbreaking research, talented workforce, and technological know-how, the United States has the distinction of having the world's most costly and inefficient health care system.[32]

Table 10-1 reveals the magnitude of preventable mortality. In total, these causes of death account for approximately 40% of all deaths occurring each year. Tobacco, diet, and sedentary lifestyles are major contributors to early mortality, yet effective medical interventions are not integrated into the practice standards that drive the delivery of medical services.[32]

Clearly, the medical and public health systems that evolved from the remarkable scientific achievements since World War I placed their emphases on tests, drugs, surgeries, vaccines, and environmental controls. Personal behaviors were considered either outside the scope of the medical care system or immutable to change. Medical insurance companies that rarely reimbursed providers for preventive services in general and behavioral counseling in particular reinforced these assumptions.

Table 10-1 Deaths from Preventable Causes, USA, Year 2000

Cause	Number	Percent of Total U.S. Deaths
Smoking	435,000	18.1
Poor Diet/Physical Inactivity	400,000	16.6
Alcohol Consumption	85,000	3.5
Motor Vehicle Crashes	43,000	1.8
Firearms	29,000	1.2
Sexual Behaviors	20,000	.08
Illicit Use of Drugs	17,000	.07
Total Preventable Deaths	1,029,000	41.35

Source: Author-created from data presented by A.H. Mokdad et al in publication, "Actual Causes of Death in the United States, 2000, Journal of the American Medical Association 291, no. 10, March 2004.

Hospital-Sponsored Public Health Activities

The market forces that have changed the structure and character of hospitals during the last 2 decades have stimulated them to initiate or expand a variety of outpatient public health–type services, including community-based and work site health promotion. This integration of outpatient medical and public health services is a direct response to the pressure placed on hospitals by third-party payers to reduce inpatient admissions and lengths of stay. In many cases, acute-care hospitals have added services such as community education on healthy behaviors and risk factor reduction, comprehensive school health programs, preventive health programs in child day care facilities, community education on chronic disease prevention and management, and occupational safety and health programs. These services have both helped their service populations and provided new sources of much-needed revenue.

Public Health Services of Voluntary Agencies

The role of volunteerism, voluntary agencies, and institutions as adjunct resources and services to those provided by governments and for-profit practices and corporations is a major theme in the evolution of health care in the United States. Private not-for-profit institutions have been the prevailing mechanism through which health care services in the United States and with the government share the responsibilities for meeting the needs of communities and special populations.[33]

In addition to this country's not-for-profit hospitals, there is a host of voluntary agencies providing nursing home care, hospice care, home care, medical and vocational rehabilitation, and other personal health care services. A variety of voluntary agencies serve the special needs of persons with specific medical conditions such as AIDS, asthma, diabetes, cerebral palsy, hemophilia, and muscular dystrophy. Similar organizations support research on conditions such as cancer, heart disease, and respiratory disorders. Others, such as the American Red Cross, Planned Parenthood, and Meals on Wheels, focus on providing specific services. Of significant importance is the fact that voluntary agencies provide many valued and effective services that are not prominent in the private medical care sector. Programs directed at health education, disease prevention, disease detection, health maintenance, rehabilitation, and terminal care have been the province of voluntary not-for-profit agencies.

The influence of large nonprofit foundations, such as the Robert Wood Johnson Foundation and the Pew Charitable Trusts, on the advancement of health care from a population perspective has been considerable. By providing funds on a competitive basis to stimulate research and innovative program demonstrations, these and other foundations have caused hospitals and other agencies, in collaboration with universities and colleges, to engage in progressive health service delivery improvements that may otherwise have been years in development. Particularly commendable is the selection of health care objectives to which those funds are dedicated.

The synergistic effect of government, private, and voluntary efforts has been both a bane and a blessing in the provision of health care in the United States. Our system's disorderly evolution as a combination of the charitable efforts of voluntary and religious organizations, multilevel government responses to community needs, and traditional U.S. free enterprise ensured the development of a complex network that is both inordinately successful in a technologic sense and plagued by costly inefficiencies, duplications, and inequities in access and quality. Nevertheless, this pluralistic approach, rather than the types of national health care systems common to other industrial societies, appears, at least for the near future, to be the only health care system strategy acceptable to the U.S. people.

Changing Roles of Government in Public Health

For decades, all three levels of government in the United States—federal, state, and local—have played significant roles in financing and regulating public health services and in maintaining agencies and systems that directly or indirectly deliver health care. The federal government surveys the population's health status and health needs, sets policies and standards, passes laws and regulations, supports biomedical and health services research, provides technical assistance and resources to state and local health agencies, helps finance health care through support of programs (such as Medicare and Medicaid), and delivers personal health care services through networks of facilities (such as those maintained by the

Department of Defense, the Department of Veterans Affairs, and the Administration on Native Americans).[34]

Public health services in the states are financed, regulated, and delivered through a variety of organizational structures. In some states, public health activities are divided among several entities, including health departments, social service, welfare, aging, and Medicaid. Many states now combine health and social service agencies to create large human service operations that join health and social services for children and youth, for people with developmental disabilities and other special populations, and for special problems such as alcoholism and drug abuse. Most states contribute heavily to the financing of Medicaid, medical education, and public health programs and to mental health through both community mental health programs and state-operated psychiatric hospitals. States also are involved in regulation through health codes, licensing of facilities and personnel, and supervision of the insurance industry.

Considerable variation exists in the organizational structure of agencies engaged in public health activities in local governmental jurisdictions. Counties, districts, and other local governments may have health, social service, environmental, and mental health departments. They can be independent or divisions of state agencies. Many cities and counties support and operate local health departments, public hospitals, clinics, and various other services. They also establish and enforce local health codes.

Rather than supporting and acknowledging the many benefits of this multilevel configuration of public health agencies that ensure safe food and water; control of epidemic diseases; and programs of care for infants, children, and adults with special needs; and, in general, improve the length and quality of life in the United States, the nation has moved toward increased privatization, withdrawn support from public health activities, and allowed the system to fall into disarray. Before the terrorist attacks of September 11, the United States appeared to have lost sight of both the goals and benefits of public health.[35]

Public Health in an Era of Privatization and Managed Care

The market forces affecting hospitals, nursing homes, voluntary agencies, and other institutions of the U.S. health care system are also significantly changing the financial base and functions of public health departments.

The declines in public health funding and the trend toward privatization of those public health services that could be delivered more efficiently outside of local bureaucracies have left many local health departments with minimal staff focused on only the most essential public health services.

Outsourcing to private providers who often had more comprehensive clinical capacity was one of several organizational strategies to contain or reduce costs while maintaining or improving the quality and efficiency of necessary public health services. Survey findings indicate that those health departments merely became smaller while cost savings were rare.[36]

With few exceptions, most health departments have maintained their responsibilities for assessing and ensuring the delivery of necessary public health services even though privatized. As might be expected, however, the reduction of health department–delivered services has made it difficult for many departments to maintain a strong community presence. In addition, negotiating with private service entities for the delivery and monitoring of public health services requires staff not customarily employed by public health departments. Health departments now find it necessary to replace service personnel with management staff knowledgeable in contracting and other business-related skills.

Future Role of Government in Promoting the Public's Health

Because the provision of medical treatment and related services accounts for approximately 99% of aggregate national health expenditures, national debate and efforts to reform the U.S. health care system have focused on financing, insurance, and cost-containment of treatment. Various estimates suggest that only about 10% of all early deaths can be prevented by medical treatment. In contrast, population-wide public health approaches have the potential to help prevent some 70% of early deaths in the United States through measures targeted to the social, environmental, and behavioral factors that contribute to those deaths.[37] Clearly, the value placed on high-technology clinical medicine by individuals, societies, and governments within the United States overwhelm consideration of the more cost-effective, but less dramatic, prevention strategies of public health. Unlike pictures of heart transplant recipients, for example, images of the hundreds of thousands of children who have not been crippled and have not died due to poliomyelitis since successful immunization programs have been instituted cannot be shown by the media.

State and local governments struggling with large deficits have considered it necessary to sacrifice the personnel and services of their public health agencies. The shortsightedness of those decisions, however, is becoming increasingly evident. Although there is continued general unhappiness with tax-supported programs and institutions, pressures for improving state and local public health services are developing outside the community of public health advocates. Leaders in business and industry connect a healthy and educated public to economic growth and development. They, and others concerned about the demise of such programs as school health, maternal and child health, water quality, community nutrition, environmental control, and disease control, are rethinking the wisdom of some of these governmental cost-cutting priorities. Private foundations and voluntary agencies are not able to fill the gaps left by the withdrawal of governmental support.

The people and political leaders of the United States are going through an unprecedented reassessment of guiding principles, core values, and funding priorities. Experience with the democratic process suggests that the voting public will respond to legislative and policy errors only after the untoward effects of faulty decisions touch on them personally and significantly.

After the terrorist assaults of September 11, 2001, lawmakers, prodded by the public, recognized that a broader public health infrastructure is required to protect Americans against chemical or biological attacks. A number of public health defense programs have been proposed that include stockpiling vaccines against anthrax, plague, and smallpox. Of particular importance is the need to prepare health care professionals, hospitals, and other agencies to respond quickly and effectively to threats or actual disasters.[38]

To that end, the largest reorganization of the federal government since World War II took place in April 2003 with the establishment of the Department of Homeland Security (DHS). Twenty-two new and existing governmental agencies that include 180,000 employees were assembled under the leadership of a newly appointed Secretary of Homeland Security. The DHS has the broad mission of strengthening this country's borders, improving intelligence analyses, infrastructure protection, and comprehensive response and recovery operations should there be a terrorist attack with chemical or biologic weapons. To help fulfill its mandate, the new department has a host of interlocking governmental relationships with other federal and state units. Among those are liaisons with the NIH, the CDC, the U.S. Public Health Service, the FDA, and other units of HHS. Most importantly, state and local health departments are expected to play principal roles in prevention of spread or in response and recovery operations should any attacks occur.[39]

That federal strategy, or lack thereof, has resulted in a series of completely disjointed public health activities and practices across 3,000 local agencies operating under 50 state health departments. Without nationally consistent plans and systems, public health responses will, as occurred during the New Orleans experience, find it difficult to coordinate with other responders such as law enforcement and transportation during disasters that cross political jurisdictions. Clearly, there is no forethought of how national health protection activities should be organized and delivered. The objective of protecting the nation against catastrophic events may have been gravely weakened by leaving local and state health departments to make up their own goals and priorities. After 4 years of preparedness funding, states and localities still lack the guidance and capabilities to develop effective preparedness capabilities.[40]

Nevertheless, the fear of bioterrorism may be a "once in a lifetime" opportunity to create a system of highly effective public health departments after years of neglect. With proper systems development, operational practices, and personnel who meet high standards of professional preparation and performance, public health departments could achieve high levels of both health promotion and health protection.

Changes are already taking place that portend significant improvements in crisis preparedness. Staff in many public health departments are being "cross-trained" to take on new responsibilities in case of public health emergencies. For many such agencies, it is the first time that an entire staff has been trained to work toward a common goal outside of their normal daily activities. While these and other efforts are a good start toward stimulating a new and more focused public health practice, there are lingering problems to be overcome.

There is little agreement over who should be responsible for what, what will be the systems of accountability, and how will performance be measured.[41] Although experts at HHS and the CDC have guidance and funding, the U.S. Constitution gives the authority for health matters to the states. State health departments establish policy and entrust the local health departments to carry it out. As a result, there are about 3,000 local agencies across 50 states with different sizes and capabilities carrying out widely divergent practices. In addition, the absence of nationally consistent systems frustrates the public health effort to coordinate with law enforcement, safety, and other responder units when disasters cross geopolitical borders.

Creation of the DHS added additional complications to intergovernmental relationships. The interrelated roles of DHS and HHS are still evolving, and state and local public health officials are trying to understand governance issues and funding streams. In addition, how the Department of Defense and the National Guard are to coordinate with public health officials are still open questions. Clearly, the responsibilities of public health in this time of security risks have been significantly increased with little realistic assessment of the resources and organizational changes to carry out these important missions adequately.[40]

The next few years will be crucial to the future of public health. If governments at every level do not seize the moment to create vibrant and effective systems of health promotion and health protection, the opportunity will be lost.

It is unfortunate that it requires a new threat or epidemic to halt the demise of organized public health and restore an effective public health structure. New public health structures may not be in the models we know, but hopefully they will receive new recognition, new support, and new leadership. If that happens, public health will, once again, demonstrate its central role in maintaining the health and well-being of the U.S. people.

References

1. Shindell S, Salloway JL, Oberembt CM, et al. *A Coursebook in Health Care Delivery*. New York, NY: Appleton & Lange; 1976:304–308.
2. Rosen G. *A History of Public Health*. New York, NY: MD Publications; 1957:82–83.
3. Rosen G. *A History of Public Health*. New York, NY: MD Publications; 1957:120–129.

4. Rosen G. *A History of Public Health*. New York, NY: MD Publications; 1957:219–233.
5. Committee for the Study of the Future of Public Health, Division of Health Care Services, Institute of Medicine. *The Future of Public Health*. Washington, DC: National Academy Press; 1988:60–61.
6. Department of Health and Human Services. *The Public Health Service: Some Historical Notes*. Washington, DC: Public Health Service; 1988:1–8.
7. Raffel MW, Raffel NK. *The U.S. Health System: Origins and Functions*. 4th ed. Albany, NY: Delmar Publishers; 1994.
8. Yerby AS. Public Medical Care for the Needy in the United States. In: DeGroot LJ, ed. *Medical Care, Social and Organizational Aspects*. Springfield, IL: Charles C Thomas; 1966:382–401.
9. Department of Health and Human Services. *The Public Health Service: Some Historical Notes*. Washington, DC: Public Health Service; 1988:1–8.
10. U.S. Department of Health and Human Services. Available from http://www.hhs.gov/budget/07budget/index.html. Accessed December 1, 2006.
11. U.S. National Institutes of Health. Available from http://www.grants.nih.gov/grants/t/indef.html. Accessed December 12, 2006.
12. Available from http//www.cms.hhs.gov/researchers/priorities/grants.asp. Accessed December 22, 2004.
13. Department of Veterans Affairs. Veterans Health Administration. Available from http://www.va.gov/About_va/orgs/vha/index.htm. Accessed August 14, 2000.
14. Department of Veterans Affairs. Veterans Health Administration. Available from http://www.va.gov./OCA/testimony/SVAC/06021600.asp. Accessed December 12, 2006.
15. Department of Veterans Affairs, Veterans Health Administration. Facts About the Department of Veterans Affairs. Available from http://www.va.gov/pressrel/vafacts.htm. Accessed September 11, 2002.
16. Asch SM, McGlynn EA, Hogan MM, et al. Comparison of Quality of Care for Patients in the Veterans Health Administration and Patients in a National Sample. *Ann Intern Med*. 2004;141:938–945.
17. Office of the Assistant Secretary of Defense (Health Affairs) and the TRICARE Management Activity. Available from http://www.tricare.mil/Factsheets/browsat03.cfm. Accessed December 12, 2006.
18. Available from www.cms.hhs.gov/statistics. Accessed December 12, 2006.
19. National Association of Public Hospitals and Health Systems. America's essential community providers. Available from http://www.naph.org/welcome.html, 1. Accessed August 4, 2000.
20. Shonick W. *Government and Health Services: Government's Role in the Development of U.S. Health Services, 1930–1980*. New York, NY: Oxford University Press; 1995:460–464.
21. Shonick W. *Government and Health Services: Government's Role in the Development of U.S. Health Services, 1930–1980*. New York, NY: Oxford University Press; 1995:98–101.

22. U.S. Department of Health and Human Services. *Public Health Service, For a Healthy Nation: Returns on Investment in Public Health*. Washington, DC: U.S. Government Printing Office; 1994:1–13.

23. Turnock BJ, Handler, A, Hall W, Potsic S, Nallori R, et al. Local health department effectiveness in addressing the core functions of public health. *Public Health Rep*. 1994;109:653–658.

24. U.S. Department of Health and Human Services, Prevention Report. *Addressing Disparities in Health*. 2000;14:1–2.

25. Committee for the Study of the Future of Public Health, Division of Health Care Services, Institute of Medicine. *The Future of Public Health*. Washington, DC: National Academy Press; 1988:17.

26. Committee for the Study of the Future of Public Health, Division of Health Care Services, Institute of Medicine. *The Future of Public Health*. Washington, DC: National Academy Press; 1988:32.

27. Available from http://content.healthaffairs.org/cgi/content/abstract/hlthaff. w3.54v1?Maxtoshow=&HITS. Accessed December 23, 2004.

28. Gebbie KM, Turnock BJ. The public health workforce, 2006: new challenges. *Health Affairs*. 2006;25:923–933.

29. Freymann JG. Medicine's great schism: prevention vs. cure: an historical interpretation. *Med Care*. 1975;13:525–536.

30. Starr P. Transformation in defeat: the changing objectives of national health insurance. *Am J Public Health*. 1982;72:78–88.

31. Avruch S, Cackley AP. Savings achieved by giving WIC benefits to women prenatally. *Public Health Rep*. 1995;110:27–34.

32. Vogt TM, Hollis JF, Lichtenstein E, et al. The medical care system: the need for a new paradigm. *HMO Pract*. 1999;12:5–12.

33. Seay JD, Vladeck BC. *Mission Matters: A Report on the Future of Voluntary Health Care Institutions*. New York, NY: United Hospital Fund of New York; 1988:13–15.

34. Committee for the Study of the Future of Public Health, Division of Health Care Services, Institute of Medicine. *The Future of Public Health*. Washington, DC: National Academy Press; 1988:7–10.

35. Committee for the Study of the Future of Public Health, Division of Health Care Services, Institute of Medicine. *The Future of Public Health*. Washington, DC: National Academy Press; 1988:19–32.

36. *Privatization and Public Health: A Study of Initiatives and Early Lessons Learned*. Washington, DC: Public Health Foundation; 1997.

37. U.S. Public Health Service. *Prevention Report*. Washington, DC: Department of Health and Human Services; 1995:1–12.

38. Suddenly, Public Health Administration Is Seen as Top Priority. *Wall Street Journal*. September 28, 2002:A16.

39. Available from www.govexec.com/homelandHSchart.hbm. Accessed April 30, 2003.

40. Salinsky E, Gursky EA. The case for transforming governmental public health. *Health Affairs*. 2006;25:1017–1028.

41. Laurie N, Wasserman J, Nelson CD. Public health preparedness: evolution or revolution? *Health Affairs*. 2006;25:935–945.

CHAPTER 11

Research: How Health Care Advances

This chapter explains the focus of different types of research and how each type contributes to the overall advances in health and medicine. Health services research, a newer field that addresses the workings of the health care system rather than specific problems of disease or disability, is described. The offices and goals of its major funding source, the federal Agency for Healthcare Research and Quality, are listed. Finally, research into the quality of medical care, the problems being addressed, and the research challenges of the future are discussed.

The last half of the 20th century saw a remarkable growth of scientifically rigorous research in medicine, dentistry, nursing, and the other health professions. The change from depending on the clinical impressions of individual physicians and other health care practitioners to relying on the statistical probability of accurate findings from carefully controlled studies is one of the most important advances in scientific medicine. No longer is the literature of the health professions filled with subjective anecdotal reports of the progress of treatment in one or more individual cases. Now readers of peer-reviewed professional journals can monitor the progress of basic science or clinical or technologic discoveries with confidence, knowing that published findings are, with only rare exceptions, based on research studies that have been rigorously designed and conducted to yield statistically credible results.

In contrast, the ever-growing volume of reports of medical developments that appears in the popular media are often premature and, depending on the source, may be cause for skepticism. The imprudent publication of inadequately or unproven therapies, the sensationalizing of minor scientific advances, and the promotion of fraudulent devices and treatments create unrealistic expectations among anxious patients and families that often result in crushing disappointments, mistreatment, and costly deceptions.

From both professional and public perspectives, the continuing research yield of new technologies and clinical advances creates ongoing challenges of evaluation, interpretation, and potential applications.

The Focus of Different Types of Research

Figure 11-1 illustrates the focus of the different types of health care research. There are clear distinctions among researchers in terms of focus, methods, and the nature of their subsequent findings. Although the kinds of information derived from each type of research may be different, each knowledge gain is an essential step in the never-ending quest to create a more efficient and effective health care system.[1]

Research in Health and Disease

Research studies conducted by those in the professional disciplines of health and disease fall into several categories. Basic science research is the

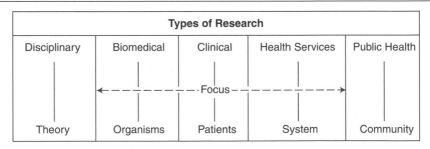

FIGURE 11-1 Variations in Research Focus.
Source: Aday et al. *Evaluating the Healthcare System: Effectiveness, Efficiency and Equity, 3rd edition.* (2004). Reprinted with permission.

work of biochemists, physiologists, biologists, pharmacologists, and others concerned with sciences that are fundamental to understanding the growth, development, structure, and function of the human body and its responses to external stimuli. Much of basic science research is at the cellular level and takes place in highly sophisticated laboratories. Other basic research may involve animal or human studies. Whatever its nature, however, basic science research is the essential antecedent of advances in clinical medicine.

Clinical research focuses primarily on the various steps in the process of medical care—the early detection, diagnosis, and treatment of disease or injury; the maintenance of optimal physical, mental, and social functioning; the limitation and rehabilitation of disability; and the palliative care of those who are irreversibly ill. Individuals in all the clinical specialties of medicine, nursing, allied health, and related health professions conduct clinical research, often in collaboration with those in the basic sciences. Much of clinical research is experimental, involving carefully controlled clinical trials of diagnostic or therapeutic procedures, new drugs, or technologic developments.

Clinical trials test a new treatment or drug against a prevailing standard of care. If no standard drug exists or if it is too easily identified, a control group will receive a placebo or mock drug to minimize subject bias. To reduce bias further, random selection is used to decide which volunteer patients will be in the experimental and control groups. In a double-blind study, neither the researchers nor the patients know who is receiving the test drug or treatment until the study is completed and an identifying code revealed.

Research studies have a number of safeguards to protect the safety and rights of volunteer subjects. Studies funded by governmental agencies or foundations are subject to scrutiny by a peer-review committee that judges the scientific merit of the research design and the potential value of the findings. Then a hospital-based or institutional review board checks for ethical considerations and patient protections. Finally, volunteer subjects must receive and sign an informed consent form that spells out in clear detail the potential risks or side effects and the expected benefits of their participation. Volunteers must weigh any potential risks against the likelihood that, by participating in research, they will receive state-of-the-art care and close health monitoring and will contribute to the advancement of science.

Epidemiology

Epidemiology, or population research, is concerned with the distribution and determinants of health, diseases, and injuries in human populations. Much of that research is observational; it is the collection of information about natural phenomena, the characteristics and behaviors of people, aspects of their location or environment, and their exposure to certain circumstances or events.

Observational studies may be descriptive or analytical. Descriptive studies use patient records, interview surveys, various databases, and other information sources to identify those factors and conditions that determine the distribution of health and disease among specific populations. They provide the details or characteristics of diseases or biological phenomena and the prevalence or magnitude of their occurrence. Descriptive studies are relatively fast and inexpensive and often raise questions or suggest hypotheses to be tested. They usually are followed by analytic studies, which try to explain biologic phenomena by seeking statistical associations between factors that may contribute to a subsequent occurrence and the occurrence itself.

Some analytic studies attempt, under naturally occurring circumstances, to observe the differences between two or more populations with different characteristics or behaviors. For instance, data about smokers and nonsmokers may be collected to determine the relative risk of a related outcome such as lung cancer or a cohort study may follow a population over time, as in the case of a Framingham, Massachusetts study. For years, epidemiologists have been studying a cooperating population of Framingham to determine associations between such variables as diet, weight, exercise, and other behaviors and characteristics related to heart disease and other outcomes. These observational studies are valuable in explaining patterns of disease or disease processes and providing information about the association of specific activities or agents with health or disease effects.

Experimental Epidemiology

Observational studies are usually followed by another major type of research: experimental studies. In experimental studies, the investigator actively intervenes by manipulating one variable to see what happens with the other. Although they are the best test of cause and effect, such studies are technically difficult to carry out and often raise ethical issues. Control populations are used to ensure that other nonexperimental variables are not affecting the outcome. Like clinical trials, such studies may raise ethical issues when experiments involve the use of a clinical procedure that may expose the subjects to significant or unknown risk. Ethical questions also are raised when experimental studies require the withholding of some potentially beneficial drug or procedure from individuals in the control group to prove decisively the effectiveness of the drug or procedure.

Other Applications of Epidemiologic Methods

Because the population perspective of epidemiology usually requires the study and analysis of data obtained from or about large-scale population samples, the discipline has developed principles and methods that can be applied to the study of a wide range of problems in several fields. Thus, the concepts and quantitative methods of epidemiology have been used not only to add to the understanding of the etiology of health and disease, but also to plan, administer, and evaluate health services; to forecast the health needs of population groups; to assess the adequacy of the supply of health personnel; and, most recently, to determine the outcomes of specific treatment modalities in a variety of clinical settings.

Advances in statistical theory and the epidemiology of medical care make it possible to analyze and interpret performance data obtained from the large Medicare and other insurance databases. Many of the findings of inexplicable geographic variations in the amount and cost of hospital treatments and in the use of a variety of health care services resulted from analysis of Medicare claims data and other large health insurance databases.

Health Services Research

Until the last 2 decades, most research addressed the need to broaden understanding of health and disease, to find new and more effective means of diagnosis and treatment, and in effect, to improve the quality and length of life. For the 2 decades after World War II, supply-side subsidy programs dominated federal health care policy. Like other subsidy programs, Medicare and Medicaid were politically crafted solutions rather than research-based strategies. Nevertheless, those major health care subsidy programs were the driving forces behind the rise of health services research. The continuous collection of cost and utilization data from these programs revealed serious deficiencies in the capability of the health care system to deliver efficiently and effectively the knowledge and skills already at hand. In addition, evidence was growing that the large variations in the kinds and amounts of care delivered for the same conditions represented unacceptable volumes of inappropriate or questionable care and too much indecision or confusion among clinicians about the best courses of treatment. Health services research was born of the need to improve the efficiency and effectiveness of the health care system and to determine which of the health care treatment options for each condition produces the best outcomes.

Agency for Health Care Research and Quality

Ever since John Wennberg documented large differences in the use of medical and surgical procedures among physicians in small geographic areas in the late 1980s, a number of similar studies brought the value of increasingly more costly health care into serious question. Wennberg noted that the rate of surgeries correlated with the numbers of surgeons and the number of hospital beds, rather than with differences among patients. He found that per-capita expenditures for hospitalization in Boston were consistently double those in nearby New Haven.[2–4] Widely varying physician practice patterns provided little direction as to the most appropriate use of even the most common clinical procedures. In addition, adequate outcome measures for specific intervention modalities generally were lacking.

The problem did not escape the attention of the 101st Congress. The development of new knowledge through research has long been held as an appropriate and essential role of the federal government, as evidenced by the establishment and proactive role of the National Institutes of Health. When it became clear that the indecision about the most appropriate and effective ways to diagnose and treat specific medical, dental, and other conditions was contributing to unacceptably large variations in the cost, quality, and outcomes of health care, federal legislation was passed to support the development of clinical guidelines. The Agency for Health Care Policy and Research (AHCPR) was established in 1989 as the successor to the National Center for Health Services Research and Health Care Technology. It is one of eight agencies of the Public Health Service within the Department of Health and Human Services.

AHCPR was responsible for updating and promoting the development and review of clinically relevant guidelines to assist health care practitioners in the prevention, diagnosis, treatment, and management of clinical conditions. Clinical guidelines are intended to enhance the quality, appropriateness, and effectiveness of health care.[5] The authorizing legislation directed that panels of qualified experts be convened by AHCPR or by public and not-for-profit private organizations. These panels were to review the literature that contained the findings of numerous studies of clinical conditions and, after considering the scientific evidence, to recommend clinical guidelines to assist practitioner and patient decisions about appropriate care for specific clinical conditions.

The agency's priority activities included extramural research through the Medical Treatment Effectiveness Program. The Medical Treatment Effectiveness Program funded two types of research projects: patient outcome research teams and literature synthesis projects or meta-analyses. Both the patient outcome research teams and the smaller literature synthesis projects identified and analyzed patient outcomes associated with alternative practice patterns and recommended changes where appropriate. During its decade-long existence, AHCPR supported studies that resulted in a prodigious array of publications focused on patient care and clinical decision making, technology assessment, the quality and costs of care, and treatment outcomes. Although no longer directly involved in producing clinical practice guidelines, the agency assists private-sector groups by supplying them with the scientific evidence that they need to develop their own guidelines.

Within the AHCPR, there was an Office of the Forum for Quality and Effectiveness in Health Care, which focused on the development and periodic review of practice recommendations. In addition, there were

Centers for Intramural and Extramural Research, an Office of Technology Assessment, and an Office for Data Development, among others.[5]

Some changes occurred in the mandate of AHCPR since its 1989 inception. The agency narrowly escaped the loss of funding and possible elimination in 1996 after incurring the wrath of national organizations of surgeons. In keeping with its original mission, AHCPR issued clinical guidelines. One such guideline discouraged surgery as a treatment for back pain on the grounds that it provided no better outcomes than more conservative treatments. Organizations of angry surgeons led a lobbying effort that convinced key members of Congress that the agency was exceeding its authority and establishing standards of clinical practice without considering the expertise and opinions of the medical specialists involved.[6]

The dispute was resolved when AHCPR agreed to function as a "science partner" with public and private organizations by simply assisting in developing knowledge that can be used to improve clinical practice. The agency would no longer produce clinical guidelines but would focus instead on funding research on medical interventions and analyzing the data that would underlie the development of clinical guidelines. The guidelines themselves would be generated by medical specialty and other organizations.

Subsequently, a Healthcare Research and Quality Act of 1999 was passed, which retitled the AHCPR to the Agency for Healthcare Research and Quality (AHRQ) and changed the title of the administrator to director. The mission of AHRQ is to (1) improve the outcomes and quality of health care services, (2) reduce its costs, (3) address patient safety, and (4) broaden effective services through establishment of a broad base of scientific research that promotes improvements in clinical and health systems practices, including prevention of disease.[7]

The agency is composed of the following components:[8]

1. Center for Delivery, Organization, and Markets
2. Center for Access, Financing, and Cost Trends
3. Center for Outcomes and Evidence
4. Center for Primary Care, Prevention, and Clinical Partnerships
5. Center for Quality Improvement and Patient Safety
6. Office of Director
7. Office of Communications and Knowledge Transfer

8. Office of Extramural Research, Education, and Priority Populations
9. Office of Performance Accountability, Resources, and Technology

A top priority of AHRQ is getting its sponsored research results and new health information into the hands of consumers. In addition to a number of consumer-oriented publications, the agency provides information to the public over the Internet. Its website, www.ahrq.gov, offers a great deal of health care information.

Building on concerns about medical errors and the quality of care, Congress and the president have increased support of the AHRQ. If that support continues during the next decade, the agency's greatest contribution to health care may be in the increases in patient care quality and reductions in costs that will result from provider acceptance of its service quality assessments and evidence-based practice recommendations.

Health Services Research and Health Policy

Health services research combines the perspectives and methods of epidemiology, sociology, economics, and clinical medicine; therefore, its curriculum is broader than the research courses taught in most medical schools. Although the basic concepts of epidemiologic research and associated statistics apply, process and outcome measures that reflect the behavioral and economic variables associated with questions of therapeutic effectiveness and cost benefit are also used. The ability of health services research to address issues of therapeutic effectiveness and cost benefit during this period of fiscal exigency contributed to the field's substantial growth and current value.

The contributions of health services research to health policy within recent years are impressive. Major examples include the Wennberg studies of small area variation in medical utilization, the prospective payment system based on diagnosis-related groups,[9,10] research on inappropriate medical procedures,[11] resource-based relative value scale research,[12–14] and the background research that supported the concepts of health maintenance organizations (HMOs) and managed care.

The RAND Health Insurance Experiment,[15,16] one of the largest and longest running health services research projects ever undertaken, began in 1971 and contributed vast amounts of information on the effects of cost sharing on the provision and outcomes of health services. Between 1974 and 1977, the project enrolled families in six sites, representing four major census regions, northern and southern rural areas, and a range of city sizes. Participating families were assigned to one of four different fee-for-service plans or to a prepaid group practice. As might have been expected, individuals in the various plans differed significantly in their rate of use, with little measurable effect on health outcomes. Although the reduced use of hospitals and specialized care by those in HMO plans did not affect their health status, those patients new to HMOs were somewhat less satisfied than the fee-for-service patients. The Health Insurance Experiment was followed by two large research studies: the Health Services Utilization Study and the Medical Outcomes Study. The findings of both have given impetus to the federal support of outcomes research.[17]

Determining the outcomes and effectiveness of different health care interventions aids clinical decision making, reduces costs, and benefits patients. If the United States is ever able to build political consensus in support of a national health policy, the findings of health services research will underpin the decisions. In the meantime, the findings related to treatment effectiveness guide the cost-containment efforts of managed care organizations.

Quality Improvement

Until the last few years, health care's impressive accomplishments made it difficult for health care researchers, policy makers, and organizational leaders to acknowledge publicly that poor quality health care is a major problem within the dynamic and productive biomedical enterprise in the United States. In 1990, after 2 years of study, hearings, and site visits, the Institute of Medicine issued a report that cited widespread overuse of expensive invasive technology, underuse of inexpensive "caring" services, and implementation of error-prone procedures that harmed patients and wasted money.[18,19]

Although these conclusions from so prestigious a body were devastating in their significance to health care reformers, they were hardly news to health service researchers. For decades, practitioners assumed that quality, like beauty, was in the eye of the beholder and, therefore, was unmeasurable except in cases of obvious violation of generally accepted standards. The medical and other health care professions had promoted the image of health care as a blend of almost impenetrable, science-based disciplines, leaving the providers of care as the only ones capable of understanding the processes taking place. Thus, only physicians could judge the work of other physicians. Such peer review–based assessment has always been difficult for reviewers and limited in effectiveness. Peer review recognizes that only part of medical care is based on factual knowledge. A substantial component of medical decision making is based on clinical judgment. Clinical judgment means combining consideration of the potential risks and benefits of each physician's internal list of alternatives in making diagnostic and treatment decisions with his or her medical intuition regarding the likelihood of success based on the condition of each patient. Under these complex and often inexplicable circumstances, physicians are repelled by the notion of either judging or being judged by their colleagues.

That is why, until recently, quality assurance, whether in hospitals or by regulatory agencies, was focused on identifying only exceptionally poor care. This practice, popularly known as the Bad Apple theory, was based on the presumption that the best way to ensure quality was to identify the bad apples and remove or rehabilitate them. Thus, during the 1970s and 1980s, quality assurance interventions only followed detection of undesirable occurrences. For example, flagrant violations of professional standards had to be in evidence before professional review organizations required physicians to begin quality improvement plans. Of course, physicians were guaranteed due process to dispute the evidence.

Focusing on isolated violations required a great deal of review time to uncover a single case that called for remedial action. In addition, it was an unpleasant duty for reviewers to assign blame to a colleague who might soon be on a committee reviewing their records. Most importantly, such an inspection of quality represented a method that implicitly defined quality as the absence of mishap. Clinician dislike of quality assurance activities during the 1970s and 1980s was well founded. The processes were offensive and had little constructive impact.

Specifying and striving for excellent care are very recent quality-assurance phenomena in the health care arena. Just as the automobile and other industries were late giving up supervision as a control mechanism and introducing "quality circles" or teamwork, so, too, were hospitals and other health care organizations that had long focused on peer-review committees, incident reports, and other negative quality monitoring activities.

Health services researchers had known for decades that health care quality was measurable and that excellent, as well as poor, care could be identified and quantified. In 1966, Avedis Donabedian[20] characterized the concept of health care as divided into the components of structure, process, and outcomes and the research paradigm of their assumed linkages, all of which have guided quality of care investigators to this day.

Donabedian suggested that the number, kinds, and skills of the providers, as well as the adequacy of their physical resources and the manner in which they perform appropriate procedures, should, in the aggregate, influence the quality of the subsequent outcomes. Although today the construct may seem like a simple statement of the obvious, at the time, attention to structural criteria was the major, if not the only, quality assurance activity in favor. It was generally assumed that properly trained professionals, given adequate resources in properly equipped facilities, performed at acceptable standards of quality. For example, for many years, the then Joint Commission on Accreditation of Hospitals made judgments about the quality of hospitals on the basis of structural standards, such as physical facilities and equipment, ratios of professional staff to patients, and the qualifications of various personnel. Later, it added process components to its structural standards. Aspects of process are the diagnostic, treatment, and patient management decisions and their appropriateness in relationship to current knowledge and practice. These quality assessments were directed to process components and did not attempt to determine what happened to the patients as the result of the medical decisions and interventions. Only recently did the Joint Commission on Accreditation of Healthcare Organizations include outcomes in its accreditation assessments.

Nevertheless, as far back as the 1950s, when Oscar Peterson and his associates at the University of North Carolina reported on a statewide study of general practice physicians, it was known that the quality of health service processes or practices may not reflect the quality of the underlying structural components of training and experience. Looking primarily at process components and using explicit practice quality criteria established in advance by a committee of general practitioners, researchers made onsite observations of each physician's practice behaviors for approximately 1 week. Forty-four percent of the physicians observed showed practice behaviors that were assessed as "below average" or "poor" in quality. Actual performance deficiencies may have been even greater because the presence of the observer may have motivated physicians to improve their usual performance temporarily.[21]

Similarly, in the early 1960s, M.A. Morehead conducted a study of the quality of care rendered to members of the Teamsters Union in New York City. At that time, the union was spending about $20 million per year for hospital services for its members and their families and wondered whether the quality of the services justified that expense. Unlike the North Carolina study, however, the criteria against which performance was measured were implicit, that is, left to the individual judgments of "expert" reviewers. Teams of various kinds of specialists reviewed samples of patient records from the large number of hospitals in New York City. Although an examination of outcomes was not part of the study, the researchers did look at the association between structure and process and found strong relationships. Both the level of specialty training of the physicians and the teaching status of the hospitals were associated strongly with high percentages of appropriate admissions and the provision of optimal care.[22]

The teams of medical experts making the judgments, however, were themselves board-certified specialists associated with teaching hospitals, and thus, the implicit personal standards they used reflected their own practice styles, values, and beliefs as to what constituted quality care. Clearly, their selection as judges biased the study in the direction of its subsequent findings—an intrinsic problem when standards are personal and not predefined.

Nevertheless, the findings of the Teamsters' study have been replicated in many others since. In another early study by Peterson et al.,[23] the percentage of pelvic surgical procedures with incorrect diagnoses was determined by analyses of the pathologists' examination of the removed tissues. Again, there was a significant difference between major teaching hospitals and other proprietary and not-for-profit institutions. There also was a difference between physicians who were members of the American College of Surgeons and those who were not.

These early landmark quality-of-care studies are noted to illustrate the difference between implicit and explicit normative or judgmental standards.

Implicit standards rely on the internalized judgments of the expert individuals involved in the quality assessment. Explicit standards are those developed and agreed on in advance of the assessment. Explicit standards minimize the variation and bias that invariably result when judgments are internalized. More current studies judge the appropriateness of hospital admissions and various procedures and, in general, associate specific structural characteristics of the health care system with practice or process variations. The previously noted small area variation studies are typical examples of such research designs.

There is another method for assessing the quality of health care practices that is based on empirical standards. Derived from distributions, averages, ranges, and other measures of data variability, information collected from a number of similar health service providers is compared to identify practices that deviate from the norms. A current popular use of empirical standards is in the patient severity-adjusted hospital performance data collected by health departments and community-based employer and insurer groups to measure and compare both process activities and outcomes. These performance "report cards" are becoming increasingly valuable to the purchasers of care who need an objective method to guide their choices among managed care organizations, health care systems, and group practices. The empirical measures of quality include such variables as:

- Timeliness of ambulation
- Compliance with basic nursing care standards
- Average length of stay
- Number of home care referrals
- Number of rehabilitation referrals
- Timeliness of consultation completion
- Timeliness of orders and results
- Patient wait times by department or area
- Infection rates
- Decubitus rates
- Medication errors
- Patient complaints
- Readmissions within 30 days
- Neonatal and maternal mortalities
- Perioperative mortalities

Normative and empirical standards are both used in studying the quality of health care in the United States. For example, empirical analyses are performed to test or modify normative recommendations. Empirical or actual experience data are collected to confirm performance and outcome improvements after the imposition of clinical guidelines derived from studies using normative standards.

Medical Errors

In November 1999, the IOM again issued a report on the quality of medical care. Focused on medical errors, the report described mistakes occurring during the course of hospital care as one of the nation's leading causes of death and disability. Citing two major studies, estimating that medical errors kill some 44,000 to 98,000 people in U.S. hospitals each year, the IOM report was a stunning indictment of the current systems of hospital care. The report contained a series of recommendations for improving patient safety in the admittedly high-risk environments of modern hospitals. Among the recommendations was a proposal for establishing a center for patient safety within the AHRQ. The proposed center would establish national safety goals, track progress in improving safety, and invest in research to learn more about preventing mistakes.[24] Congress responded by designating part of the increase in the budget for the AHRQ for that purpose.

Evidence-Based Medicine

Evidence-based medicine is defined as "the systematic application of the best available evidence to the evaluation of options and decisions in clinical practice, management and policy-making."[25] Although that statement may appear to be a description of the way physicians and other health care providers have practiced since the inception of scientific medicine, it reflects a spreading concern that quite the opposite is true. The wide range of variability in clinical practice, the complexity of diagnostic testing and medical decision making, and the difficulty that physicians have in keeping up with the overwhelming volumes of scientific literature suggest that a significant percentage of clinical management decisions are not supported by reliable evidence of effectiveness.

Although it is generally assumed that physicians are reasonably confident that the treatments they give are beneficial, the reality is that medical practice is fraught with uncertainty. In addition, the ethical basis for clinical decision making allows physicians to exercise their preferences for certain medical theories or practices that may or may not have been evaluated to link treatment to benefits.[26]

Proponents of evidence-based medicine propose that if all health services are intended to improve the health status and quality of life of the recipients, then the acid test is whether services, programs, and policies improve health beyond what could be achieved with the same resources by different means or by doing nothing at all. Evidence is the key to accountability; the decisions made by health care providers, administrators, policy makers, patients, and the public need to be based on appropriate, balanced, and high-quality evidence.[27]

The evidence-based approach to assessing the acceptability of research findings considers the evidence from randomized clinical trials involving large numbers of participants to be the most valid. Evidence-based medicine advocates dismiss outcomes research that uses large data files created from claim records, hospital discharges, Medicare, or other sources because the subjects are not randomized. "Outcomes research using claims data is an excellent way of finding out what doctors are doing, but it's a terrible way to find out what doctors should be doing," stated Thomas C. Chalmers, MD, of Harvard School of Public Health, Boston.[26]

In general, most of the investigations reported in the peer-reviewed medical literature have been preliminary tests of innovations and served science rather than providing guidance to practitioners in clinical practice. Only a small portion of those efforts survive testing well enough to justify routine clinical application.[27]

The situation is changing rapidly, however. Articles on evidence-based medicine are appearing with increasing frequency in the medical literature.[28] Cost-control pressures that encourage efforts to ensure that therapies have documented patient benefit, growing interest in the quality of patient care, and increasing sophistication on the part of patients concerning the care that they receive have stimulated acceptance of the concepts of evidence-based medical practice.[29]

Outcomes Research

Given the huge investment in U.S. health care and the inequitable distribution of its services, do the end effects on the health and well-being of patients and populations justify the costs? Insurance companies, state and federal governments, employers, and consumers are looking to outcomes research for information that will help them make better decisions about what kinds of health care should be reimbursed, for whom, and when.

Because outcomes research evaluates results of health care processes in the real world of physicians' offices, hospitals, clinics, and homes, it contrasts with traditional randomized controlled studies that test the effects of treatments in controlled environments. In addition, the research in usual service settings, or "effectiveness research," differs from controlled clinical trials, or "efficacy research," in the nature of the outcomes measured. Traditionally, studies measured health status, or outcomes, with physiological measurements—laboratory tests, complication rates, recovery, or survival. To capture health status more adequately, outcomes research measures a patient's functional status and well-being. Satisfaction with care also must complement traditional measures.

Functional status includes three components that assess patients' abilities to function in their own environment:

1. Physical functioning
2. Role functioning—the extent to which health interferes with usual daily activities, such as work or school
3. Social functioning—whether health affects normal social activities, such as visiting friends or participating in group activities

Personal well-being measures describe patients' senses of physical and mental well-being—their mental health or general mood, their own view of their general health, and their general sense about the quality of their lives. Patient satisfaction measures the patients' views about the services received, including access, convenience, communication, financial coverage, and technical quality.

Outcomes research also uses meta-analyses, a technique to summarize comparable findings from multiple studies. More importantly, however, outcomes research goes beyond determining what works in ideal circumstances to assessing which treatments for specific clinical problems work best in different circumstances. Appropriateness studies are conducted to determine circumstances in which a procedure should and should not be performed. Even though a procedure is proven effective, it is not appropriate for every patient in all circumstances. The frequency of inappropriate clinical interventions is one of the major quality-of-care problems in the system. Research is also under way to develop the tools to identify patient preferences when treatment options are available. Although most discussions about appropriateness stress the cost savings that could be achieved by reducing unnecessary care and overuse of services, it is important to remember that outcomes research may be just as likely to uncover underuse of appropriate services.

It is important to recognize that the ultimate value of outcomes research can be measured only by its ability to incorporate the results of its efforts into the health care process. To be effective, the findings of outcomes research must first reach and then change the behaviors of providers, patients, health care institutions, and payers. The endpoint of outcomes research, the clinical practice guidelines intended to assist practitioners and patients in choosing appropriate health care for specific conditions, must be disseminated in acceptable and motivational ways. With the health care industry in a state of rapid and generally unpredictable change, the need to make appropriate investments in outcomes research has become increasingly apparent. The conclusion is now inescapable that the United States cannot continue to spend over $1.5 trillion a year on health care without learning much more than is now known about what that investment is buying.[30]

Patient Satisfaction

Patient satisfaction has become an important component of the quality of care. Although the subjective ratings of health care received by patients may be based on markedly different criteria from those considered important by care providers, they capture aspects of care and personal preferences that contribute significantly to perceived quality. It has become increasingly important in the competitive market climate of health care that the providers' characteristics, organization, and system attributes important to the consumers be identified and monitored. In addition to caregivers' technical and interpersonal skills, such patient concerns as waiting times for appointments, emergency responses, helpfulness and communication of staff, and the facility's appearance contribute to patient evaluations of health services delivery programs and subsequent satisfaction with the quality of care received.

A number of instruments have been devised to measure patient satisfaction with health care, and most managed care plans, hospitals, and other health service facilities and agencies have adopted one or more to assess patient satisfaction regularly. Some, such as the Patient Satisfaction Questionnaire developed at Southern Illinois University School of Medicine, are short, self-administered survey forms.[27] Others, such as the popular patient satisfaction instruments of the Picker Institute of Boston, Massachusetts, may be used as self-administered questionnaires mailed to patients after a health care experience or completed by interviewers during telephone surveys.[31] Whether by mail, direct contact, or telephone interview, questioning patients after a recent health care experience is an effective way to both identify outstanding service personnel and uncover fundamental problems in the quality of care as defined by patients. It not only serves the purpose of providing humane and effective care, but it is also good marketing to do everything possible to increase patient satisfaction, maintain patient loyalty, and enhance patient referrals.

Research Ethics

In the 6 decades since World War II, the federal government has invested heavily in biomedical research. The ensuing public–private partnership in health has produced some of the finest medical research in the world. The growth of medical knowledge is unparalleled, and the United States can take well-deserved pride in its research accomplishments.

However, many, if not most, of the sophisticated new technologies address the need to ameliorate the problems of the patients who already have the condition or disease under treatment. Both the priorities and the profits intrinsic to the U.S. health care system focus on remedial rather than preventive strategies. Only in the case of frightening epidemics, such as that of polio in the 1940s or AIDS in the 1990s, have there been the requisite moral imperatives to fund adequately abundant research efforts that address public health problems. Clearly, much of the recent funding for medical research has failed to fulfill the generally held belief that the products of taxpayer-supported research should benefit not only the practice of medicine, but also the community at large.[32]

The increasing amount of research funding emanating from pharmaceutical companies is of growing concern. Pharmaceutical companies that pay researchers to design and interpret drug trials have been accused of spinning the results or suppressing unfavorable findings. The conflicts that arise in the testing of new drugs and publishing the results are deepened as more and more of these studies are shifted from academic institutions to commercial research firms.[33]

To compound the problem further, the Federal Drug Administration (FDA), which regulates about a fourth of the U.S. economy, has been without a permanent director for several years. The lack of permanent leadership plus the federal legislation, which shifted the FDA's funding from the government to the same pharmaceutical companies it is supposed to monitor, has had a damaging effect. Political and pharmaceutical pressures have caused the FDA to stray from its science-based public health mandate. At this writing, the FDA is embroiled in controversy over its alleged failure to monitor adequately the risks of widely advertised and commonly used drugs for the treatment of arthritis.[34]

Commercialism, with its accompanying ethical concerns, has invaded the research laboratory in a big way with the unfolding of the human genome. The scientific importance of being able to read the 3 billion DNA "letters" of the human body is being overshadowed by visions of the technology's commercial potential. The completion of the DNA sequence will revolutionize medicine by giving scientists unprecedented insights into the workings of the human body. Although the benefits of these genetic breakthroughs are years away, debates over whether the technology will stay in the public domain and strategies for profiting from the ability to treat medical conditions through gene manipulation are already under way. Clearly, the admirable advances in understanding and technology resulting from sophisticated medical research are increasingly accompanied by less-than-commendable bending of ethical precepts.

Future Challenges

Much, if not most, of U.S. health care research has been directed toward improving the health care system's ability to diagnose and treat injury, disease, and disability among those who seek care from the health care providers in the vast and complex array of existing health services. For decades, health care has been a complaint and response system, with most patient and provider interactions initiated by ailing patients. Physicians and other health professionals have maintained the mindset that their major, if not sole, duty was to resolve patient problems as expeditiously as possible. Now, largely because of the influences of managed care, research studies are increasingly focused on identifying and improving the health status of populations. Research priorities are shifting from an individual patient perspective to a population orientation and toward continuous scrutiny of the efficiency and effectiveness of the care delivered.

Basic science research will continue to contribute to the diagnostic and therapeutic efficacy of health care by adding to the knowledge about the human body and its functions. In small but critically important increments, basic science research will unlock many of the secrets of aging, cell growth regulation, mental degradation, and other mysteries of immunology, genetics, microbiology, and neuroendocrinology. The propensity of medicine to use newly obtained knowledge to alter certain physiologic processes, as in the several forms of gene manipulation, will produce new ethical, legal, and clinical issues that then will require further research and adjudication.

Massive databases of gene and protein sequences and structure/function information have made possible a new worldwide research effort called bioinformatics. Bioinformatic research probes those large computer databases to learn more about life's processes in health and disease and to find new or better drugs. It is considered the future of biotechnology.

Of particular interest is research in genomics, the study of genetic material in the chromosomes of specific organisms. The sequencing of the human genome will reshape biology and medicine and lead to significant improvements in the diagnosis of disease and individual responses to drugs.[35]

Similarly, certain advances in clinical medicine and the other health disciplines will result in new and particularly disturbing moral dilemmas. Medical achievements, such as those that permit the maintenance of life in otherwise terminal and unresponsive individuals or the transplantation of organs in short supply that require choosing among recipient candidates when those denied will surely die, generate extremely complex ethical, economic, religious, personal, and professional issues. Thus, much of the basic and clinical research that solves yesterday's problems relating to individual patient care will create new problems to be addressed in the never-ending cycle of discovery, application, and evaluation.

Medical researchers and clinicians are becoming increasingly concerned that health care in the United States is entering a "postantibiotic" era in which bacterial infections will be unaffected by even the most powerful of available antibiotics. Evidence is accumulating that a growing number of microbes, including strains of staphylococcus and streptococcus bacteria, are becoming resistant to common antimicrobials.[36]

Staphylococcus bacteria are the major cause of hospital infections. According to the Centers for Disease Control and Prevention, these infections are responsible for about 13% of the 2 million infections that occur in U.S. hospitals each year. Overall, those hospital infections result in the deaths of 60,000 to 80,000 patients.[32]

Although epidemiologists and clinicians specializing in infectious disease have warned for decades that misuse and overuse of antibiotics would result in a host of deadly drug-resistant pathogens, it appears that neither physicians nor patients took the warnings seriously. Apparently, there was a widespread belief that the constant development of new antimicrobial drugs would keep medicine a step ahead of bacterial resistance. Although the limited development of new antibiotic drugs has failed to keep step with antibiotic resistance, scientists see a promising alternative in bacterial genetics. Introducing synthetic genes into bacteria appears to turn off the bacteria's ability to resist antibiotics.[32]

While researchers address the problems of treatment of these lethal infections, hospitals strive to prevent them. Because bacteria can be transmitted on blankets, clothing, walls, medical equipment, and by hand, hospitals are implementing rigorous infection control and surveillance policies and new education programs for both providers and patients.

Health services research, on the other hand, will continue to focus on the performance of the health care system as the basis for proposing or evaluating health policy alternatives. It is interdisciplinary, value-laden research concerned with the effectiveness or benefits of care, the efficiency or resource cost of care, and the equity or fairness of the distribution of care. As the U.S. health care system goes through its wrenching adjustment to the competitive, market-driven reforms, health services research becomes more and more central to the development of a logical, well-documented rationale for future health care policies and delivery systems.

At present, clinical uncertainty is pervasive in the health care industry as it defines illness, selects among treatment options, and tries to determine the probabilities of desired and unintended results and to judge the quality of individual outcomes.

Documenting the influence of financial incentives that affect both patient and provider, understanding the important relationships of socioeconomic status to health and health care, determining the effects of the training and experience of the health care team and the ability of the members to work together, and understanding how these many influences interact are basic to improving the quality of care. Reducing the monumental quandaries in medicine and health care about what works well in what situations is the challenge of health services research and the key to a more effective, efficient, and equitable health care system.

Managed care companies and groups of consumers and businesses are supporting an effort to develop national performance measures for health plans that will help consumers and payers compare plans on measures other than cost. Insurers are increasingly using outcomes research results to refine and improve their reimbursement systems. Hospitals, HMOs, and other organized care systems are incorporating results of outcomes research into their quality review and improvement practices. Results not only provide guidance on what constitutes good care, but also form the basis for discussion among providers and managers about ways of designing more efficient delivery systems.

Public health research is a related research arena that deserves to receive higher priority and significantly increased political support. If health care is ever to develop a true population perspective rather than an individual patient perspective and reap the health and economic benefits of preventive rather than curative medicine, then epidemiology and public health research must be charged with finding ways to better understand and resolve the huge differences in health, health behaviors, health care, and health system effectiveness among communities and the population groups within them. Epidemiology, the core discipline of public health research, relates the health problems and use of health care resources to defined populations. It identifies groups that do not present themselves for health care, as well as those that do. Thus, epidemiology can assess the health problems and the provision of health care for the total population rather than just those who are in contact with health services. Surveillance and monitoring of health conditions and assessing the effect of health care measures on the entire population are important factors in formulating health policy, organizing health services, and allocating limited resources.[37] The strategy for identifying and dealing with real or suspected biological attacks on citizens of the United States will depend heavily on the ability of epidemiologists to identify the common source of such outbreaks, the patterns of transmission, and the outcomes of preventive and remedial efforts.

As health care adds to its traditional focus on theories, disease, and individual patient care, the performance of the health care system and the health status of populations, public health, and health services research assume increasing relevance and importance. No matter how well the health care system performs for some of the people, it will never be fully satisfactory until it can provide a basic level of care for all.

References

1. Aday LA, Lairson DR, Balkrishnan R, et al. *Evaluating the Medical Care System: Effectiveness, Efficiency, and Equity.* Ann Arbor, MI: Health Administration Press; 1993:4.

2. Wennberg JE, Freeman JL, Culp WJ, et al. "Are hospital services rationed in New Haven or over-utilized in Boston?" *Lancet.* 1987;1:1185–1189.

3. Wennberg JE. Which Rate Is Right? *N Engl J Med.* 1986;314:310–311.

4. Wennberg JE, Freeman JL, Shelton RM, et al. Hospital use and mortality among Medicare beneficiaries in Boston and New Haven. *N Engl J Med.* 1989;321:1168–1173.

5. Agency for Health Care Policy and Research, U.S. Department of Health and Human Services. *AHCPR Program Note.* Rockville, MD: Public Health Service; 1990:1–5.

6. Stephenson J. Revitalized AHCPR pursues research on quality. *JAMA.* 1997; 278:1557.

7. AHRQ Fiscal Year 2003 Budget in Brief, Agency for Healthcare Research and Quality, Rockville, MD. Available from http://www.ahrq.gov/about/cj2003/budbrf03.htm. Accessed August 28, 2002.

8. Agency for Healthcare Research and Quality. Available from http://www.ahrq.gov. Accessed September 19, 2006.

9. Mills R, Fetter RB, Riedel DC, et al. AUTOGRP: an interactive computer system for the analysis of health care data. *Med Care.* 1976;14:603–615.

10. Berki SE. DRGs, incentives, hospitals and physicians. *Health Affairs*, Winter 1985;4(4):70–76.

11. Chassin MR, Kosecoff J, Park RE, et al. Does inappropriate use explain geographic variations in the use of health care services? A study of three procedures. *JAMA*. 1987;258:2533–2537.

12. Hsiao WC, Stason WB. Toward developing a relative value scale for medical and surgical services. *Health Care Finan Rev*. 1979;1:23–28.

13. Hsiao WC, Braun P, Yntema D, et al. Results and policy implications of the resource-based relative value study. *N Engl J Med*. 1988;319:881–888.

14. Hsiao WC, Braun P, Yntema D, et al. *A National Study of Resource-Based Relative Value Scale for Physician Services: Final Report to the Health Care Financing Administration*. Boston, MA: Harvard School of Public Health; 1988.

15. Newhouse JP. A design for a health insurance experiment. *Inquiry*. 1974; 11:5–27.

16. Newhouse JP, Keeler EB, Phelps CE, et al. The findings of the RAND health insurance experiment—a response to Welch et al. *Medical Care*. 1987; 25:157–179.

17. Newhouse JP. Controlled experimentation as research policy. In: Ginzberg E. ed. *Health Services Research: Key to Health Policy*. Cambridge, MA: Harvard University Press; 1991:162–194.

18. Lohr KN. *The Institute of Medicine. Medicare: A Strategy for Quality Assurance. Vol 1*. Washington, DC: National Academy Press; 1990:1–19.

19. Palmer RH. Considerations in defining quality of health care, part I. In: Palmer RH, et al, eds. *Striving for Quality in Health Care: An Inquiry into Policy and Practice*. Ann Arbor, MI: Health Administration Press; 1991:1–4.

20. Donabedian A. Evaluating the quality of medical care. *Milbank Mem Fund Q*. 1966;44:166–206.

21. Peterson O. An analytic study of North Carolina general practice. *J Med Educa Suppl*. 1956;4:18–24.

22. Morehead MA. The medical audit as an operational tool. *J Public Health*. 1967;57:1643–1656.

23. Peterson O, Barsamion EM, Eden NN, et al. A study of diagnostic performance: a preliminary report. *J Med Educ*. 1966;41:797–803.

24. Kohn LT, Corrigan JM, Donaldson MS, et al. *To Err is Human: Building a Safer Health System*. Washington DC: Institute of Medicine; 1999:74–77.

25. Ware, JE Jr, Snyder MR, Wright R, et al. Defining and measuring patient satisfaction with medical care. *Eval Plan*. 1983;6:247–263.

26. Watanabe M. A call for action from the National Forum on Health. *Canad Med Asso J*. 1997;156:999–1000.

27. Marwick C. Federal agency focuses on outcomes research. *JAMA*. 1993; 270:164–165.

28. Castiel LD. The urge for evidence based knowledge. *J Epidemiol Commun Health*. 2003;57:482.

29. Hooker RC. The rise and rise of evidence-based medicine. *Lancet*. 1997; 349:1329–1330.

30. Reinhardt UE, Hussey PS, Anderson GF, et al. U.S. health care spending in an international context. *Health Affairs*. 2004;23:10–25.

31. Gerteis M, Edgman-Levitan S, Daley J. *Through the Patient's Eyes: Understanding and Promoting Patient-Centered Care*. San Francisco, CA: Jossey-Bass Publishers; 1993:1–15.

32. Constantine LM. *Healthcare Providers Confront Rise in Resistant Pathogens. Report of Medical Guidelines and Outcomes Research 8, no. 21*. Boston, MA: Capitol Productions; October 16, 1997:1–5.

33. Stevens R. *In Sickness and in Wealth*. New York, NY: Basic Books; 1989:48.

34. Available from http://msnbc.com/id/6733148. Accessed December 20, 2004.

35. The George Washington University Medical Center. Available from http://www.gwumc.edu/bioinformatics, 3. Accessed August 27, 2002.

36. Bodenheimer T. Uneasy alliance-clinical investigators and the drug industry. *N Engl J Med*. 2000;342:1516–1518, 1539–1544.

37. Ibrahim MA. *Epidemiology and Health Policy*. Gaithersburg, MD: Aspen Publishers; 1985:6.

12

The Future of Health Care

This concluding chapter provides some forecasts about the future of various components of the U.S. health care system. It outlines the changes that have occurred among health care organizations, services, and facilities and among physicians, nurses, and other personnel, and then it projects those trends into the future. The chapter also sketches the corporate growth in health care and the impact of technologic advances, managed care, academic health centers and federal and state governmental initiatives and draws conclusions about the future of America's health care system.

In the previous chapters, we have presented a mix of facts, expert opinions, findings of published studies, and historical background. Although the selection of content and the interpretations of historical events undoubtedly reflect our own public health or population perspective, we have tried to provide a balanced view of the health care system and its evolution, strengths, and weaknesses. When discussing the future, however, we are entering uncharted territory, progressing from the current structure and conduct of health care to conjecture about its reformation. Looking ahead is far more hazardous than looking back, and we acknowledge that the predictions that follow represent only our personal educated guesses about the directions our health care system will take in the coming years. Even the most thoughtful forecasts, founded on carefully studied trends and database projections by reputable authorities, will be affected by unforeseeable and rapid changes in the health care environment.

According to chaos theory, "A small change in input can quickly translate into overwhelming differences in output,"[1] and as has been demonstrated already, the health care system is particularly sensitive to input changes. In the past, every tinkering effort to address one of the three basic problems of the health care system—costs, quality, and access—has resulted in significant changes in one or both of the others. Improving access to health care for low-income populations and older adults through Medicaid and Medicare had a significant inflationary effect on costs. Containing costs through managed care now raises questions about quality and access. Similarly, seemingly small changes within a health care institution, such as a leadership response to an outside financial, technologic, or market development, may result in unanticipated pressures on the operations within the organization. Thus, many of the recent organizational machinations of the institutions and agencies struggling to cope with health care reforms may, in the long run, turn out to be counterproductive overreactions.

The Paradox of U.S. Health Care

It is unfortunate that the extraordinary successes of the U.S. health care system and the technologic accomplishments that brought worldwide acclaim to U.S. scientists are offset by the system's persistent and increasingly evident deficiencies. The policy decisions of health care leadership after World War II are duly credited with medicine's impressive advances, its prestige, and its wealth. Those health care policies led the National Institutes of Health and the National Science Foundation to invest heavily in the potential of our nation's universities and medical schools to develop basic and applied research and to dedicate federal and state funds to the expansion of academic medical centers. The burgeoning health care industry prompted the initiation of federal programs that significantly expanded the number and size of U.S. hospitals and led to an exponential increase in the size of the health care workforce. Those health care policies that produced the financial incentives in the health care reimbursement system encouraged specialization among physicians and other health care practitioners.

Those policies also contributed to long-standing health care problems of inequitable access, variable quality, and runaway costs. The success of the health care industry, the growth of its workforce, its astounding physical and technologic infrastructure, its impressive outcomes, and its unfettered revenues must be weighed against its failure to recognize a social mission broader than addressing the individual needs of those who accessed its services. Until recently, the technology-oriented, can-do culture that pervades health care, and medicine in particular, appeared to have mesmerized the consuming public and health care providers into thinking that more dramatic medical marvels would solve the ills of the system. For many years, the public that supported the rising costs of health care had equally ascending expectations for what medicine could accomplish.

Now, however, there is growing discontent with a system that cannot deliver even a basic level of health care to significant portions of the public, that cannot control costs that have increased at twice the rate of other commodities, and that provides some services of doubtful necessity and therapeutic benefit. Nothing has shaken the public's previously durable faith in medicine as much as the growing awareness that many of the new technologies that yield economic benefits to providers may be of only marginal value in the diagnosis and treatment of patients.

The Major Challenges Facing Health Care

Regardless of widespread criticism of America's system of health care, the public and political clamor for fundamental reform waned for a few years after its peak in the mid-1990s. The competitive managed care systems that followed the demise of national health care reform were somewhat effective in containing health care costs. That influence was short-lived, however, and rising costs and several other very serious problems continued to plague the system. Those problems, described over a decade ago as "major forces reshaping the health care system industry," remain unaddressed and are as relevant today as they were then. Both the consumers and the providers of health care are increasingly concerned that the negative consequences of social, technical, and economic forces impacting the health system are resulting in a more disordered and less trustworthy health care system. Major forces reshaping health care are outlined in Table 12-1.[2]

Table 12-1 Key Forces Influencing the Health Care System

Forces	Implications and Issues
· Growing number of uninsured	· Creation of basic benefits package · State-level experimentations · What does the country want to afford?
· Demand for greater accountability—fiscal and clinical	· Search for value (greater quality for a given cost or lower cost for a given level of quality) · What works?
· Technological growth and innovation	· New diagnostic and treatment modalities · Growth of outpatient care · Increased issues involving prolongation of life
· Changing population composition: growth of elderly and ethnically heterogenous population	· Changes in demand for care · Increased number of ethical issues · Increased social morbidity
· Changing professional labor supply	· Shortages of key health professionals · Redefinition of professional roles · Productivity and quality issues
· Globalization of the economy	· Increased scrutiny of health care costs
· Changing composition of the delivery system: consolidations and mergers—horizontal and vertical	· Increased potential for managing a continuum of care · Increased potential for providing care to defined populations
· Information management	· Facilitates accountability · Tool for increased productivity · Direct clinical applications · Opportunity to actively manage clinical care

Source: Reprinted with permission: Shortell SM and Reinhardt UE, eds., Creating and Executing Health Policy in the 1990s, in: Shortell SM and Reinhardt UE, eds. *Improving Health Policy and Management: Nine Critical Research Issues*, pp 3–36 ©1992 Health Administration Press.

The Growing Number of Uninsured

The population of uninsured Americans is a constantly changing, heterogeneous group that includes the full range of annual incomes. The sluggish economy, receding governmental budgets, and rising health care costs have dissuaded an increasing number of middle- and upper-income people to forgo health insurance. Many are self-employed or retired early without insurance benefits. Findings from the latest survey of the U.S. Bureau of the Census indicate that much of the most recent increase in the number of uninsured was due to a significant decline in employer-sponsored health insurance. Employers, deterred by double-digit inflation in health insurance premiums, are finding ways to break away from paying for employee health insurance.[3]

Two other groups make up the balance of the uninsured. Many low-income uninsured are eligible for Medicaid or State Children's Health Insurance Programs (SCHIPs) but are unaware of either their eligibility or the enrollment process. The other uninsured group is made up of low-income people who do not qualify for public programs. According to the National Institute for Health Care Management, about 9 million people fall into this category. Many of these people are employed full- or part-time in low-paying jobs without health benefits or in transition after losing a job. Still others have been dropped from Medicaid after moving into the workforce. These transition gaps are the reason for the constantly changing composition of the uninsured population.

Addressing the huge problem of uninsured Americans always raises the political issues that swirl around the concept of a national health insurance or single payer system. Yet, small segments of the problem have been addressed quite successfully by governments through Medicaid, SCHIP, and a number of innovative state programs. They are limited, however, to low-income groups. The major impediment to insuring most of the over 46.6 million uninsured Americans is affordability. Nevertheless, the uninsured do get health care. As might be expected, that care is delayed, more expensive, episodic, and incomplete.[4] The care is provided by clinics, hospitals, physicians, and other providers who either absorb the costs or receive some general support from government or private funds.

Comprehensive health care coverage is simply too expensive for most small businesses and low- to moderate-income individuals. If health care costs continue to rise at unacceptable rates, more and more people will find health insurance unaffordable. The concept of medical savings accounts in which people simply set aside money, tax-free, to cover medical expenses and each year roll over unspent funds may become more attractive.

Demand for Greater Accountability, Fiscal and Clinical

The health care system, apart from the advances in clinical practice, has a built-in resistance to change. Entrenched interests, the many professions, employers, employees, and service, financial, and educational institutions have repeatedly demonstrated the capability of exercising the power necessary to maintain the status quo. As a consequence, the long and escalating problems of health care costs and unconscionable rates of unacceptable clinical quality have remained unabated for decades. Because there are no single solutions to these complex problems and little likelihood that all or most of the vested interests would support a set of simultaneously applied solutions, the problems continue. Anything more than tinkering with the system would have a negative effect on at least one of the major players capable of nullifying the proposed changes.

The failed attempts to address the issue of the variable quality of clinical care illustrate a facet of the problem. Concerns about the quality of health care, both anecdotally and empirically, have been expressed for decades. Because there were always small numbers of patients involved in medical errors in any individual hospital, physicians and hospital executives tended to overlook the problems. Finally, in 1999, the credible, widely publicized assessment of the problem by the Institute of Medicine (IOM) entitled, *To Err is Human: Building a Safer Health System*, produced a brief flurry of discussion in Congress and then moved far down on the list of U.S. concerns. When 3,000 people died on September 11th, 2001, the United States went to war. When over 3,000 people die every 2 weeks as a result of medical errors, the silence is incomprehensible and discouraging.

The lack of immediate response by physicians and policy makers reflects the generally held assumption that the medical profession effectively polices itself. The esteemed position of physicians in society and the confidentiality of the interactions between doctors and their patients have long shielded medicine from the sweeping reforms that corrected abuses in other industries. Nevertheless, the truth is that the medical profession has only recently begun to exercise the leadership necessary to correct the longstanding medical care system deficiencies that the IOM report identified.

Michael L. Millenson, author of the 1997 book *Demanding Medical Excellence: Doctors and Accountability in the Information Age*, published by the University of Chicago Press, described that shortcoming in the journal *Health Affairs*.[5]

> *The blunt answer is that professionalism alone has consistently failed to protect patients. Rather, it has been professionalism pushed into action by pressure from the press, public, politicians, and the pocketbook. For example, anesthesiologists finally acted to improve patient safety only after a television exposé of anesthesia accidents. Rising malpractice premiums—an economic incentive— provided an extra sense of urgency. Similarly, the "sign your site" protocol came*

in reaction to a nationally publicized incident in which a Florida surgeon amputated the wrong foot of a diabetic man in 1995. The People's Medical Society, a consumer group, had suggested a "sign your site" initiative a decade before, only to be met by indignation and ridicule on the part of surgeons. In mid-2002, the provider-dominated Joint Commission on Accreditation of Healthcare Organizations (JCAHO) finally proposed rules requiring hospitals to reduce wrong site surgery—seven years after the scandal and seventeen years after the consumer group had suggested such a move. Even with this delay and even with the utter simplicity of the act of signing one's name, 20–40 percent of surgeons continue to resist efforts to get them to sign voluntarily, a past president of the orthopedic academy admitted to the Washington Post.

In fairness, physicians and other providers are beset by so many individual problems that they willingly leave the more global problems of clinical practice to their organizational leadership. They are caught between patient demands, their own uncertainties as to the best course of treatment, and the need to constrain costs. In addition, the steady production of new drugs, devices, and procedures makes current knowledge quickly obsolete. The time and effort required to remain current with clinical developments place a heavy burden on busy practitioners. They readily admit that they find it impossible to keep up with their voluminous literature and attend even the most relevant continuing professional education courses. That many practitioners become outmoded, despite their best efforts, contributes to the quality chasm.

Although achieving system-wide improvements in health care quality depends on resolving complex, multidimensional issues, there are some hopeful signs on the horizon. Continuously rising health care costs encourage purchasers of health care coverage, individuals, employers, and state and federal governments to become more involved in assessing and improving the quality of care. Nothing is more expensive nor wasteful than the cost of inappropriate or error-prone care and its sequelae.

The federal Agency for Healthcare Research and Quality is helping to pierce the culture of silence that seems to surround medical errors by establishing the first peer-reviewed, Web-based medical journal, www.webmm. ahrq.gov, to stimulate discussion of medical errors in a blame-free environment.[6] Physicians and other health professionals submit medical errors cases to the site for interactive discussion and analysis. Contributors may remain anonymous if they prefer.

In addition, the Department of Health and Human Services is participating in the Hospital Quality Information Initiative, a joint effort with the leadership of the nation's hospitals to provide the public with information on the quality of care. A similar effort was launched in 2002 that involved providing quality measures of nursing home care. These concepts are different from the contentious issue of a proposed national mandatory, or even voluntary, error reporting system. The federal government's strategy is clearly moving away from assigning blame and toward educating both providers and consumers to function as full partners.

As previously described, the successful "100,000 Lives Campaign" of the Institute for Healthcare Improvement and its subsequent "5 Million Lives Campaign," sponsored principally by the Blue Cross and Blue Shield health plans, have the potential to make huge gains in patient safety by inducing hospitals to institute critically important and long-ignored safety interventions.[7]

With the capability of the Internet to dispense knowledge that used to be available only to the few "insiders," previously thwarted consumers, purchasers, legislators, and other interested parties are driving the demand for information. When purchasers of health care services have the information and performance measures that allow them to identify high-quality, safe medical care based on scientific evidence of effectiveness, poor-performing providers and institutions will be forced to shape up or lose their market to higher quality competitors. Clinical practice guidelines, evidence-based medicine, and other mechanisms for improving the practice of medicine will find greater acceptance among service facilities and practitioners.

Health Care Costs

Like the long-standing "quality of care" problem, the comparable dilemma of escalating health care costs has received only infrequent and generally ineffective attention. The sweeping takeover of health care in the United States by managed care organizations had only a temporary impact on the rate of national health care spending. There has been a rapid acceleration of health spending since 1998 and no promising measures in sight to curb spending growth.[8]

In fact, no initiatives in the last 30 years, either regulatory or voluntary, have had other than a temporary impact on this nation's health care costs; however, the current war on terrorism and its ripple effects on federal and state budgets and the economy, in general, make runaway health care costs a far more critical problem. On one side, new and costly drugs and procedures continue to proliferate and add to medicine's already impressive capability. On the other, the aging population and others with persistent medical care needs are increasingly finding the high cost of drugs and other medical services beyond their means. The problem intensifies as the economy weakens and governmental support and personal budgets decline.

All of the potential remedies to the problem of health costs are painful. The U.S. health care system has long enjoyed unrestrained demand and exercised every incentive to do all that is possible for every patient regardless of cost. For the most part, patients, unless uninsured, have been protected from any significant out-of-pocket costs associated with those procedures. Until recently, employers, the major purchasers of health insurance coverage, considered that employee benefit a reasonable addition to wages and salaries. Now that health care costs have increased beyond acceptable levels, however, many people must choose between forgoing other goods and services or living without health insurance and some treatments and drugs. State and federal programs are reducing benefits, and employers are turning more of the costs of employee health insurance back to their workers. In the current environment of unrestrained wartime expenditures, there appears to be little political will to take the drastic actions that would be necessary to curb health care spending. As was evident in the approach to the problems of health quality, governmental initiatives during this period of economic turmoil are likely to be uncoordinated strategies that nibble at the margins of the problem.

The increasing use of the Internet to obtain health information by the public reflects the will and ability of Americans to understand complex issues and make informed decisions about their health care. It is increasingly evident that judgments about the consumption of medical services, formerly the province of providers with compliant patients, will be made in the future by more knowledgeable consumers who are concerned about the economic consequences of those decisions. If and when assertive users of health care services take charge of their medical care, market forces will begin to function on the basis of cost and quality as they do in other service areas.

The alternative to reducing excessive costs is a single-payer system that eliminates the substantial amount of health care dollars that are wasted on the administration of multiple insurance plans and the huge burden of their required paperwork. Nothing in the current political environment, however, portends interest in reducing the largess of big corporate insurers with impressive lobbying capability.

Technologic Growth and Innovation

Growth of Home, Outpatient, and Ambulatory Care

The changes occurring in hospital care and the demographics of aging have produced rapid growth of home care in recent years. In fact, home health care has been the fastest growing segment of the health care industry since 1989. Spending for home health services increased 60% between 1993 and 1994, whereas the health care industry overall increased by only about 8%. Lacking any major change in Medicare (which still reimburses home health care on a retrospective basis), growth within the home care industry is expected to continue rapidly over the next few years.[9]

A number of factors are responsible for the most recent extraordinary growth in the number of medical and surgical procedures performed in outpatient and ambulatory settings. Advances in diagnostic technology, anesthesiology, and surgery have combined to make same-day surgery possible for procedures that formerly required hospital inpatient admissions. Third-party payers were quick to recognize the considerable cost savings of ambulatory surgery and began producing an ever-lengthening list of diagnostic and surgical procedures that would no longer be reimbursed if patients were admitted to hospitals as inpatients unless there were extenuating medical circumstances.

With federal and state incentives to encourage the development of more outpatient and ambulatory facilities and broad consumer acceptance, every service possible is now being provided in outpatient or ambulatory settings. These include cancer treatment, kidney dialysis, diagnostic imaging, rehabilitation services, urgent care, wellness and preventive medicine activities, and sports medicine, in addition to surgery. With the care comparable to, if not better than, that received in hospitals and provided at far lower cost, it is clear that ambulatory care will reduce the mission of hospitals to serving only those patients in need of intensive nursing and medical interventions.

Technology

A revealing example of the coercive power of glamorous and expensive technologic developments over thoughtful considerations of cost benefit to patients is the medical popularity of magnetic resonance imaging (MRI) scanners. More than 2,000 of these very profitable, high-technology imaging devices have been installed in hospitals and outpatient facilities across the country. At an average cost of about $1.5 million each, the national investment in them is nearly $3 billion. Each of these machines is paid for by charging patients $900 to $1,200 per MRI scan, generating upward of another $3 billion in health care costs. How has this huge investment in admittedly superior diagnostic capability paid off in terms of medical care improvements? An extensive literature search published in the American College of Physicians' *Annals of Internal Medicine* in 1994 could not find a single study that documented a change in patient outcomes. Although the diagnostic information the MRI scan provided was considered clearer and a truer demonstration of the disease or the anatomy, neither controlled comparisons of diagnostic accuracy or changes in therapeutic choices documented patient benefits.[10] It is particularly discouraging that in many communities the number of MRI scanners installed near each other exceeds any reasonable estimate of population need or service requirement. They are only adding to the costs of health care as redundant entrepreneurial ventures.

Similarly, the technology that permits physicians to save the lives of extremely low birthweight babies (1 to 2 pounds), only to have them suffer from lifelong neurosensory impairments, behavior problems, and learning disorders, raises serious questions about the role of technology in modern medicine. With all of America's impressive neonatal technology, infant mortality is worse than that of at least 24 other countries.[11] Because most of the infant deaths occur among very low-weight infants, the problem relates to the lack of prenatal instruction and care. Clearly, the health care value system does not give high priority to such a low-tech, relatively low-cost solution. As a result, an infant born in Cuba has a statistically better chance of surviving than an infant born in the United States.

The ability to prolong the life of advanced Alzheimer's patients and other seriously demented and terminally ill patients, in many cases over the objections of family members who would rather their loved ones die peacefully, is another example of the dominant role of technology in medical practice.

It is becoming increasingly clear that technologic progress in health care has been a mixed blessing. The impersonal, if not inhumane, imposition of high-technology medicine between patients and practitioners has changed both the image and the mission of the health care enterprise. The complex social problems that affect access to health care; the geographic, economic, and other demographic inequities in the value and availability of care; and the serious discrepancies in the quality of care are issues that cannot be remedied by technologic means.

Changing Population Composition

As was previously discussed, the U.S. population is growing older and will continue to do so for decades. The older population will not only increase in size relative to younger groups, but a growing number of older adults will survive to very advanced ages. In addition, the number of large, intact families capable of housing and caring for aged relatives has diminished rapidly. Families raise fewer children, and those children often migrate to other locations when they attain maturity. Consequently, the health care needs of the larger population of the more frail older adults are expected to place increasing demands on the health care system. Those demands will focus particularly on the chronic care component of the U.S. system, a sector that has not been particularly attractive to health care providers. In addition, much of the long-term care capability in the United States is in the hands of the private, for-profit sector, which has an uneven record for the quality of its services.

The health care needs of this growing adult population will also be influenced by its changing racial and ethnic diversity. The major changes occurring in the total U.S. population will be reflected in the older population. Minority groups and Hispanics in particular will become larger proportions of the older population. These changes have important implications for medical care. There are significant differences in mortality rates, chronic conditions, service preferences and use, and attitudes toward medical care across racial/ethnic groups. For instance, Hispanics have lower rates of diseases such as hypertension and arthritis than whites and higher rates of conditions such as diabetes. Blacks are more likely to require treatment for hypertension, cerebrovascular disease, diabetes, and obesity than whites and have persistently higher mortality rates.[12]

The increased demands on the health care system posed by population changes coupled with the problems of health care workforce supply portend serious staffing problems ahead. The growth in demand for nurses, nursing aides, various types of therapists, and aides in the acute-care sector and the relative unattractiveness of long-term facilities as employment sites for those service personnel have left many chronic-care facilities dangerously understaffed. At the moment, there are neither the funds available in the long-term care system to attract those difficult-to-recruit service personnel nor alternative plans for meeting the residential needs of the Medicaid-dependent older population.

The chronically ill who do not require placement in the long-term care facility also have problems with a health care system that retains its historical focus on acute illness or injury and those conditions that are amendable to remediation. The current system does not deal well with the aged chronically ill who present persistent symptoms, increasing disability, psychosocial sequelae, and difficult lifestyle adjustments. Although small gains have been made by managed care organizations addressing specific chronic conditions, effective chronic illness care would require a major change in health service priorities. Simply adding new geriatric services to a system focused on acute care does not solve the basic problem.[13]

In addition to the need to change organizational designs and services, obstacles to improving the care of the chronically ill also include changing the personal values and clinical behaviors of physicians, nurses, and other health professionals. Educated for and trained in acute-care facilities, it requires a major shift in mindset and practice behaviors for clinicians to accept the less dramatic, multidisciplinary nature of geriatric practice. As a result, health care reform as it relates to the chronically ill aged will be slow and will not keep pace with the more dramatic advances in other areas of clinical practice.

Changing Professional Labor Supply

Health care workers, other than physicians, have generally been ignored in the debates over health care policy and reforms. Nevertheless, the economic and other forces reducing the size and services of the hospital industry, shifting inpatient procedures to outpatient settings, and producing other organizational changes are likely to result in significant disruptions in the established employment practices of many classes of health care workers. Although the health care industry always will employ a significant portion of the U.S. workforce, the number and kinds of employees and the sites of their employment will be in transition during the next several years as the health care system adjusts itself.

Health economist Uwe E. Reinhardt lists several reasons that predicting the size or composition of the future health workforce is ill advised.[14] He points out that health care providers are exercising considerable flexibility in assigning tasks to the various health professions. He expects that staffing patterns of health institutions will be sensitive to the relative cost of different types of providers. In the quest for efficiency, Reinhardt expects a great deal of experimentation and variation in staffing patterns across health care systems and regions in the United States. In addition, scientific advances constantly provide new opportunities to substitute technology for human labor. Other technologic advances create needs for new types of health personnel. Under all of these disparate and evolving circumstances, it would be imprudent, indeed, to predict a future surplus or shortage for any type of health professional. It is likely, however, that whatever health care staffing patterns eventually result, the impact of health care reforms on the health care workforce will be considerable.

Physicians

Nothing has been more dramatic during health care reforms than the reduction in power, prestige, and independence of physician specialists. In the 1990s, managed care limitations on the number of specialists that could join their systems and on the frequency and circumstances of their use temporarily altered their positions in the health care hierarchy. In contrast, the demand for primary care practitioners increased as more people enrolled in managed care plans. There was a critical need for physicians who could provide primary care, serve as gatekeepers to limit access to more expensive specialists, and emphasize preventive medicine and health promotion. As the supply of primary care physicians increased and managed care organizations relaxed their more stringent restrictions on specialist care, however, the ratio of specialists to generalists began returning to its former levels.

Clearly, the predictions of the last 2 decades have not materialized. In contrast, current market indicators suggest that, rather than a surplus, a shortage of physicians will exist in major regions of the country.

In addition, less desirable practice locations such as inner city and rural areas continue to suffer from an undersupply of both primary care and specialty physicians. It is now apparent that those who believed that physician distribution problems would be solved by producing more physicians did not reckon with the ability of newly trained physicians to start up busy practices and earn satisfactory incomes in areas already well served.

In the absence of medical workforce policies or government intervention, market forces will continue to reconfigure the system on the basis of economic concerns, with little or no regard for considerations of quality or access. Quality and access are public and professional concerns, not market concerns, and are the issues that governments and health organizations should be addressing. Even in geographic areas where physicians are in adequate supply, too many individuals remain without access to medical care, and too many hospitals depend on graduates of foreign medical schools to provide essential inpatient services.

Major gaps in the availability of primary care physicians have been filled by substitution of NPs and PAs. In addition, the increasing popularity of chiropractors, acupuncturists, and other alternative practitioners reflects public dissatisfaction with the complexity and impersonal nature of today's medical care. The increasing number of substitutes for traditional medical practitioners presents a formidable problem for health policy planners that could have severe economic, public, and professional consequences. If nothing is done, the profession of medicine is likely to find itself competing with an ever-increasing array of nonphysician practitioners.[15]

New Physician Roles

Two relatively new roles have emerged for physicians in the changing health care system. The first is the hospitalist, who provides all of the care to the hospital inpatients of office-based physicians. Because these physicians are constantly in hospitals and are more familiar with their inner workings, they are considered to be more efficient and more capable of continually monitoring and managing inpatient care than are office-based physicians. More and more hospitals are employing hospitalists to gain the benefits of shorter lengths-of-stay, decreased complications, and increased patient satisfaction.

The second promising role for physicians is that of medical manager or administrator. Physicians, many with additional management or administration training, are entering the medical management area through employment in pharmaceutical companies, managed care organizations, hospitals, or large group practices. The demand for physicians with advanced training in management or administration is expected to increase as the corporatization of health care continues. At the same time, physicians, frustrated by the changes wrought in private practice by managed care, see health care administration as a highly regarded alternative to patient care.

Health Professions

As noted earlier, the health reforms taking place are being driven by market forces. Fiscal exigency is forcing reorganizing and restructuring of health care facilities and services. Addressing the social mission of health care is a completely different and far more demanding challenge to health care professionals. For providers to be socially responsive, they have to be broadly educated to identify and understand the needs and workings of society.

Roger J. Bulger, president of the Association of Academic Medical Centers, has urged a major reorientation of health professional education:[16]

> *Health professionals need to understand the anthropology of healing and the social meaning of the whole health enterprise, from primary through the most high-tech tertiary care. Forces have been unleashed over the last decade with which the health professions have collaborated, but which in my view have seriously eroded the public trust in the so-called serving health professions and seem to threaten the very foundations of these professions. Thus our students and faculties must become more sophisticated in their thinking about the nature and role of professions and the proper functions of the university in the post-modern, post-industrial society.*

A significant change in the philosophies of the health professions must occur before the U.S. health care system can understand and adopt a more community health-oriented, less disease-oriented mission and embrace a perspective that is oriented toward populations rather than individuals. The institutions and organizations of the health professions must mature beyond their conservative and self-protective policies and become more effective at leading rather than obstructing the inevitable system changes that will take place. The health professions must make a concerted effort to demonstrate to an increasingly skeptical public that they understand and are concerned about the need to provide more equitable financial access to health care for all. Providers can do much to restore the eroding public trust in the health care enterprise by showing a collective social responsiveness to the best interests of the public, as well as the professions. Clearly, clinicians must refocus from their narrow identification with a single profession or specialty to their obligations to the larger community. This means that health professionals must become more deeply involved with helping the political and other societal leaders work through the health policy issues at every level.

As long as health care providers see themselves as highly trained skilled experts in narrow technical fields that are part of a mosaic of narrow health care specialties, they will be unlikely to understand or be capable of applying a population perspective. Thus, only the most optimistic believe that current efforts to correct the imbalance between specialists and generalists and the primary care focus of managed care organizations will bring a new community focus and health promotion perspective to health care.

Nevertheless, the public perception of the health professions is changing. In the future, it will not be enough for health care providers to serve and comfort one individual at a time. An effort will have to be made to teach and exercise compassion for groups of people, which will have a beneficial impact on the public's health. The education of all health professionals should enhance their potential to address the problems of unequal access to competent care and promote accountability for the effectiveness of their therapies. By virtue of their elite position in society, health professionals are held to a higher standard of performance than the average wage earner. Health professionals will be expected to contribute to the public good and to perform their professional duties responsibly. They will be expected to bring their salient knowledge and problem-solving skills to bear on relevant social problems. In its highest expression, medicine and health care are a calling to public service irrespective of the patients' economic or political position. It is the exercise of that professional obligation for which health care providers are rewarded and from which their special status is derived.

Nurses

In many ways, nurses are the most qualified to respond to the changes that have occurred in the health system. Nurses' training focuses more on the behavioral and preventive aspects of health care than does physician education. Their skills are as relevant to outpatient care as they are to inpatient care. Nurses are important members of health care teams and have experience in managing lesser-trained caregivers. Nevertheless, the radical changes occurring in both the organization and delivery of health care are particularly disconcerting to the nursing profession. The financial pressures on acute-care hospitals and the major movements to managed care and integrated health care systems profoundly affected the over 2.2 million registered nurses who constitute the largest component of the health professions. Throughout the last decade, two thirds of all employed nurses were employed in hospitals.[17] Increased case-mix severity, decreased nurse–patient ratios, and delegation of traditional nursing duties to lesser-trained personnel have given hospital nurses reason to be concerned over the quality of patient care that has long been their responsibility. That this large proportion of the health care workforce is singularly vulnerable to the staff reductions that must accompany the declining admission and occupancy rates of acute-care hospitals is of major concern to nursing leaders and educators.

With mounting evidence that pervasive understaffing of hospital nurses is resulting in preventable complications and patient deaths, provider, public, and governmental pressures to improve the hospital nursing environment and give inpatient nurses reason to, once again, take pride and pleasure in their work are increasing. The number of entrants to schools of nursing is growing. More men are entering the field, and an influx of foreign-trained nurses is relieving some of the pressures.

Much will have to change, however, to improve the circumstances of hospital nursing. Excessive paperwork, inefficient communication systems, managerial responsibilities, and supervision of lesser-trained aides require an inordinate amount of time spent in functions other than providing direct patient care. Combined with long work hours and other difficulties, they contribute to low job satisfaction and frustrating work environments.

Nursing is of vital importance to hospitals, and hospitals need to improve their overall relationships with the nursing profession. The future ability of hospitals to serve the needs of the growing population of older patients, to improve the quality of care, and to serve the latest advances in medicine and its technology depends on an adequate workforce of well-prepared and competent nurses. Solving the multiple problems presented to nurses by hospitals in times of fiscal constraints will require strong commitment to quality improvement, work redesign, and building strong, respectful relationships between the hospital and its nurses. The future of both hospitals and the nursing profession depends on it.[18]

Nurse Practitioners and Physician Assistants

Nurse practitioners (NPs) and physician assistants (PAs), described in detail in Chapter 6, are in great demand and will be increasingly important in the provision of primary health care. Public satisfaction with the services provided by NPs and PAs is high, and demand for their services will continue as they fill niches where physician services are in short supply. Estimates suggest that there could be as many as 110,000 clinically active NPs and PAs in the next several years, representing one-sixth of the total U.S. medical providers.[19] It is realistic to expect that NPs and PAs, supported by effective practice guidelines and computerized treatment protocols, could become the patient's first point of entry into the health care system.[20]

The Future of America's Health Insurance Systems

For over 50 years, employer-sponsored health insurance protected the majority of Americans from overwhelming medical expenses. Although weakened by employer reluctance to absorb the increasing costs of health insurance premiums, the insurers themselves are enjoying a period of strong financial growth. Although there are increasing calls for expanding publicly sponsored programs, such expansions are more likely to benefit rather than harm commercial insurers. Most recently, the health insurance industry has gained by diversifying into Medicare and Medicaid. State and federal programs are increasingly outsourcing to commercial insurers the difficult tasks of managing care and dealing with taxpaying beneficiaries.[21] Clearly, whether it is employment-based or governmentally sponsored health insurance, the commercial insurers have managed to maintain their primary profit-making roles. Although they add significantly to the costs of America's annual health care bill, it would be unwise to predict that anything less than conversion to a single payer health care system will diminish the costly role of commercial health insurers.

Although physicians have always been vehemently opposed to what they call "universal health care," no one would be happier to see the demise of managed care insurers than physicians. Angered by ever more stringent cost-containment tactics that reduced their incomes and autonomy and subjected them to continuing disputes over service decisions, physicians have built public and legislative pressure to correct perceived abuses. In addition, many physicians have changed practice patterns in response to loss of income. They formed coalitions that increased their clout when contracting with managed care organizations and reduced the number of alternative sources of care with which managed care organizations could contract. "Any-willing-provider" laws, which require managed care organizations to open their networks to any physician who wants to join, also increased physician power.

Patients, too, are gaining more control in their relationships with physicians, hospitals, and insurers because of widespread dissemination of health information about alternative treatments and sources of care in the media and on the Internet. The result has been a more equitable balance of power among managed care organizations, physicians, and patients.[22]

Patients' Rights Legislation

Legislators at both the state and the federal level are showing a growing interest in protecting consumers from perceived or potential problems with managed care plans. At the same time, they are concerned with predictions that government involvement will cause managed care plans to increase premium costs and/or ration care. Because consumer protection legislation is generally opposed by a coalition of large employers and managed care organizations, production of a "Patients' Bill of Rights" has been stalled in the U.S. Congress.[23] Frustrated by years of congressional inaction, over 40 states have already passed their own version of a "Patients' Bill of Rights."

It is important to note that advocates of patients' rights legislation take the popular and persuasive position that such protections are necessary to "shift power . . . from managed-care companies, insurance companies, and health care facilities to patients and their physicians."[24] Because patients' rights legislation protects and empowers physicians as much as consumers, the American Medical Association is increasing the pressure on lawmakers to pass "real" rights legislation.

New Health Insurance Plans

There are at least three new types of health insurance that provide alternative insurance opportunities for employers, employees, and individuals alike. They are consumer-controlled health plans that involve both benefits and risks. Health savings accounts (HSAs) were created by the federal legislation that revised Medicare in 2003. It allows consumers to save pretax dollars for future medical expenses. First, however, HSAs require individuals to acquire a high-deductible insurance plan, at least $1,000 for individuals and $2,000 for families, to cover exceptional medical expenses. Then employers contribute a set amount, say $2,000, into a personal care account for each employee. Workers can then use that money any way they want for health care expenses. Any money that is unspent at the end of the year is carried over into their account for the next year. Self-employed individuals can establish the same plan by buying the high-deductible insurance and setting aside pretax dollars for medical expenses. Because the Internal Revenue Service allows unspent funds to be carried over into future years, it is possible for healthy individuals to accumulate thousands of dollars in their personal accounts. The unspent funds can also be used to purchase additional insurance policies to cover their deductibles.

Health reimbursement accounts are similar to HSAs in that they are also paired with high-deductible insurance; however, employees are not allowed to put their own funds into the plan, and employers may keep the money if an employee quits.

The third option is also similar to an HSA. It is a flexible spending account (FSA), which allows employees to set aside pretax dollars for medical expenses. Unlike an HSA, the money unspent in a flexible spending account expires at the end of the year.[25]

The new plans are expected to reduce medical expenses by providing a strong incentive for employees to avoid minor health care services and make more cost-effective medical decisions. Aware for the first time of the true costs of medical procedures, employees are expected to become wiser users of health care services.

Consumer-driven health insurance plans have not been in effect long enough to judge their effectiveness in controlling the costs of employer or employee health benefits or satisfaction with the method. Although the innovation has the potential of making a major change in the health insurance market, the response to date has been limited.

Changing Composition of the Delivery System

Hospitals, although still critically important to medical care, are no longer the hub of the health care system. Although occupancy rates for many facilities are improving, they have not returned to the levels of more than a decade ago, nor is an occupancy rebound likely to occur. The growing development of privately owned ambulatory surgery centers, diagnostic facilities, and now specialty hospitals has the potential to cause traditional acute-care hospitals to become a combination of high-level intensive care units and full-service facilities for those with more serious conditions, the uninsured, and the indigent. Regardless of excess hospital capacity, a variety of business, political, and social reasons will make hospital closings very difficult.[26] More importantly, almost all hospitals are now part of for-profit or not-for-profit corporate networks. Where many separate and competing hospitals once served a particular geographic area, now a somewhat smaller number of institutions divided among a few health care networks are meeting regional needs.

Given the many important relationships of hospitals with the other components of the health care system and the strong community support that most hospitals enjoy, it is unlikely that rapid change will occur in the rate of hospital closures. It will be much easier to close hospital beds and convert the space to other types of service. An increasing number of services can be provided by hospitals without using inpatient beds. One such development that hospitals are employing with great success is the use of subacute-care units to get around the diagnosis-related group cost controls. Instead of discharging patients when initial treatments are finished, hospitals are shifting those patients to newly developed subacute-care units where they receive skilled nursing and rehabilitative services. Thus, patients are better prepared to go home and hospitals collect an additional daily rate for their subacute care. Unfortunately, most hospital investments in new and more profitable services and associated marketing efforts will contribute to rising health care costs.

Corporate Growth in Health Care

In the last few years, stakeholders in health care have been scrambling to find the right template of size and service to remain competitive in the rapidly changing health care marketplace. The pervasive influence of managed care, the reductions in state and federal financial support, and the ever-increasing sophistication of health care technology have combined to offer remarkable opportunities to break away from outdated traditions and take venturesome risks.

The results have been disappointing. There is little evidence to date that many communities have benefited from the service efficiencies and improvements that institutional mergers and acquisitions were supposed to achieve. Rather, recent data suggest that such consolidations added market power and increased prices for hospitals, but did not translate into improved services or quality of care.[27]

With considerable success, the more entrepreneurial for-profit health care corporations have built their own integrated health service systems to improve their market positions. Unfortunately, experience has demonstrated that the introduction of large for-profit conglomerates into the health care arena increases the risk that corporate growth and profit will have higher priority among corporate executives than patient care and community service.[28]

This should not deter the not-for-profit sector from aggressively pursuing more contemporary business and service plans. To survive the health care reformation, voluntary hospital systems must free themselves from the cultural inertia that has made implementing lasting change so time-consuming and difficult and, instead, emulate those highly successful private sector companies that thrive on the flexibility to make strategic choices and redefine corporate goals in opportunistic ways. To cope with new challenges, voluntary hospitals will require the same clarity of purpose, flexibility, and determination to make strategic choices as for-profit companies do. They will need unequivocal plans that spell out the relative importance of competing priorities and guide decisions about personnel, resources, and service delivery. Those hospitals that become essential components of vertically integrated systems will take part in the future of health care. Those that do not will remain part of its past and eventually disappear.

Information Management

The growing numbers of new and efficient technologies for managing and transferring volumes of data allow providers and health plans to replace voluminous and often disorganized medical records with standardized, reliable, and clinically relevant information. Opportunities for transcription mistakes, misinterpretation of handwriting or medication orders, and other common errors of information transfer are minimized.

Although the technology for management of data, once collected, is at a high level of sophistication, there are serious obstacles to obtaining and assembling complete health information about individual patients. Because most patients obtain health care services from a number of providers and facilities, the information about their care is divided among the various settings and sites. The still unmet information management challenge is dealing with fragmentation of patient information, as those patients move through a disorganized treatment system.[29]

Originators of seamless health information systems that allow sharing of patient diagnostic, treatment, and outcome information face other problems as well. There are incredibly complex confidentiality, compatibility, and transferability issues that have challenged system designers for years. Nevertheless, the critical role of advanced information and communications technologies in evidenced-based assessments of clinical practice, physician report cards, clinical guidelines, patient education, and a large number of other uses is recognized by everyone concerned with the future of health care. As with other obstacles to health service advances, the growing need to solve those intrinsic system problems will drive information experts to develop acceptable solutions.

In the meantime, the importance of those health information technologies has alerted the business community to the promise of an emerging health information infrastructure. Although much of the current information system development has been the result of the academic medical researchers and developers, a number of private health information technology industries are already engaged in the building of the technical components of that hardware and software infrastructure. Other private companies are working on paperless solutions to recording and monitoring clinical procedures. It appears that the free-enterprise system is augmenting, if not supplanting, the years of information systems development by in-house designers employed by hospitals and academic institutions. Whether harmonious or competitive, it appears that the common interests of the clinical communities and the profit-motivated commercial sector will eventually result in a new era of health care information technology. It will be a giant step forward in advancing the efficacy, efficiency, and safety of medical care.[30]

Government's New Role in Public Health

The terrorist attack of September 11th was the stimulus for a national examination of the numerous, inconsistent, and outdated public health laws in the United States. Suddenly, the protection of the public's health in case of any one of a number of possible attacks became an immediate priority. Out of the crisis came the political and legislative will to ensure coordinated responses among federal, state, and local agencies in case of a public health emergency. The long overdue effort resulted in the drafting of the Model State Emergency Health Powers Act (MSEHPA). The act assists states in reviewing their emergency health powers and provides governors with the authority to declare a public health emergency and implement an adequate response. That response may involve the allocation of health resources and the implementation of actions to safeguard public health such as isolation and quarantine.[31]

In addition to addressing the basic public health functions of preparedness, disease surveillance, management of property, communication, and individual protection, the MSEHPA seeks to reconcile various antiquated and inconsistent public health statutes. Many were written before modern disease-prevention methods existed.[32]

The evident lack of public health preparedness at the time of the September 11th attack made it apparent that clear and effective communication with the public in crisis situations is an essential component of public health practice. The U.S. Department of Health and Human Services, Centers for Disease Control and Prevention responded by addressing the crisis preparedness education of health professionals and developing a more comprehensive information dissemination system for the public.[33]

It is a reflection of this country's health care priorities that it took a devastating terrorist attack to draw attention to the fact that the U.S. public health system is poorly funded, fragmented, and ill-prepared to provide an effective health defense system—even when the routine public health functions of offering credible health information, safeguarding air quality, protecting and educating workers, and ensuring food safety were basic elements of the called-for response. If anything positive results from the ill-fated September 11th experience, it will be that the public of the future will have public health safeguards appropriate to the latest high-technology health care expertise.

The long accepted, but often unfulfilled, core functions of regional and local public health agencies now must be enhanced with a broad array of protections and services. Achievement of those new responsibilities, however, will require a major restructuring of local and regional resources, procedures, staffing, and communication systems. New and more forceful leadership, effective planning, communication, working relationships among different levels of government, and adequate resource allocations will be basic to meeting threats to the public's health in times of crisis.

Whether the system will reform itself to create a vibrant public health structure capable of meeting new demands while serving traditional needs is still an open question. The importance of the outcome, however, in case of potential disasters, should not be underestimated.[34]

Conclusion

The period from 1990 to 2006 marked a major reformation in the U.S. health care system. The social and economic changes affecting society during that period altered public perceptions and expectations of health care and prepared Americans for sweeping reforms in both the organization and delivery of health care services. Although tensions exist between the advocates of major and immediate system revisions and those who prefer more limited, incremental changes, all agree that the health care industry is in a period of unprecedented instability and transition.

Although concerns about costs are prompting new examinations of the allocation of resources and the assignments of health personnel, there also are new perspectives on the value and quality of health care services. There are strong pressures on providers to analyze and document the outcomes and effectiveness of their health care interventions.[35]

The continuing presence of over 46 million uninsured Americans reflects the nation's reluctance to decide whether the federal government should assure health coverage for all its citizens or only fill the gaps for those without the means to obtain their own. Other nations have long considered health care a right of citizenship and provide the subsidies necessary to give everyone reasonable access to basic care.

Repeatedly in the history of health care in the United States, however, the public has been persuaded to instruct its representatives that health care is a "good" that should be supplied privately with as few exceptions as possible. That the system costs more and has large gaps, illogical redundancies, and inexplicable variations in quality and access is countered by the prevailing belief that its scientific and technologic superiority makes up for its deficiencies.

The need for industry restructuring to remedy the deficiencies in the health care system, however, is the overriding concern of those who believe the United States should develop a more socially responsible system of health care and end its embarrassing distinction as the only Western democracy that permits a sizable percentage of its population to live without health insurance coverage. Given that health care in the United States evolved out of the professional and economic objectives of providers rather than consumer needs and has been financed by a convoluted system of private insurance augmented by inadequately managed and inflationary public sector programs, it is not surprising that the resulting system is characterized by escalating costs and glaring gaps in coverage. Clearly, the problems cannot be solved satisfactorily without major structural revisions.[36]

Physicians, who historically have been rewarded generously for their work, are already distressed and will be increasingly frustrated by being forced to participate in systems they believe violate their professional prerogatives. To them, their changing role signifies the decline of medicine as a profession. The autonomy that physicians enjoyed in their work and the feeling that their profession constituted a special brotherhood devoted to a higher purpose are diminished. Physicians now see themselves more as workers in the health service machine rather than occupants of a lofty position in society.[37]

Patients, too, have changed. Keenly aware of the variability in the quality of care, they no longer consider medicine as a kind of mystical art that only physicians and nurses can understand. Patients now educate themselves on health matters, increasingly challenge medical decisions, and turn to alternative providers and treatments if they are dissatisfied with their care. The Internet and other medical information sources have empowered patients and are rapidly turning them into educated consumers. As such, their dissatisfactions with health care can no longer be ignored by either health care providers or governments.

To summarize, the basic questions facing the stakeholders in the health care industry today are as follows:

- What is society's obligation to ensure access to a basic level of health care for all its citizens, and how can this be accomplished?
- How can an acceptable quality of health care be ensured?
- How can the costs of health care be kept affordable for both individuals and society?
- How can the ethical dilemmas produced by technologic advances and limited resources be resolved?

The idealized solutions to the problems of huge variations in costs, treatments, and outcomes; fragmented services; episodic treatment of illness; and badly distributed overcapacity all have general support as concepts but engender opposing views on how to resolve them. Among the most frequently voiced suggestions are these:

- Alter the health care focus from diagnosing and treating illness to maintaining wellness and preventing illness.

- Expand the health care system's accountability from the health status of individual patients to that of defined populations.
- Change the health services' emphasis from acute episodic care to continuous comprehensive care and chronic disease management.
- Eliminate the financial incentives to provide more services and fill hospital beds, and substitute incentives to provide appropriate care at an appropriate level.
- Assume universal access to health care.
- Change from merely coordinating the delivery of services to actively managing the quality of processes and outcomes.
- Add a serious commitment to the resolution of community and public health issues.

Current trends suggest that the future of health care in the United States will include more reforms at the state level. As individual state experiments show positive results, other states will adopt the changes. Many of those state reforms will support the expansion of managed care. That support, however, will be contingent on a series of patient protection standards that hold managed care organizations responsible for faulty decisions. The ability of managed care organizations to contain costs by limiting expensive and discretionary specialist use and by exercising cost-based oversight of ineffective or marginally beneficial interventions is tremendously attractive to states and other purchasers of health care.

The managed care backlash, however, has made patients more aggressive and less trusting. The wide publicity given to the Institute of Medicine's report on the frequency of medical errors has increased public concerns about patient safety in medical environments. Managed care disputes with physicians over reimbursement for certain procedures have created doubts about the appropriateness of those procedures. Access to ubiquitous medical information on the Internet has given the public a better understanding of the breadth of choice faced by physicians in making clinical judgments and medical decisions. These factors combined with the increasing costs of health care are, once again, producing a surge of interest in increased governmental involvement in health care reforms.

Health care reforms can make the systems of care different, but they cannot make the care better. Only the providers working in concert with supportive systems can improve health care outcomes. Freed from many of the disincentives of fee-for-service medicine, providers may emphasize wellness and prevention and reduce unnecessary interventions. They may become as effective in improving the health status of entire populations as they have for patients they formerly treated on an individual basis.

It is anticipated that the public and purchasers will be aided in choosing from among competing providers and managed care plans by having access to a great deal of timely performance information. Unlike the selective secrecy that has characterized health care in the past, it is expected that future health care organizations will be required to provide annual quality performance "report cards" for public and purchaser scrutiny. Some institutions and managed care organizations already produce these.

Hospitals face a harsh short-term future. Unrelenting economic pressures in the face of reduced occupancy rates will undoubtedly result in a significant number of closings, and those that survive will be different institutions from those that presently exist. Hospitals are likely to be just one component of a vertically integrated system of care that includes long-term as well as ambulatory care and a variety of community-based services. Because many of the acute-care services will be provided in ambulatory settings, the major role of hospitals probably will be in the provision of intensive patient care and, perhaps, the diagnosis and management of the chronically ill.

The relationship of hospitals to physicians will take on increasing importance as the old assumptions about medical care and surgery continue to undergo profound change. The future of hospitals depends on the future of medicine. The future of medicine is grounded in the scientists and clinicians developing the cutting-edge advances in medicine and surgery. Thus, it behooves hospitals to convene and respond to those whose combined expertise and judgment can formulate solutions to deficits in quality and patient satisfaction and can anticipate the service modalities of the future.

The changing demographics in the United States will compel a major expansion of long-term care facilities and services. Long-term care will become an increasingly complex array of services integrated into vertical systems. Of all the problems facing the future health care system, the aging of the population, with its attendant burden of chronic disease and disability, presents the most formidable organizational and economic challenge. Needless to say, those facilities and services striving mightily to survive the more immediate challenges have yet to develop longer range plans to cope with that future inevitability.

The growing demand for support of chronic care is likely to force a major change in the structure and financing of health care in the United States. Unlike the acute-care system, chronic care is unplanned and often insensitive to desperate situations. For example, regardless of type, the insurance coverage for the extraordinary care provided in a hospital to save a life often abruptly ceases when the patient is brought home. Although essential patient services such as feeding, bathing, transferring from bed to wheelchair, and preventing bedsores are considered "medically necessary" when provided by skilled nurses in institutions, those same services are dismissed as "custodial care" when delivered at home.

As more and more middle-aged Americans find themselves faced with the care of aged and functionally limited relatives, the demand for expanded support of chronic care services will increase. Public awareness of the deficiencies of the current system will grow and bring considerable pressure for change in public and private financing mechanisms.

People with chronic conditions already consume almost 70% of the nation's expenditures on personal care, mostly for physician and hospital services, a reflection of the system's focus on acute incidents.[38] Clearly, there is a monumental challenge in this era of severe economic constraint to create and finance a chronic care system that meets social as well as medical needs. Until that can be accomplished, the aged and chronically ill and their caregivers will be required to meet their home care, transportation, social support, and other needs however they can.

Although the health care system itself is in turmoil, the sciences within health care are making extraordinary progress. Medical technology is a major driver of the health care system, and the system quickly absorbs new devices and pharmaceuticals. Just as clinicians and researchers embraced the use of new imaging techniques, so too will they adopt new devices for minimally invasive surgery, gene mapping and therapy, new vaccines, artificial blood, and other advances that will transform the practice of medicine.

These dramatic advances, however, will be accompanied by new and vexing problems of cost, accessibility, inadequate training, and professional ethics. Practicing physicians are already overwhelmed with the profusion of new knowledge. Currently, there are 10 million citations on the computerized scientific literature resource, Medline, and 3,000 more are added to the popular bibliographic database each month. The availability of new knowledge also vastly exceeds the capacity of the institutions that deliver and finance health care to access and use it. It is difficult for these hierarchical organizations to respond to past problems, much less adapt to new developments. The fact that thousands of deaths were reported to occur each year as a result of medical errors in hospitals and that neither the public nor the health care community seemed aware of the magnitude of the problem is a reflection of the size, complexity, and disorder that characterizes the system. Compare that fact with the response to a single airplane crash, after which every fragment of evidence is collected to determine the cause and prevent its reoccurrence.

The enormous potential for good that the U.S. health care system enjoys comes with deep concerns. How will the recipients of new technology be chosen? Who will address the ethical dilemmas that lie behind the ability to genetically alter human beings? When will the need to set stricter standards of competence when people's lives are at stake be faced by the medical profession? When will the government rein in the unlimited profits of pharmaceutical firms that price their drugs beyond the means of those who need them the most? These and similar issues are central to a constructive reformation of the U.S. health care system.

The public and the stakeholders in the health care system have expressed a generalized dissatisfaction with the manner in which health care has been delivered—the inexplicable variation in how patients are treated, the resultant costs, and the increasing number of people without access to at least a minimum level of basic care. Similar dissatisfaction exists among health care providers, but for quite different reasons. Although the causes of the problem are easily identifiable, they do not lend themselves to simple, uncomplicated solutions. Experience has demonstrated that changes in public policy that threaten U.S. commitment to social diversity and the preservation of individual autonomy inevitably fail. The vested interests in the traditional modes of health care delivery have repeatedly demonstrated their ability to generate political opposition to serious legislative challenges to the health care status quo. On the other hand, those same interests, including the powerful health care political lobbies, seem ineffectual in the face of apparently overwhelming market forces. Rather than change occurring as a result of public policy, economic forces are driving a combative health care system reformation that is altering the roles of many traditional health care institutions. The end result, however, is expected to be a more comprehensive, coordinated, and cost-efficient system.

These are exciting times for students of health care. Never has so large a change in so important an industry so intimately affected so many people. It is a time for introspection regarding one's values, circumspection regarding one's advocacy for any one position, and careful inspection of any experimental changes that come about. Will the health care reforms now in progress resolve or worsen the key issues of access, costs, and quality? Can we possibly achieve an ideal health policy scenario, such as that proposed by Stephen Shortell et al., in which there is fiscal and clinical accountability for defined populations, resources allocated according to a region's consumer needs, and up-front negotiations among all relevant parties about what services will be delivered to what people at what price?[39] Only time and skilled leadership will tell.

References

1. Gleick J. Chaos: Making a New Science. In: Sifonis JG, Goldberg B, eds. *Corporation on a Tightrope: Balancing Leadership, Governance, and Technology in an Age of Complexity.* New York, NY: Viking; 1987:1–19.
2. Shortell SM, Reinhardt UE. Creating and executing health policy in the 1990s. In Shortell SH, Reinhardt UE, eds. *Improving Health Policy and Management: Nine Critical Research Issues for the 1990s.* Ann Arbor, MI: Health Administration Press; 1992:5–6.
3. Available from http://www.census.gov/Press.Release/www/releases/archives/income-wealth/002484.html. Accessed January 12, 2005.
4. Hadley J, Holahan J. How much medical care do the uninsured use, and who pays for it? *Health Affairs.* 2003;22:23.
5. Millenson ML. The silence. *Health Affairs.* 2003;22:103–112.
6. Clancy CM, Scully T. A call to excellence. *Health Affairs.* 2003;22:113–115.
7. Institute for Healthcare Improvement. Available from http://www.ihi.org/ihi/aboutus/people.aspx. Accessed December 6, 2006.
8. Hefler S, Smith S, Won G, et al. Health spending projections for 2001–2011: The latest outlook. *Health Affairs.* 2002;21:207–218.
9. *The Comparative Performance of U.S. Hospitals: The Sourcebook, 1996.* Baltimore, MD: Health Care Industry Analysts, Inc; Chicago, IL: Deloitte and Touche; 1996:25.
10. Kent DL, Haynor DR, Longstreth WT, et al. The clinical efficacy of magnetic resonance imaging. *Ann Int Med.* 1994;120:856–875.
11. Starfield B. U.S. child health: what's amiss, and what should be done about it? *Health Affairs.* 2004;23:165–170.

12. Wolf DA. Population change: friend or foe of the chronic care system? *Health Affairs*. 2001;20:64–78.

13. Wagner EH, Austin BT, Davis C, et al. Improving chronic illness care: translating evidence into action. *Health Affairs*. 2001;20:28–42.

14. Reinhardt UE. The economic and moral case for letting the market determine the health workforce. In: Osterweis M, et al., eds. *The U.S. Health Workforce: Power, Politics, and Policy*. Washington, DC: Association of Academic Health Centers; 1996:3–13.

15. Cooper RA, Getzen TE, McKee HJ, Laud P. Economic and demographic trends signal an impending physician shortage. *Health Affairs*. 2002;21:140–154.

16. Bulger RJ. If a rose is a rose, then what is an academic health center? Paper presented at Millard Fillmore Hospitals' Annual Vital Issues in Health Care Symposium, April 18, 1991; Buffalo, NY.

17. Aiken LH, Buchan J, Sochalski J, et al. Trends in international nurse migration. *Health Affairs*. 2004;23: 69–77.

18. Buerhaus P, Needleman J, Mattke S, et al. Strengthening hospital nursing. *Hosp Affairs*. 2002;21:123–132.

19. Hooker RS, Berlin LE. Trends in the supply of physician assistants and nurse practitioners in the United States. *Health Affairs*. 2002;21:174–180.

20. Amara R, Bodenhorn K, Cain M, et al. Health and healthcare 2010: the forecast, the challenge. In: Engehart JK, ed. *The Institute for the Future* 15, no. 2. San Francisco, CA: Jossey-Bass Publishers; 2000:73–84.

21. Robinson JC. The commercial health insurance industry in an era of eroding employer coverage. *Health Affairs*. 2006;25:1475–1486.

22. Grembowski DE, Cook KS, Patrick DL, et al. Managed care and the U.S. health care system: a social exchange perspective. *Social Sci Med*. 2002; 54:1167–1180.

23. Aston G. Employers oppose house bill creating federal standards for managed care plans. *Am Med News*. 1997;3–4.

24. Annas GJ. A national bill of patients' rights. *N Engl J Med*. 1998;338:695–699.

25. Rubenstein S. Employers lag in offering policies health savings accounts require. *Wall Street Journal*. January 12, 2005:D4.

26. Draper DA, Hurle RE, Lesser CS, et al. The changing face of managed care. *Health Affairs*. 2002;21(1):11–23.

27. Cuellar AE, Gertler PJ. How the expansion of hospital systems has affected consumers. *Health Affairs*. 2005;24:213–219.

28. HCA Sews Up Fraud Lawsuit for $95.3M. *Nashville Business Journal*. December 14, 2000. Available from http://nashville.bizjournals.com/Nashville/stories/2000/12/11/dail. Accessed August 29, 2002.

29. Kleinke JD. Clinical information technology in the real world. *Health Affairs*. 1998;17:23–38.

30. Bell DS, Marken RS, Meili RC, et al. Rand electronic prescribing expert advisory panel. *Health Affairs*. 2004:305–317.

31. Department of Health and Human Services, Centers for Disease Control and Prevention, Public Health Guidance for Community Level Preparedness and Response to Acute Respiratory Syndrome, Version 2 (June 8, 2004). Available at www.publichealthlaw.net/MSEHPA/MSEHPA2.pdf. Accessed December 10, 2004.

32. Matthews JW. Legal preparedness for bioterrorism. *J Legal Med Ethics*. 2002; 30:52–53.

33. Parvanta CF, Freimuth V. Health communication at the Centers for Disease Control and Prevention. *Am J Health Behav*. 2000;24:337–347.

34. Salinsky E, Garsky EA. The case for transforming governmental public health. *Health Affairs*. 2006;25:1017–1028.

35. Gelijns AC, Brown LD, Magnell C, et al. Evidence, politics, and technological change. *Health Affairs*. 2005;24:29–40.

36. Haislmaier E. A cure for the health care crisis. *Issues Sci Technol*. 1990; 6:59–63.

37. Dworkin RW. The cultural revolution in health care, the public interest. *Nat Affairs*. 2000;35–49.

38. Hoffman C, Rice D, Sung HY, et al. Persons with chronic conditions, their prevalence and costs. *JAMA*. 1996;276:1473–1479.

39. Shortell SM, Morrison EM, Friedman B, et al. *Strategic Choices for America's Hospitals: Managing Change in Turbulent Times*. San Francisco, CA: Jossey-Bass Publishers; 1990:301–327.

Abbreviations and Acronyms

AACN	American Association of Colleges of Nursing
AAFP	American Academy of Family Physicians
AAMC	Association of American Medical Colleges
AAN	American Academy of Nursing
AARP	American Association of Retired Persons
ACEHSA	Accrediting Commission on Education for Health Services Administrators
ACF	Administration on Children and Families
ACGME	Accreditation Council for Graduate Medical Education
ACHE	American College of Healthcare Executives
ACP	American College of Physicians
ACR	Advanced Certified Rolfer
ACS	American College of Surgeons
ACYF	Administration for Children, Youth, and Families
ADAMHA	Alcohol, Drug Abuse, and Mental Health Administration
ADD	Administration on Developmental Disabilities
ADLs	Activities of Daily Living

AFDC	Aid to Families with Dependent Children
AFL-CIO	American Federation of Labor and Congress of Industrial Organization
AHA	American Hospital Association
AHC	Academic Health Center
AHCPR	Agency for Health Care Policy and Research (formerly Agency for Healthcare Research and Quality)
AHP	Accountable Health Plan
AHRQ	Agency for Healthcare Research and Quality (formerly Agency for Health Care Policy and Research)
AHSR	Association for Health Services Research (formerly Academy for Health Services Research and Health Policy)
AID	U.S. Agency for International Development
AIDS	Acquired Immune Deficiency Syndrome
ALOS	Average Length of Stay
AMA	American Medical Association
AMC	Academic Medical Center
ANA	Administration for Native Americans; American Nurses Association
AoA	Administration on Aging
APA	American Psychiatric Association; American Psychological Association
APEX/PH	Assessment Protocol for Excellence in Public Health
APHA	American Public Health Association
APTA	American Physical Therapy Association
ASAHP	Association of Schools of Allied Health Professions
ASH	Assistant Secretary for Health

ASHED	AIDS School Health Education Database
ASHP	Adolescent and School Health Programs
ASIM	American Society of Internal Medicine
ASSIST	American Stop Smoking Intervention Study
ASTHO	Association of State and Territorial Health Officials
ATF	Bureau of Alcohol, Tobacco, and Firearms
ATSDR	Agency for Toxic Substances and Disease Registry
AUPHA	Association of University Programs in Health Administration
BAC	Blood Alcohol Concentration
BBA	Balanced Budget Act of 1997
BC/BS	Blue Cross and Blue Shield
BCHS	Bureau of Community Health Services
BHP	Bureau of Health Professions
BHRD	Bureau of Health Resources Development
BIA	Bureau of Indian Affairs
BLS	Bureau of Labor Statistics
BPHC	Bureau of Primary Health Care
BRFSS	Behavioral Risk Factor Surveillance System
CAH	Critical Access Hospital
CAM	Complementary and Alternative Medicine
CAT	Computerized Axial Tomography (scanner)
CBER	Center for Biologics Evaluation and Research
CCN	Community Care Network; Critical Care Nurse
CCRC	Continuing Care Retirement Community
CDC	Centers for Disease Control and Prevention
CDER	Center for Drug Evaluation and Research

CDF	Children's Defense Fund
CDRH	Center for Devices and Radiological Health
CEO	Chief Executive Officer
CEU	Continuing Education Unit
CFO	Chief Financial Officer
CFSAN	Center for Food Safety and Applied Nutrition
CHAMPUS	Civilian Health and Medical Program of the Uniformed Services
CHAP	Child Health Assurance Program
CHC	Community Health Center
CHID	Combined Health Information Database
CHP	Comprehensive Health Planning
CME	Continuing Medical Education
CMHC	Community Mental Health Center
CMMS	Center for Medicare and Medicaid Services (formerly HCFA, the Health Care Financing Administration)
COBRA	Consolidated Budget Reconciliation Act
COGME	Council on Graduate Medical Education
CON	Certificate of Need
CPI	Consumer Price Index
CPR	Customary, Prevailing, and Reasonable (fees)
CPSC	Consumer Product Safety Commission
CPT	Current Procedure Terminology
CPT-4	Current Procedural Terminology, 4th edition
CQI	Continuous Quality Improvement
CRCC	Commission on Rehabilitation Counselor Certification
CT	Computed Tomography

CTP	Certified Trager Practitioner
CVM	Center for Veterinary Medicine
DC	Doctor of Chiropractic
DHEW	Department of Health, Education, and Welfare
DHHS	Department of Health and Human Services
DME	Durable Medical Equipment
DNR	Do Not Resuscitate
DNS/DNSc	Doctor of Nursing Science
DO	Doctor of Osteopathy
DOE	Department of Education
DOI	Department of Interior
DOJ	Department of Justice
DOL	Department of Labor
DOT	Department of Transportation
DRG	Diagnosis-Related Group
DVA	Department of Veterans Affairs
EACH	Essential Access Community Hospital
EAP	Employee Assistance Program
ECA	Epidemiologic Catchment Area
ECF	Extended Care Facility
EMS	Emergency Medical Services
EPA	Environmental Protection Agency
EPO	Epidemiology Program Office
EPSDT	Early and Periodic Screening, Diagnosis, and Treatment
ER	Emergency Room
ERISA	Employee Retirement Income Security Act

ESRD	End-Stage Renal Disease
FAHS	Federation of American Health Systems
FAS	Fetal Alcohol Syndrome
FDA	Food and Drug Administration
FDIR	Food Distribution Program on Indian Reservations
FEHBP	Federal Employee Health Benefits Program
FEMA	Federal Emergency Management Association
FFS	Fee for Service
FHSR	Foundation for Health Services Research
FHWA	Federal Highway Administration
FIC	Fogarty International Center
FMG	Foreign Medical Graduate
FNS	Food and Nutrition Service
FQHC	Federally Qualified Health Center
FSAs	Flexible Spending Accounts
FTC	Federal Trade Commission
FTE	Full-Time Equivalent
FY	Fiscal Year
GDP	Gross Domestic Product
GHAA	Group Health Association of America
GHC	Group Health Cooperative
GHI	Group Health Insurance
GME	Graduate Medical Education
GMENAC	Graduate Medical Education National Advisory Committee
GNP	Gross National Product
HACCP	Hazard Analysis Critical Control Point

HANES	Health and Nutrition Examination Survey
HBCU	Historically Black Colleges and Universities
HBV	Hepatitis B Virus
HCA	Hospital Corporation of America
HCFA	Health Care Financing Administration
HCV	Hepatitis C Virus
HDL	High-Density Lipoprotein Cholesterol
HEDIS	Health Plan Employer Data and Information Set
HETC	Health Education and Training Center
HEW	Health, Education, and Welfare
HHS	Health and Human Services (Department of)
HIAA	Health Insurance Association of America
HIP	Health Insurance Plan
HIPPA	Health Insurance Portability and Accountability Act
HIS	Health Interview Survey
HIV	Human Immunodeficiency Virus
HMO	Health Maintenance Organization
HNIS	Human Nutrition and Information Service
HPDP	Health Promotion and Disease Prevention
HPEAA	Health Professions Educational Assistance Act
HRA	Health Resources Administration
HRAs	Health Reimbursement Accounts
HRQL	Health-Related Quality of Life
HRSA	Health Resources and Services Administration
HSA	Health Systems Agency
HSAs	Health Savings Accounts

HTPCP	Healthy Tomorrows Partnership for Children Program
HUD	Department of Housing and Urban Development
IADLs	Instrumental Activities of Daily Life
ICD	International Classification of Diseases
ICD-9-CM	*International Classification of Diseases,* 9th Revision, Clinical Modification
ICU	Intensive Care Unit
IDDM	Insulin-Dependent Diabetes Mellitus
IHPO	International Health Program Office
IHS	Indian Health Service
IMGs	International Medical Graduates
IMR	Infant Mortality Rate
INPHO	Information Network for Public Health Officials
IOM	Institute of Medicine
IPA	Individual Practice Association
IPN	Integrated Provider Network
IPO	Independent Practitioner Organization
Joint Commission	Joint Commission on Accreditation of Healthcare Organizations
LCME	Liaison Committee on Medical Education
LDL	Low-Density Lipoprotein Cholesterol
LIHEAP	Low-Income Home Energy Assistance Program
LOS	Length of Stay
LPN	Licensed Practical Nurse
LTC	Long-Term Care
MBHCC	Managed Behavioral Health Care Company

MCHB	Maternal and Child Health Bureau
MCN	Migrant Clinicians Network
MCO	Managed Care Organization
MD	Medical Doctor
MDC	Major Diagnostic Category
MDS	Minimum Data Set
MEDLARS	Medical Literature Analysis and Retrieval System
MEDTEP	Medical Treatment Effectiveness Program
MEHP	Minority Environmental Health Program
MHTS	Minority Health Tracking System
MLP	Midlevel Practitioner
MRI	Magnetic Resonance Imaging
MSA	Metropolitan Statistical Area; Medical Savings Account
MSEHP	Model State Emergency Health Powers Act
MSHA	Mine Safety and Health Administration
MSO	Management Services Organization
MVP	Medicare Volume Performance
NACAA	National Association of Consumer Agency Administrators
NACHM	National Advisory Commission on Health Manpower
NACHO	National Association of County Health Officials
NAHC	National Association for Home Care
NAIEP	National AIDS Information and Education Program
NAM	National Association of Manufacturers
NAMCS	National Ambulatory Care Survey

NAMHC	National Advisory Mental Health Council
NAMI	National Alliance for the Mentally Ill
NAPO	National AIDS Program Office
NCADI	National Clearinghouse for Alcohol and Drug Information
NCAI	National Congress of American Indians
NCCAN	National Center on Child Abuse and Neglect
NCCDPHP	National Center for Chronic Disease Prevention and Health Promotion
NCEH	National Center for Environmental Health
NCHGR	National Center for Human Genome Research
NCHS	National Center for Health Statistics
NCHSR	National Center for Health Services Research
NCI	National Cancer Institute
NCID	National Center for Infectious Diseases
NCIPC	National Center for Injury Prevention and Control
NCPIE	National Council on Patient Information and Education
NCPS	National Center for Prevention Services
NCQA	National Committee on Quality Assurance
NCRR	National Center for Research Resources
NCTR	National Center for Toxological Research
ND	Doctor of Naturopathy; Doctor of Nursing
NEI	National Eye Institute
NF	Nursing Facility
NHDS	National Hospital Discharge Survey
NHE	National Health Expenditures

NHIC	National Health Information Center
NHIS	National Health Interview Survey
NHLBI	National Heart, Lung, and Blood Institute
NHSC	National Health Service Corps
NIA	National Institute on Aging
NIAAA	National Institute on Alcohol Abuse and Alcoholism
NIAID	National Institute of Allergy and Infectious Diseases
NIAMS	National Institute of Arthritis and Musculoskeletal and Skin Diseases
NICHD	National Institute of Child Health and Human Development
NIDA	National Institute on Drug Abuse
NIDCD	National Institute on Deafness and Other Communication Disorders
NIDDK	National Institute of Diabetes and Digestive and Kidney Diseases
NIDR	National Institute of Dental Research
NIDRR	National Institute on Disability and Rehabilitation Research
NIEHS	National Institute of Environmental Health Sciences
NIGMS	National Institute of General Medical Sciences
NIH	National Institutes of Health
NIMH	National Institute of Mental Health
NINDS	National Institute of Neurological Disorders and Stroke
NINR	National Institute of Nursing Research

NIOSH	National Institute of Occupational Safety and Health
NLM	National Library of Medicine
NLN	National League for Nursing
NLTN	National Laboratory Training Network
NMIHS	National Maternal and Infant Health Survey
NMR	Nuclear Magnetic Resonance
NQF	National Quality Forum
NVSS	National Vital Statistics System
OAM	Office of Alternative Medicine
OASIS	Outcomes and Assessment Information Set
OBRA	Omnibus Budget Reconciliation Act
OCS	Office of Community Services
OCSE	Office of Child Support Enforcement
ODPHP	Office of Disease Prevention and Health Promotion
OECD	Organization of Economic Development
OEO	Office of Economic Opportunity
OFA	Office of Family Assistance
OHTA	Office of Health Technology Assessment
OIH	Office of International Health
OMB	Office of Management and Budget
OMH	Office of Minority Health
ORHP	Office of Rural Health Policy
ORT	Operation Restore Trust
OSH	Office of Smoking and Health
OSHA	Occupational Safety and Health Administration
OT	Occupational Therapy

OTA	Office of Technology Assessment
OWH	Office on Women's Health
PA	Physician Assistant
PAC	Political Action Committee
PACE	Program of All-Inclusive Care for the Elderly
PAR	Preadmission Review
PCP	Primary Care Provider; Primary Care Physician
PET	Positron Emission Tomography
PGP	Prepaid Group Practice
PharmD	Doctor of Pharmacy
PHO	Physician–Hospital Organization
PHP	Prepaid Health Plan
PHS	Public Health Service
PIRC	Preventative Intervention Research Center
PMPM	Per Member Per Month
PMPY	Per Member Per Year
POE	Point of Enrollment
PORT	Patient Outcomes Research Team
POS	Point of Service
PPA	Preferred Provider Arrangement
PPCM	Primary Care Case Management
PPHA	Pennsylvania Public Health Association
PPO	Preferred Provider Organization
PPRC	Physician Payment Review Commission
PPS	Prospective Payment System
PRO	Peer Review Organization

ProPAC	Prospective Payment Assessment Commission
PSO	Provider Service Organization; Provider-Sponsored Organization
PSQ	Patient Satisfaction Questionnaire
PSRO	Professional Standards Review Organization
PT	Physical Therapy
PTMPY	Per Thousand Members Per Year
QA	Quality Assurance
RAPs	Radiologists, Anesthesiologists, and Pathologists
RBRVS	Resource-Based Relative Value Scale
RMP	Regional Medical Program
RN	Registered Nurse
RPCH	Rural Primary Care Hospital
RPP	Registered Polarity Practitioner
RRA	Registered Records Administrator
RRC	Residency Review Committee
RSPA	Research and Special Programs Administration
RUG	Resource Utilization Group
RVS	Relative Value Scale
RVUs	Relative Value Units
SAMHSA	Substance Abuse and Mental Health Services Administration
SCHIP	State Children's Health Insurance Program
SEIU	Service Employees International Union
SHMO	Social Health Maintenance Organization
SMI	Supplemental Medical Insurance
SNF	Skilled Nursing Facility

SSA	Social Security Administration
SSI	Supplemental Security Income
STD	Sexually Transmitted Disease
TEFRA	Tax Equity and Fiscal Responsibility Act
Title XVIII	Medicare
Title XIX	Medicaid
TPA	Third-Party Administrator
TPN	Total Parenteral Nutrition
TQM	Total Quality Management
UCR	Usual, Customary, and Reasonable Reimbursement
UR	Utilization Review
USDHEW	United States Department of Health, Education, and Welfare
USDHHS	United States Department of Health and Human Services
USFMG	United States Foreign Medical Graduate
USPHS	United States Public Health Service
VA	Veterans Administration; Department of Veterans Affairs
VNA	Visiting Nurses Association
WHO	World Health Organization
WIC	Special Supplemental Food Program for Women, Infants, and Children

Websites

U.S. Government

Agency for Healthcare Research and Quality: www.ahrq.gov.

Centers for Medicare and Medicaid Services: www.medicare.gov.

Department of Health and Human Services: www.HHS.gov.

Department of Veterans Affairs, Veterans Health Administration: http://www.va/gov/health_benefits.

National Center for Complementary and Alternative Medicine: http://www.nccam.nih.gov.

National Center for Health Statistics: http://www.cdc.gov/nchs.

National Guideline Clearinghouse: www.guideline.gov.

National Institutes of Health: www.nih.gov.

National Library of Medicine: http://clinicaltrials.gov and http://www.nlm.nih.gov/medlineplus.

Office of Disease Prevention and Health Promotion: www.healthfinder.gov.

State Children's Health Insurance Program: http://cms.hhs.gov/schip.

U.S. Administration on Aging: http://www.aoa.dhhs.gov.

U.S. Centers for Disease Control and Prevention: http://www.cdc.gov.

U.S. Congressional Budget Office: http://www.cbo.gov.

U.S. Department of Health and Human Services: http://www.hhs.gov.

U.S. Department of Labor, Bureau of Labor Statistics: http://stats.bls.gov.

U.S. Food and Drug Administration: http://www.fda.gov.

Other Organizations

Alliance for Quality Health Care: www.nyhealthfinder.com.

American Academy of Family Physicians: www.familydoctor.org.

American Accreditation Healthcare Commission: www.urac.org.

American Association of Health Plans: http://www.aahp.org.

American Association of Retired Persons: www.aarp.org/health.

American Board of Medical Specialties: www.certifieddoctor.org.

American Cancer Society: www.cancer.org.

American Health Care Association: http://www.ahca.org.

American Heart Association: www.americanheart.org.

American Lung Association: www.lungusa.org.

American Medical Association: www.ama-assn.org/aps/amahg.htm.

Annals of Long Term Care: http://www.mmhc.com.

The Commonwealth Fund: http://www.cmwf.org.

Families USA: http://www.familiesusa.org.

Health Care Careers and Jobs Center: http://www.healthcarejobs.org.

Internet Collection of Reviewed Articles: www.medscape.com.

Joint Commission on Accreditation of Healthcare Organizations: www.jcaho.org.

Kaiser Family Foundation and Health Research and Educational Trust: http://www.kff.org.

Long-Term Care Provider.com News & Analysis: http://www.longtermcareprovider.com.

Mayo Clinic: www.mayoclinic.com.

Medscape: http://www.medscape.com.

Modern Healthcare: http://www.modernhealthcare.com.

National Alliance for Caregiving: http://www.caregiving.org.

National Alliance for the Mentally Ill: http://www.nami.org.

National Association for Home Care: http://www.nahc.org.

National Center for Assisted Living: http://www.ncal.org.

National Committee for Quality Assurance: www.ncqa.org.

National Council on Aging: www.HealthCareCoach.com.

Index

Note: Page numbers followed by italicized letters *f* and *t* indicate figures and tables respectively.